27-50

This book is to be returned on or before
the last date stamped below.

28 SEP 1992

Nicholls, P. A.

HOMOEOPATHY AND THE MEDICAL PROFESSION

HOMOEOPATHY
—— and the ——
Medical Profession

PHILLIP A. NICHOLLS

CROOM HELM
London • New York • Sydney

© 1988 Phil Nicholls
Croom Helm Ltd, Provident House, Burrell Row,
Beckenham, Kent, BR3 1AT
Croom Helm Australia, 44-50 Waterloo Road,
North Ryde, 2113, New South Wales

Published in the USA by
Croom Helm
in association with Methuen, Inc.
29 West 35th Street
New York, NY 10001

British Library Cataloguing in Publication Data

Nicholls, Phil
    Homeopathy and the medical profession.
    1. Homeopathy
    I. Title
    615.5'32   RX71
    ISBN 0-7099-1836-4

Library of Congress Cataloging-in-Publication Data

Nicholls, Phil.
    Homoeopathy and the medical profession.
    "Published in the USA by Croom Helm in association with
Methuen, Inc." — T.p. verso.
    Includes bibliographies and index.
    1. Homoeopathy — Great Britain — History. 2. Social
medicine — Great Britain — History. I. Title. [DNLM:
1. Homoeopathy. WB 930 N615h]
RX51.N53 1988 615.5'32'0941 87-20043
ISBN 0-7099-1836-4

Printed and bound in Great Britain
by Billing & Sons Limited, Worcester.

CONTENTS

Preface
Acknowledgements

PREFACE

This book has a long history. It began life as a doctoral thesis, which was eventually submitted in 1984. I was then encouraged to publish, and Croom Helm were kind enough to back the process of substantial revision and additional research required to bring the project to fruition.

The main objective was to write a history of homoeopathy in Britain from the nineteenth century to the present day, and thus to fill a gap in the literature. Hopefully, I have managed to achieve this result. Hopefully, too, it will be of some interest to the medical community, to historians and sociologists of medicine, and to the lay-person interested in holistic medicine. Being of a sociological background myself, however, an opportunity has been taken to develop some more esoteric points concerning the social forces affecting the nature and institutionalisation of medical knowledge and practice, and the manner in which the division of medical labour is constructed and controlled (hence, partly, the comparative chapter on the United States). Probably I have fallen between two stools: these issues will perhaps be felt to be too underplayed and/or imperfectly developed ('theorised', to use the ugly term) by social scientists, and too obtrusive for the reader with no theoretical axes to grind. I can only hope that each audience will tolerate the interest of the other.

Many people have helped in the writing of this book. Undoubtedly, without the forbearance and support of family and friends the research would not have been completed. I should also like to thank my colleagues at the North Staffordshire Polytechnic who generously rearranged their timetables so that I could find time to write and research, the staff at the Faculty of Homoeopathy in London who provided me with such cheerful and ready assistance, Christine Burton who typed an infuriating manuscript, and Tim Hardwick for editorial guidance. My indebtedness to the ideas of others is obvious from the notes and references to each chapter: but all errors of interpretation, and of judgement in the text are, as the saying goes, my own.

Perhaps no one who finishes a substantial piece of research is fully satisfied with the result. This certainly holds true for me. Given the chance, I would probably write the book differently. Fortunately, nobody is likely to give me the chance: writing and thinking, after all, are hard work, and as the Hippocratics observed, 'Life is short, science is long ...'

Phil Nicholls
Department of Sociology
North Staffordshire Polytechnic

For Jean, Peter and Paul Nicholls

Tut, man, one fire burns out another's burning,
One pain is less'ned by another's anguish;
Turn giddy, and be holp by backward turning;
One desperate grief cure's with another's languish.
Take thou some new infection to thy eye,
And the rank poison of the old will die.

(Benvolio to Romeo, Act I, Scene II)

ACKNOWLEDGEMENTS

The quotations from Hahnemann in chapter six have been reprinted by permission of E. Hamlyn (ed.), The Healing Art of Homoeopathy, The Organon of Samuel Hahnemann (Beaconsfield Publishers Ltd., Beaconsfield, 1979); those from Hippocrates in chapters two and three by permission of G.E.R. Lloyd (ed.), Hippocratic Writings, Translated by J. Chadwick and W.N. Mann (Pelican, Harmondsworth, 1978). The cover cartoon, 'The Great Fight' has been reproduced by permission of Punch Publications Ltd., from Punch, vol. XLIV (Jan. 28th 1888) p. 38.

Part I

THE ILL-FAVOURED HOMILY: HOMOEOPATHIC
MEDICINE FROM HIPPOCRATES TO HAHNEMANN

Chapter One

THE SIMILE IN MEDICINE

The successful treatment of illness, according to homoe-opathy, involves the adoption of particular therapeutic principles. First among these, and occupying a position of central importance in the homoeopathic perspective, is the principle of 'the simile'. Dr Ronald Livingston, writing for the British Homoeopathic Association, explains what this entails:

> Homoeopathy is based on the observation made by Dr Samuel Hahnemann, its founder, that if a dose of a substance is administered artificially to a patient, the effects of which sufficiently simulate the illness from which the patient is known to be suffering, the original illness disappears. This might be described colloquially as treatment by analogy or mimicry. What needs to be done in treating a patient is to observe all the essential details of the illness and then seek out the nearest possible group of substances producing clinical effects which can be found to correspond, and to give the patient suitable immunizing doses of these substances.[1]

Homoeopathy, then, is a therapeutic system which argues that in the domain of illness and its treatment, a causal relationship obtains between similars: the administration of a drug, known to produce a symptom complex identical with that manifested in an individual case of illness, will restore the patient to health. To use Hahnemann's own aphorism, homoeopathy declares 'similia similibus curentur' - let likes be treated by likes. In contrast, regular medicine generally prescribes allopathically, i.e. treatment is based on principles other (from the Greek 'allos') than symptom similarity. Typically, allopathic medicine tries to remove or oppose disease causes, and to suppress or palliate symptoms.

At different points in its evolution, this perspective has variously understood disease as some peccant humour in the blood, to be evacuated by bleeding, purging and sweating; as an excess of acidity, to be neutralised by alkalies; as a contraction or relaxation of tissues or organs, to be cured by relaxants and astringents; as debility or irritability to be treated with tonics or sedatives; or as a phlogistic phenomenon to be attacked with antiphlogistics; and more recently as the product of germ infection, to be treated with antiseptics (carbolic acid being among the first) and later antibiotics.

In reality, however, the division between modern homoeopathic and allopathic medicine is not as absolute as the rules of 'similarity' and 'opposition' might suggest. Homoeopathic doctors often resort to allopathic drugs, such as antibiotics, where appropriate; and allopathic practitioners often use treatments based on a simile principle - vaccination, allergy desensitisation, and the use of radiation in cancer treatment, are among the obvious examples. However, while modern homoeopaths often prescribe drugs from allopathy's materia medica, regular practitioners do not reciprocate. Although there is some overlap between the two pharmacopoeias, the indications for use, dose size and technique of remedy preparation suffice to make homoeopathic medicines anathema to allopathic practice. Given that homoeopathic medicines are produced by a process which, through a series of dilutions, may leave no physically detectable trace of the original remedy, this is not perhaps surprising.[2]

Allopaths therefore tend to regard most homoeopathic medicines as pharmacologically inactive - as nothing more than placebos. This has been a charge levelled against homoeopathy ever since doctors, after the publication of Hahnemann's Organon of Rational Healing in 1810, began to adopt his system.[3] Placebo therapy or not, however, patients in Europe and America (and subsequently in many other countries), were well satisfied: homoeopaths flourished in the nineteenth century, and in so doing called forth not only much criticism from their regular colleagues, but also an eventual moderation of the heroic therapy fashionable at the time.

Ironically, since the danger and violence of nineteenth century therapeutics had almost certainly been responsible for much of homoeopathy's popularity, this result meant that homoeopathy had helped to sow the seeds of its own decline. Today, however, demand for homoeopathy is rising, and outstrips the number of medically qualified practitioners available to prescribe it - a phenomenon whose probable origins can be traced, as in the nineteenth century, to the condition of conventional therapeutics. The profile of disease characteristic of most modern industrial societies is now relatively resistent to medical amelioration and drug induced mortality and morbidity has reached serious proportions. Together, these phenomena appear to have stimulated a revivification of public interest in the safer more holistic approach of alternative therapies such as homoeopathy.[4]

Identification of the simillimum, the objective of a
homoeopathic consultation, is a time consuming process. An
hour can easily be spent in developing a precise symptom
picture presented by a patient. Importantly, the symptom
picture aimed for is a holistic one, including both physical
and mental features. Considerable skill and experience is then
required to match the patient's individual symptom complex
with the intricate and subtle 'drug pictures' in the homoeopathic pharmocopoeia. Clients tend to appreciate the degree of
individual attention that homoeopathic prescribing demands,
and doctors are usually quite open about the therapeutic
benefit for their patients of the consultation itself. There is,
then, a placebo effect involved in any improvement derived
from homoeopathic remedies. The longer and more intense the
consultation, and the greater the degree of patient expec-
tation of improvement, the more powerful is the effect likely
to be.

Importantly, however, this observation holds true
irrespective of the therapeutic allegiances of the physician
involved. The placebo effect is by no means unique to homoeo-
opathy. On the contrary, it is present whenever social interaction between doctor and patient leads to diagnosis and
prescription: homoeopaths may simply magnify the effect
because they are prepared to spend more time with their
patients - some of whom will, in addition, already have high
expectations of improvement, born of a long-standing commitment to homoeopathic treatment. Besides, it is easy enough to
control for placebo influence through double-blind techniques,
and where these have been used to evaluate the therapeutic
effect of homoeopathic remedies, some positive results have,
in fact, been reported.[5]

The confidence of the healer and client in the treatment
decided upon thus plays its own role in the promotion of the
healing process. This is the case whether medicine itself is
grounded in magical, religious or metaphysical systems,
empirical folk wisdom, or a scientific paradigm. The contemporary physician thus has a tenuous link with the shaman,
despite the gulf which separates their approach to diagnosis
and treatment.

For the homoeopath, however, this link is marginally
stronger. It will be recalled that Livingston indicated that
homoeopathy 'might be described colloquially as treatment by
analogy or mimicry' - and it is magic which provides probably
the earliest instances of the therapeutic simile in action. Sir
James Frazer, in his classic work The Golden Bough writes:

If we analyse the principles of thought on which magic is
based, they will probably be found to resolve themselves
into two: first, that like produces like, or that an effect
resembles its cause; and second, that things which have
once been in contact with each other continue to act on

each other at a distance after the physical contact has
been severed. The former principle may be called the
Law of Similarity, the latter the Law of Contact or
Contagion. From the first of those principles, namely the
Law of Similarity, the magician infers that he can
produce any effect he desires merely by imitating it:
from the second he infers that whatever he does to a
material object will affect equally the person with whom
the object was once in contact, whether it formed part of
his body or not. Charms based on the Law of Similarity
may be called Homoeopathic or Imitative Magic. Charms
based on the Law of Contact or Contagion may be called
Contagious Magic.[6]

As Frazer points out, although the conceptual distinction
between homoeopathic and contagious magic is clear enough,
in practice they share the underlying assumption that things
'... act on each other at a distance through a secret sympathy'[7] Thus '... the two branches are often combined; or,
to be more exact, while homoeopathic or imitative magic may
be practised by itself, contagious magic will generally be
found to involve an application of the homoeopathic or
imitative principle.'[8]

Homoeopathic magic, then, can be used to 'produce' any
number of effects through a ritualistic imitation of the result
desired. Frazer gives examples which demonstrate its employment in helping to ensure good harvests, the success of
hunting or fishing expeditions, courage and good fortune in
war, rainfall, fertility, and the death of enemies.[9] The list
could go on. Indeed logically it is open to indefinite extension, since the principle involved implies that any culturally
valued result can be achieved through its magical imitation.

The treatment of sickness has been an inevitable concern
of all cultures. Theories of disease in many pre-industrial
societies have often involved notions of soul loss, enchantment
or witchcraft, or some form of object or spirit intrusion.
Predictably, the imitative potency of the magical simile has
been widely employed in such instances to restore health. For
example: a person falls sick; morbid material may have been
magically implanted in the patient by a witch; homoeopathic
magic can help to remove it. Or, working with an object that
had once been in contact with the suspected witch, homoeopathic magic can be used against the offender in order to
encourage the latter to remove the sick-making spell. Frazer
gives another example:

A Dyak medicine man, who has been fetched in a case of
illness, will lie down and pretend to be dead. He is
accordingly treated like a corpse, is bound up in mats,
taken out of the house, and deposited on the ground.
After about an hour the other medicine men loose the

pretended dead man and bring him to life; and as he recovers, the sick person is supposed to recover too.[10]

Examples of this kind are fairly common in the anthropological literature on small-scale, pre-industrial societies. The magical simile, however, is also a principle of great antiquity in medicine. References to its application can be found in texts surviving from the ancient civilisations of Egypt, Mesopotamia and India. In Mesopotamia, for example, an intrusive demon might be:

... transferred through magic formulae into a pot of water, which was then broken so that the water was spilled. Or he was drawn into a little boat, which then sailed away; or he was tied into magic knots, or an onion was peeled and one peel after the other was thrown into the fire while the priest recited the appropriate incantation.[11]

Often, too, remedies which were selected for specific complaints show the influence of simile thinking. Typically, their administration would be accompanied by a magical or religious incantation: in Egypt, egg of ostrich was advised for fractures of the skull; a raven's egg or blood from the horn of a black ox for greyness of the hair; hedgehogs' quills for baldness; ground pigs' eyes for blindness: in Mesopotamia, turmeric was advised for yellow teeth; mustard for coughs where yellowish phlegm was expectorated; the shell of ostrich egg for kidney stones: and in India, the treatment of dropsy, jaundice, and of pale spots on the skin - characteristic of the early stages of leprosy - all invited simile remedies and ritual.[12]

Throughout history, then, many cultures have employed the magical simile in the fight against sickness and disease. Though in one sense magic is, as Frazer argues, 'false science', it is insensitive to link this - as he does - to 'the crude intelligence' of 'ignorant and dull witted people'.[13] Magic is more than that. It is, variously, an expression of support and sympathy, a source of reassurance, and a way of coping with doubt and uncertainty. In the treatment of sickness, magic helps to reassure the patient by providing an explanation of the malady and by the claim that something can be done to relieve it; moreover the ritual involved in magical therapy helps to instil confidence in the efficacy and expertness of the treatment, as well as providing an overt demonstration of general social concern and support for the sick individual.

Expressed through the magical simile, these features of the encounter between healer and patient have a therapeutic benefit in their own right, and in so far as these same

7

features are inherent in the encounter between modern homoeopaths and their clients, then it is legitimate to press the analogy of the magical and the homoeopathic simile. In effect, however, this is to concede very little, for part of the efficiency of any form of treatment - including orthodox scientific medicine - depends on the confidence of the patient in the physician's ability to provide help.

The magical and homoeopathic simile are, then, connected: but the connection is one which turns on recognition of the socially structured similarities present in all therapeutic encounters which elicit placebo response, rather than on any identity of the actual principle employed. For as far as the assumptions of the two cognitive systems which incorporate the simile hypothesis are concerned, homoeopathy and magic very clearly part company.

There is, after all, an important difference between the selection of a medicine on the basis of its ability to reproduce, in a healthy person, the symptom complex manifested by a patient, and the selection of a medicine on the basis of some physical resemblance between it and the organ affected, a symptom of the disease, or the therapeutic effect desired. Again, there is a crucial difference between the homoeopathic method of symptom reproduction and the symbolic or ritual acting out of the curative process. The one is a precise and recognisable scientific procedure, the other is ad hoc and magical - an expression of concern that a cure will be effected, and that action can be taken, in situations where the materia medica generated by collective experience is perhaps devoid of measures more certain.

Boyd summed up the point well in 1936:

> The magic simile states: Euphrasia [the plant Eyebright] is useful in eye diseases because the flower looks like an iris. The modern simile in its most elementary form states: if a substance, for example, Euphrasia is demonstrated pharmacologically to possess the property of evoking ocular phenomena, it can be considered therapeutically in eye diseases which involve the same structures. What is the relationship between two doctrines, when one states opium is useful in diseases of the 'head' because it possesses a 'crown', the other that pharmacological proof that opium affects the cerebrum is an indication of its field of therapeutic activity?[14]

And he went on to conclude that:

> ... the unsupportable statement alleging the identity of the magic and modern simile, falls to the ground since they embody fundamentally different doctrines. One is a dogma based upon the arbitrary selection of some incidental external property as the sole means of deter-

mining the domain of drug activity. The other idea is diametrically opposed since its basic implication belies any selection founded on inference and relies solely upon experimentation.[15]

The 'experimentation' to which Boyd refers is known as 'proving'. As indicated, the therapeutic domain of any drug in homoeopathy is determined through its administration to healthy volunteers, who then record over a specified period all the mental and physical symptoms which they experience.[16] The resulting data constitute a drug picture which, if matching the symptom complex exhibited by a patient, shows that the drug is the appropriate one for the case in question.

By the time Hahnemann died in 1843, he had supervised the proving of 99 medicines. The idea that this would identify the therapeutic domain of each drug, however, had apparently occurred to Hahnemann around 1790. In that year, he had been translating (into German) William Cullen's Treatise of the Materia Medica,[17] and in so doing found himself in disagreement with the author's comments on the efficacy of Peruvian bark (Cinchona officinalis) which contains quinine. Cullen was anxious to explain how 'the bark' worked in order to remove its empirical status as a specific for fever (actually, it is a specific for malarial fever only, then a widespread disease in Europe). Cullen attributed the bark's pharmacological activity to its astringent and bitter qualities which, he believed, helped to restore normal 'tone' to the system. In Hahnemann's translation, he appended the following comment:

... by combining the strongest bitters and the strongest astringents we can obtain a compound which, in small doses, possesses much more of both of these properties than the bark, and yet in all eternity no fever specific can be made from such a compound. The author should have accounted for this. This undiscovered principle of the effect of the bark is probably not very easy to find.

Hahnemann, however, pointed out that certain substances - such as arnica (Arnica montana) and arsenic - which were capable of producing fever, also seemed able to control it, and he investigated the matter further by taking:

... for several days, as an experiment, four drams of good china [i.e. cinchona bark] twice daily. My feet and finger tips, etc. at first became cold; I became languid and drowsy; then my heart began to palpitate; my pulse became hard and quick; and intolerable anxiety and trembling (but without a rigor); prostration in all the limbs; then pulsation in the head, redness of the cheeks, thirst; briefly all the symptoms usually associated with intermittent fever appeared in succession, yet without the actual rigor ... This paroxysm lasted from two to three hours every time, and recurred when I repeated the dose, and not otherwise. I discontinued the medicine and I was once more in good health.[18]

Hahnemann's reasoning is obvious enough. Cullen's explanation of the efficacy of cinchona must be wrong, since substances more bitter and astringent than the bark could be made, and yet they would prove ineffective against malarial symptoms. However, cinchona is known to be effective in such cases; it also produces the symptoms of intermittent fever when administered to a healthy person; ergo that which produces certain symptoms in a healthy person should be used to restore health to a person who exhibits them in sickness. (Actually, cinchona could only relieve malarial symptoms - quinine does not cure the disease itself.)

Hahnemann waited some time before giving vent to these ideas. The Essay on a New Principle for Ascertaining the Curative Power of Drugs, which provided a formal statement and defence of the principles of proving and similarity, did not appear until 1796.[19] And a further fourteen years passed before the first edition of the Organon appeared - years spent in careful refinement, evaluation and elaboration of the homoeopathic doctrine.[20] By that time, all the cardinal features of the homoeopathic system were in place: similia similibus curentur (not 'sanantur', which represents the stronger claim that 'likes are cured by likes),[21] the proving of medicines on healthy subjects, the single remedy, and the minimum (minute) dose. Since conventional remedies at this time were often complex and powerful - not least because of the vested interest of the pharmacists - Hahnemann was to succeed in adding their ire to that of the medical profession, whose theory and practice was so decisively rejected by the Organon.

Indeed, much of Hahnemann's career after 1810 was spent in defending himself and homoeopathy from the hostility of the regular profession. These experiences echoed the difficulties of his early career.[22] Born in 1755 in Saxony, Hahnemann's schooling and medical education had suffered from constant interruption due to financial hardship. He eventually graduated in 1779 and two years later established a small practice in Dessau, where he found ample time to supplement his income by translating various texts on chemistry - a discipline he began to study with increasing seriousness. In 1782, Hahnemann married the daughter of the local apothecary. Thereafter, his career entered a phase of itinerant hardship and uncertainty. By the time he settled in Torgau in 1805, he had moved at least seventeen times. His desire to provide financial support for his family conflicted powerfully with a growing conviction that to do so via the practice of the medicine in which he had been trained could only jeopardise the health of his patients:

> My sense of duty would not easily allow me to treat the unknown pathological state of my suffering brethren with these unknown medicines ... The thought of becoming in this way a murderer or a malefactor towards the life of my fellow human beings was most terrible to me, so terrible and disturbing that I wholly gave up my practice in the first years of my married life ... and occupied myself solely with chemistry and writing.[23]

From 1782 until 1796 Hahnemann earned a meagre living through work as a translator, writer and chemical researcher. The problem of founding medicine upon a safer and more reliable basis, however, continued to be a preoccupation – one no doubt exacerbated by the experience of sickness among his own children. As described above, the break through came in the 1790s. Hahnemann then returned to the role of physician – and, in propagating his system, earnt the opposition of the regular profession.

In 1812, he gained a lectureship at the University of Leipzig, and hoped to win support for homoeopathy among a new generation of physicians. But his secluded life did not prove to be fitting preparation for pedagogy, and his students found themselves more captivated by his eccentric style of delivery than by his ideas.[24] His audiences dwindled: eventually, Hahnemann ceased to lecture and instead gathered round him a group of sympathisers interested in the proving required to develop the homoeo-pathic pharmacopoeia.

Homoeopathy, meanwhile, was recording its first practical successes: first, in the typhus epidemic of 1813, then against cases of scarlet fever, and then again, in 1831 and 1832, against Asiatic cholera. Establishment opposition began to intensify. Hahnemann responded in kind, bitterly denouncing the treatment of the orthodox profession, especially its fascination with repeated and copious bleedings. Pharmacists, too, were opposed to homoeopathy on the grounds of Hahnemann's insistence that since they could not be trusted to prepare the remedies conscientiously, homoeopathic physicians should prepare their own. The potential threat to the livelihood of the pharmacists was obvious. Legislation ensued, the pharmacists were successful, and Hahnemann was obliged to leave Leipzig for Koethen, where he arrived, at the invitation of the Duke, in 1821. Nine years later, his wife died. In 1835, he remarried and, having moved to Paris where he established a flourishing practice, remained there until his death in 1843.

Although the translation of Cullen's Treatise appears to have been a crucial turning point in Hahnemann's thought, he was neither the first to have suggested the medical simile - as he admitted - nor was its presence entirely absent from his own thinking prior to 1790.[25] John Hunter's 1786 essay, Treatise on the Venereal Diseases,[26] in which he observed the effects of venereal inoculation, seems to have been influential. Certainly, Hunter's work is mentioned by Hahnemann in his own publication of 1789, Instructions for Surgeons Respecting Venereal Diseases,[27] and indications of the subsequent direction of Hahnemann's ideas, realised in the New Principle essay of 1796, may be found here.

One of the most immediate precursors of Hahnemann was Anton von Stoerck (1731-1803) who, in the 1760s, suggested the treatment of diseases with poisons according to the principle of similars. For example, according to von Stoerck, 'If Stramonium [Thornapple] makes the healthy mentally sick through a confusion of the mind, why should one not determine whether it gives mental health in that it disturbs and alters the thoughts and sense in mental disease?'[28] Since Hahnemann had studied medicine under Joseph von Quarin at Vienna, who in turn had studied under von Stoerck, one of the more proximate sources of Hahnemann's thinking is perhaps indicated here.

In the introduction to the Organon Hahnemann, concerned to find additional support in previous medical writing, cites a number of authors who had also advocated homoeopathic principles.[29] Among those mentioned are Hippocrates and von Stoerck; John Hunter, Thomas Sydenham, Benjamin Bell and Edward Kentish, who had recommended heating remedies for burns; and the Danish army physician Stahl. Hahnemann quoted the latter:

> The rule generally acted on in medicine to treat by means of oppositely acting remedies is quite false ...; I am, on the contrary, convinced that diseases will yield to, and be cured by, remedies that produce a similar affection - burns by exposure to the fire, frost-bitten limbs by the application of snow ...; inflammation and bruises by distilled spirits; ... acidity of the stomach by a very small dose of sulphuric acid ...[30]

Hahnemann also drew attention to the homoeopathic action of some well-known remedies, such as rhubarb (Rheum officinale) for diarrhoea and senna (Cassia senna) for colic. The examples of quinine for intermittent (malarial) fever, and of mercury for syphilis, were also obvious ones to Hahnemann. Finally, he was not slow to recognise Edward Jenner's innovative work on vaccination, published in 1798, as confirmation of the simile principle.[31]

One of the authors mentioned by Hahnemann, however, merits particular attention - Hippocrates - for it is in the collection of works which bear his name that the underlying principles of the homoeopathic and allopathic paradigms first appeared in Western medical thought. This issue provides the major focus for Chapter Two.

NOTES

1. R. Livingston, Homoeopathy, Born 1810 - still going strong (The British Homoeopathic Association, London, 1973), p. 2.

2. Strictly, the process involves serial dilution with succussion (shaking) at each stage - a process known homoeopathically as 'potentisation' or 'dynamisation'. For a fuller account of the procedure, see Chapter Six.

3. C.F.S. Hahnemann, Organon of Rational Healing (Arnold, Dresden, 1810). The Organon went through six editions. A useful English rendition is: S. Hahnemann, Organon of Healing, 2nd. Indian edition. Translated from the fifth edition by R.E. Dudgeon MD, with Additions and Alterations as per sixth edition translated by William Boericke MD (Roy Publishing House, Calcutta, 1970).

4. S. Fulder and R. Munro, The Status of Complementary Medicine in the United Kingdom (Threshold Foundation Bureau Ltd., London, 1982).

5. R.G. Gibson et al., 'Homoeopathic Therapy in Rheumatoid Arthritis: Evaluation by Double-Blind Clinical Therapeutic Trial', The British Journal of Clinical Pharmacology, vol. 9, no. 5 (May 1980) pp. 453-9.

6. J.G. Frazer, The Golden Bough, A Study in Magic and Religion, 3rd edition, 12 vols. (Macmillan and Co., London, 1907-15) vol. 1, p. 52.

7. Ibid., p. 54.

8. Ibid.

9. Ibid., chapters III-V.

10. Ibid., p. 84.

11. H.E. Sigerist, A History of Medicine, 2 vols. (Oxford University Press, New York, 1951 and 61) vol. 1, p. 471.

12. For these and many other examples, see the appropriate discussions in H.E. Sigerist, op.cit., vol. 1.

13. J.G. Frazer, op.cit., vol. 1, pp. 53-4.

14. L.J. Boyd, A Study of the Simile in Medicine (Boericke and Tafel, Philadelphia, 1936) p. 3. Original italics.

15. Ibid., p.6. The philosophy and sociology of science has moved on since Boyd's day. Clear lines of demarcation between magic and science are not so easily drawn as criteria such as controlled experimentation and falsifiability might suggest. This issue merits a book in itself. Unfortunately, it

cannot be this one. It is, however, at least worth drawing
attention to Feyerabend's iconoclastic discussions, and to
point out that experimental documentation of the placebo
effect confirms one of the assumptions of magic - that the
spoken word can affect the physiological environment. On the
magic and science issue see P. Feyerabend, Against Method
(New Left Books, London, 1975) and Science in a Free
Society (New Left Books, London, 1978).
  16. There is an obvious weakness in this method, since
over any extended period not all reported symptoms may be
due to drug action. A check is provided by using more than
one prover, and by reproving medicines. It is also worth
recording that contemporary provings also include clinical
symptoms, i.e. symptoms known to have been removed by
homoeopathic drugs during treatment.
  17. W. Cullen, Treatise of the Materia Medica (Charles
Elliot, Edinburgh, 1789).
  18. Quoted in R. Haehl, Samuel Hahnemann: His Life
and Work. Translated by Marie L. Wheeler and W.H.R.
Grundy, edited by J.H. Clarke and F.J. Wheeler. 2 vols.
(Homoeopathic Publishing Co., London, 1931), vol. I. Both
passages from p. 37.
  19. S. Hahnemann, 'Essay on a New Principle for
Ascertaining the Curative Power of Drugs' in S. Hahnemann,
The Lesser Writings of Samuel Hahnemann. Collected and
translated by R.E. Dudgeon MD (W. Headland, London, 1851)
pp. 295-352.
  20. See R. Haehl, op.cit., vol. I, chapters V-IX.
  21. See R.E. Dudgeon, 'What is homoeopathy?', The
British Medical Journal, vol. II (1899) p. 816.
  22. For a detailed guide to Hahnemann's career, see R.
Haehl, op.cit. A more recent, but briefer, biography is T.M.
Cook, Samuel Hahnemann (Thorsons, Wellingborough, 1981).
  23. Quoted by G. Ruthven Mitchell, Homoeopathy: The
First Authoritative Study of its Place in Medicine Today
(W.H. Allen, London, 1975) p. 12.
  24. See the report of the amused onlookers in R.
Haehl, op.cit., vol. II, p. 98.
  25. Isolated instances of the simile in the history of
medical thought are quite frequent. See the discussion in
L.J. Boyd, op.cit. For the similar remedy as an expression of
the empirical tradition in medicine, the following work is
unique: H.L. Coulter, Divided Legacy, a History of the
Schism in Medical Thought, 3 vols. (Wehawken Book
Company, Washington, 1973-7).
  26. J. Hunter: 'Treatise on the Venereal Diseases' in
J.F. Palmer (ed.), The Works of John Hunter, 4 vols.
(Longman, London, 1835-7) vol. II, pp. 131-488.
  27. S. Hahnemann, 'Instructions for Surgeons Respecting Venereal Diseases' in S. Hahnemann, The Lesser Writings,
op.cit., pp. 1-188. See esp. pp. 25-6.

28. Quoted by L.J. Boyd, op.cit., p. 19. Original italics.

29. See, for example, the Dudgeon-Boericke translation of the 5th and 6th editions, S. Hahnemann, Organon of Healing, op.cit., pp. 72-4.

30. Ibid., p. 74.

31. See S. Hahnemann, The Organon of Medicine, 6th edition. Introduction by James Krauss (Roysingh and Co., Calcutta, 1962), section 46 and note 47. Smallpox inoculation had a long history, possibly being practised in India as long ago as 1000 BC. See R.H. Major, A History of Medicine, 2 vols. (Blackwell Scientific Publications, Oxford, printed in the USA, 1955) vol. I, p. 78. See also E. Jenner, Inquiry into the Causes and Effects of the Variolae Vaccinae (Printed for the author, London, 1798).

Chapter Two

THE SCHISM IN MEDICAL THOUGHT

In the Hippocratic text Of the Places in Man, probably
written around 350 BC, the writer holds that the general
therapeutic rule is 'contraria contrariis curentur', but notes
'Another type is the following: through the similar the disease
develops and through the employment of the similar the
disease is healed'. For example, 'If one gives much water to a
man who is suffering from vomiting, so the material causing
the vomiting will be removed by the vomiting. So the vomiting
is stopped by an emetic'.[1]
  Hippocrates, the most famous of all Greek practitioners
and teachers of medicine, was born about 460 BC. Though he
was possibly the author of some of the 70 odd texts comprising the Hippocratic Treatises, it is really impossible to
identify the 'genuine works'. Mostly written between 430 and
330 BC, they are all anonymous. The texts embrace a wide
variety of medical topics - ranging through surgery and
ethics to diagnosis, prognosis and treatment - but have as a
unifying theme a strikingly modern approach to the understanding of health and disease. Magical and metaphysical ideas
are deliberately eschewed in favour of scientific and
theoretical explanations. The text on The Sacred Disease,
which develops a very effective critique of magico-religious
accounts and treatments of epilepsy, is one of the more
striking examples of this new approach.
  If, however, the Hippocratic writers were modern in
terms of their preference for theory, this does not mean that
the various authors were by any means agreed about which
particular theory was correct. Indeed, the texts reveal
debates between rival theorists representing different schools
of Greek medical thought.
  Careful examination of the texts discloses two entirely
different therapeutic perspectives at work. It should be
emphasised, however, that none of the individual writings
fully articulate either position, and that some - as in Of the
Places in Man - contain elements of both. Nevertheless, by
abstracting and combining points discussed by authors of

similar persuasion, two opposing models emerge with a fair degree of clarity. The first argues for a holistic appreciation of the human organism, with the physician helping to promote the curative (vitalistic) response of the body as it finds expression through signs and symptoms. This suggests the use of 'similar' remedies. The second approach argues for a more particularistic physiology, with symptoms viewed pathologically, and an emphasis on the correction of bodily imbalances through opposing medicines. The homoeopathic-allopathic therapeutic disjuncture thus originates, as does the modern scientific perspective in Western medicine, with the physicians of Ancient Greece.

Harris Coulter's detailed and persuasive research - presented in the three volumes of Divided Legacy - suggests that this 'schism in medical thought' has structured all subsequent debates about the appropriate paradigm for medicine.[2] Though both perspectives are present in the Hippocratic Corpus, it has been the allopathic approach, Coulter points out, which has been historically dominant. This invites sociological explanation.

After all, the long-term appeal of allopathic practice cannot be fully explained in terms of therapeutic superiority. It only has to be remembered that for much of medicine's history, the number of genuinely curative measures within the materia medica was extremely small, and that the doctrine of treatment by opposition could easily - and often did - incite a vigorous medical style which increased the risk of iatrogenic damage. If anything, in the virtual absence of effective drugs, simply helping nature to take its course would, in many cases, have promised as good, and perhaps better results, than those achieved by active intervention. Clearly, something other than the clinical record of allopathic practice has to be involved in understanding its historical appeal to the medical profession.

More detailed consideration of this issue, however, is reserved for Chapter Three. Meanwhile, the Hippocratic writings themselves deserve closer examination. This helps to locate Hahnemann's work within the evolution of Western medical thought and, importantly, rescues his contribution from marginalisation as a mere eighteenth century idiosyncrasy (a status which it is customarily assigned in the history of medicine). Coulter's admirable analysis of the Hippocratic texts provides the inspiration for the ensuing discussion.

It is worth remarking at the outset that Hippocratic medicine in general was strictly limited in terms of ideas about disease causation, methods of patient examination and range of treatments. Most of the texts are agreed that illness was related either to environmental factors - such as seasonal changes, climate, winds, temperature and the nature of local water or soil - or to individual excesses of diet, exercise, alcohol or sexual activity. Similarly, the writers evinced a collective concern with the examination of various patient evacuations (blood, sweat, faeces, urine, phlegm, vomit) in diagnosis and prognosis, and refer to a similar materia medica: emetic and purging drugs, enemas and suppositories, massage and friction with various unguents and oils, warm water, careful regulation of food and drink, bleeding and exercise.

These superficial similarities, however, concealed fundamental disagreements about the nature and constitution of the body, about the interpretation of signs and symptoms, the objective and rationale of treatment, the role of the physician, the number of disease types, and about the action, use and nature of remedies. The allopathic interpretation of these issues is illustrated in the text on The Nature of Man.[3]

The author commenced by arguing that just as those philosophers who suggested that the physical world was composed of one primordial substance (either air, fire or water) were misguided, so those physicians who claimed that the basic constituent of the body was either blood, bile or phlegm were also in error. 'Generation', he suggested (and we may be sure it was a 'he', a point to which it will be necessary to return in Chapter Three) 'cannot arise from a single substance':[4]

> Man is not a unity but each of the elements contributing to his formation preserves in the body the power which it contributed. It also follows that each of the elements must return to its original nature when the body dies; the wet to the wet, the dry to the dry, the hot to the hot and the cold to the cold.[5]

So far, the view is that people, in common with the material environment, are composed of four basic natural elements - earth, air, fire and water - each of which contributes characteristic qualities: water, coldness and wetness; fire, heat and dryness and so on. In the body, however, these elements and qualities combine in the form of various humours. 'The human body contains blood, phlegm, yellow bile and black bile. These are the things that make up its constitution and cause its pains and health'.[6]

The relationship among these four humours, health and morbidity is explained as follows:

> Health is primarily that state in which these constituent substances are in the correct proportion to each other, both in strength and quantity, and are well-mixed. Pain occurs when one of the substances presents either a deficiency or an excess, or is separated in the body and not mixed with others.[7]

The resulting distress was characterised as local:

> It is inevitable that when one of these is separated from the rest and stands by itself, not only the part from which it has come, but also that where it collects and is present in excess, should become diseased, and because it contains too much of the particular substance, cause pain and distress.[8]

And the type of disease resulting from this morbid process could be defined in terms of the qualities associated with the particular humour in question, for 'They are dissimilar in their qualities of heat, cold, dryness and moisture'.[9]

The relationship among humours, their qualities and disease is further elaborated by the introduction of a climatic and seasonal variable. Having already established that morbidity was due to humoural excess, the author then noted that '... the quantity of phlegm in the body increases in winter because it is the bodily substance most in keeping with the winter, seeing that it is the coldest'.[10] Spring, however, promoted an excess of blood: 'This part of the year is most in keeping with blood because it is wet and hot'.[11] Just as 'Black bile is strongest and preponderant in the autumn',[12] so yellow bile was prone to excess in the summer. In sum:

> ... as the year is governed at one time by winter, then by spring, then by summer and then by autumn; so at one time in the body phlegm preponderates, at another time blood, at another time yellow bile and this is followed by black bile.[13]

The appeal of this model lay in its economy, and in the way in which it articulated the various concerns of Greek cosmology with a theory of disease. Phlegm corresponded to winter and water on the qualitative basis of coldness and wetness; blood to spring and air (warmth and moisture); yellow bile to summer and fire (heat and dryness); and black bile to autumn and earth (cold and dryness). The writer also hinted at a connection between humoural excess and kinds of constitutions, arguing that black bile produced melancholy diseases.[14] Galen's subsequent elaboration of phlegmatic, sanguine and choleric constitutional types, i.e. of individuals with a natural predisposition for the excess of particular humours remained implicit here, however.

If, then, disease was a phenomenon of humoural excess, deficiency or separation, on what basis should the physician plan treatment? The author of The Nature of Man was in no doubt:

To put it briefly: the physician should treat disease by
the principle of opposition to the cause of the disease
according to its form, its seasonal and age incidence,
countering tenseness by relaxation and vice versa. This
will bring the patient most relief and seems to me to be
the principle of healing.[15]

Other Hippocratic physicians demonstrated agreement
with this general allopathic principle. In The Sacred
Disease,[16] the writer argued that the correct approach to
illness was to:

Wear it down by applying the remedies most hostile to
the disease and those things to which it is unaccustomed. A malady flourishes and grows in its
accustomed circumstances but is blunted and declines
when attacked by a hostile substance. A man with the
knowledge of how to produce by means of a regimen
dryness and moisture, cold and heat in the human body
could cure this disease too provided that he could
distinguish the right moment for the application of the
remedies.[17]

The author of Regimen IV concurred.[18] In discussing dreams as diagnostic indicators, he remarked 'To
dream of diving into a lake, the sea or rivers is not a good
sign as it indicates an excess of moisture. It is advisable to
use a dehydrating regimen and more exercise'.[19] Or 'If the
dreamer flies in fright from anything, this means an obstruc-
tion to the blood as a result of dehydration. It is then wise
to cool and moisten the body'.[20] In the text Airs, Waters,
Places,[21] the advice was that if a patient's '... stomach is
soft, moist and full of phlegm, the hardest and saltiest waters
are best since these will best dry it up'.[22]. And A Regimen
for Health[23] suggested the following:

People with a fleshy, soft or ruddy appearance are best
kept on a dry diet for the greater part of the year as
they are constitutionally moist.[24]

The softest and most moist diets suit young bodies best
as at that age the body is dry and has set firm. Older
people should take a drier diet most of the time, for at
that age bodies are moist, soft and cold.[25]

Women do best on a drier diet as dry foods are most
suited to the softness of their flesh ...[26]

During the winter a man should eat as much as possible,
drink as little as possible and this drink should be wine
as undiluted as possible. Of cereals, he should eat

THE SCHISM IN MEDICAL THOUGHT

bread, all his meat and food should be roasted and he
should eat as few vegetables as possible during winter
time. Such a diet will keep the body warm and dry,[27]
[but] During the summer he should live on soft barley-
cake, watered wine in large quantities and take all his
meat boiled. Such a diet is necessary in summer to make
the body cool and soft, for the season, being hot and
dry, renders the body burnt up and parched ...[28]

Overall, this group of texts suggests the following
medical paradigm: the body consists of a discrete number of
humours of characteristic qualities (significantly, the
arguments in defence of this proposition, as in The Nature of
Man, are largely of a logical and a priori nature); disease
ensues through humoural excess, deficiency, or separation,
and is localised; given the four basic qualities, and the
antipathy of opposites, there are really only four main classes
of disease (cold/wet, warm/wet, cold/dry, hot/dry), and
signs and symptoms represent the visible but morbid appearance of these underlying and unchanging categories of
morbidity; the principle of treatment is to oppose the qualitative tendency of the illness through the selection of
remedies on the basis of their heating, drying, moistening or
cooling effects; and the physician is presented as a person of
theoretical expertise, possessed of an abstract and esoteric
body of knowledge not available to patients, which allows
decisive diagnosis, despite the apparently bewildering variety
of disease phenomena, and the identification of an un-
ambiguous programme of treatment.
But other Hippocratic authors had little sympathy with
these views. They were, many felt, too simple: medical
problems could not be solved with geometrical precision. The
first and most famous of the Aphorisms,[29] for example,
stated bluntly that 'Life is short, science is long; opportunity
is elusive, experiment is dangerous, judgement is difficult'.[30] Tradition in Medicine (sometimes referred to as On
Ancient Medicine)[31] underlined the complexity of the medical
task:

One aims at some criterion as to what constitutes a
correct diet, but you will find neither number nor
weight to determine what this is exactly, and no other
criterion than bodily feeling. Thus exactness is difficult
to achieve and small errors are bound to occur.[32]

This author was particularly concerned to criticise the
kind of position defended in The Nature of Man, and it is
worthwhile following this argument at some length. 'I wish
now', he said:

21

... to return to those whose idea of research in the science is based upon the new method: the supposition of certain postulates. They would suppose that there is some principle harmful to man: heat or cold, wetness or dryness, and that the right way to bring about cures is to correct cold with warmth, or dryness with moisture and so on.

This position was then simply, but very effectively, debunked:

... let us consider the case of a man of weak constitution. Suppose he eats grains of wheat as they come straight from the threshing-floor and raw meat, and suppose he drinks water. If he continues with such a diet I am well aware that he will suffer terribly ... What remedy, then, should be employed for someone in this condition? Heat or cold or dryness or wetness? It must obviously be one of them because these are the causes of disease, and the remedy lies in the application of the opposite principle according to their theory. Really, of course, the surest remedy is to stop such a diet and to give him bread instead of grains of wheat, cooked instead of raw meat and wine to drink with it. Such a change is bound to bring back health so long as this has not been completely wrecked by the prolonged consumption of his former diet. What conclusion should we draw? That he was suffering from cold and the remedy cured him because it was hot, or the reverse of this? I think this is a question which would greatly puzzle anyone who has asked it. What was taken away in preparing bread from wheat; heat, cold, moisture or dryness? Bread is subjected to fire and water and many other things in its preparation, each of which has its own effect.[33]

The real situation, he argued, was much more complicated. Firstly, rather than articles of diet affecting specific humoural qualities, foodstuffs acted on the whole person – 'Each one of the substances of a man's diet acts upon his body and changes it in some way and upon these changes his whole life depends ...'[34] Secondly, the effect of foodstuffs was complex. Bread, for example, varied in its effect:

... according as it is made from pure flour or meal with bran, whether it is prepared from winnowed or unwinnowed wheat, whether it is mixed, over-baked or under-baked, and countless other points besides.[35]

Thirdly, exactly the same articles of diet did not always have the same effect on all individuals, as people's constitutions varied. 'Cheese ... is not equally harmful to all. Some

can eat their fill of it without any unpleasant consequences
... on the other hand, there are some who have difficulty in
digesting it'.[36] Fourthly, the body itself was not resolvable
into four simple humours. On the contrary:

> There exists in man saltness, bitterness, sweetness,
> sharpness, astringency, flabbiness and countless other
> qualities having every kind of influence, number and
> strength.[37] [And] similarly, the foods which are
> unsuitable for us and harm us if eaten, all have some
> such characteristic ...[38]

How were these points articulated in an alternative
theory of disease and treatment? Essentially, disease was
attributed '... to some factor stronger and more powerful
than the human body which the body could not master'.[39]
The factors were humoural. As the author of Tradition in
Medicine made clear, however, these humours were many and
varied. 'When ... properly mixed and compounded with one
another, they can neither be observed nor are they harmful.
But when one is separated out and stands alone it becomes
both apparent and harmful'.[40] This harmfulness continued
as long as the body's own natural reaction to morbidity 'could
not master' the problem.

The vitalistic response involved here was one of
'digestion' of peccant or harmful humours (the analogy of
fruit ripening in the sun - making it more palatable - or of
cooking food to make it more digestible, were probably influential in the formation of this idea). Thus:

> Those humours which affect the eyes are very acrid and
> cause sores upon the eyelids ... Pain, heat and swelling
> obtain until such time as the discharges are 'digested'
> and become thicker and give rise to a serum. The
> process of 'digestion' is due to their being mixed and
> diluted with one another and warmed together.[41]

The physician's programme of treatment, then, was
guided - where treatment was necessary - by the curative
processes initiated by the body. For example '... when the
body is chilled, warmth is spontaneously generated by the
body itself so there is no need to take special measures, and
this is true both in health and disease'.[42] Indeed, ignoring
the homoeostatic activity of the human organism, and applying
the principle of treatment by opposites (in effect, sub-
stituting the wisdom of the physician for the 'wisdom' of the
body), could lead to iatrogenic complications:

> If people get their feet, hands or head frozen by
> walking through snow or from exposure to cold, think of
> what they suffer from burning and irritation at night

23

when they are wrapped up and come into a warm place; in some cases blisters come up like those formed by a burn.[43]

Other Hippocratic physicians endorsed these general principles. The author of Epidemics I[44] showed the degree of detail with which the progress of disease, and the body's reaction to it, was monitored:

... we must consider [the patient's] speech, his mannerisms, his silences, his thoughts, his habits of sleep or wakefulness and his dreams, their nature and time. Next, we must note whether he plucks his hair, scratches or weeps. We must observe his paroxysms, his stools, urine, sputum and vomit. We look for any change in the state of the malady, how often such changes occur and their nature, and the particular changes which induce death or a crisis. Observe, too, sweating, shivering, chill, cough, sneezing, hiccough, the kind of breathing, belching, wind, whether silent or noisy, haemorrhages and haemorrhoids. We must determine the significance of all these signs.[45]

For this physician, signs were significant in that they indicated how the process of coction (digestion) of a raw or crude humour was proceeding:

Whenever there is danger, watch out for all ripe discharges that flow from every part of the body at their due times and for favourable and critical abscess formation. Ripeness shows that the crisis is at hand and that recovery is certain. On the other hand, what is raw and immature, as well as unfavourable abscess formation, denotes the failure to reach a crisis, pain, prolongation of the malady, death or relapse.[46]

The author went on to express his views on a fundamental rule of treatment, and on the appropriate relationship between patient and doctor:

Practise two things in your dealings with disease: either help or do not harm the patient. There are three factors in the practice of medicine: the disease, the patient and the physician. The physician is the servant of the science, and the patient must do what he can to fight the disease with the assistance of the physician.[47]

The case notes in Epidemics III[48] record many examples of the coction process. Case eight concerned one Anaxion who had 'a high fever'. By the seventeenth day, he '... began to expectorate a small quantity of ripe sputum, and his condition improved'. On the twenty-seventh day, the fever had returned, but again the patient '... brought up much ripe matter' after which 'His thirst was lost and his respiration became normal'.[49]

The author of Prognosis[50] also shared the view that evacuation of well-mixed, concocted humours was a positive sign that a resolution of the illness was in prospect, whereas the elimination of crudenesses indicated a worsening of the condition:

The most helpful kind of vomiting is that in which the matter brought up consists of phlegm and bile, as well-mixed as possible ...[51]

In all diseases which affect the lungs and sides, sputum should be brought up early and, in appearance, the yellow matter should be thoroughly mixed with the sputum.[52]

So long as the urine is thin and yellowish-red, the disease is not ripened. If the illness is prolonged and the urine remain of that colour, there is a danger that the patient may not last out till ripening occurs.[53]

Fever was usually felt to be a good sign: its heat was an indication of the body's attempts to concoct. For example, one of the Aphorisms observed that 'Fever, succeeding a convulsion or tetanus, ends the illness'.[54] Fever accompanied by the evacuation of raw humours, however, meant that the body's attempts to concoct were failing, and this invited the intervention and assistance of the physician. Regimen in Acute Diseases[55] advised that in cases of pneumonia:

... bathing [in warm water] soothes pain in the side and chest ... It also causes the sputum to ripen and aids its expectoration; it promotes good respiration and relieves fatigue. It also relaxes the joints and softens the skin; it promotes the secretion of urine, cures headache and makes the nose moist.[56]

The same point recurred in the Aphorisms:

To the head, warmth relieves headaches ... It is useful in the treatment of ulcers on the head ... Similar advantage from warmth is observed in cases of ulceration of the anus, the private parts, the womb and the bladder.[57]

Other important comments on treatment are found in the same text:

The progress of a disease should be so guided, where guidance is needed, so that it develops in the most favourable manner according to its natural tendency. [58]

In acute diseases employ drugs very seldom and only at the beginning. Even then, never prescribe them until you have made a thorough examination of the patient. [59]

It is dangerous to disturb the body violently whether it be by starvation or by feeding, by making it hot or cold, or in any way whatsoever. All excesses are inimical to nature. It is safer to proceed a little at a time, especially when changing from one regimen to another. [60]

Overall, these texts present an approach which contrasts markedly with the theory advocated by authors of the first group. This second approach may be summarised as follows: the body consists of an indefinite number of humours of many varying qualities; disease occurs when humours become raw, or 'detached' from the even blend characteristic of health, and it is implied that the whole organism is affected by the resulting 'crudity'; disease is individualistic, in the sense that the same pathogens have varying effects on different people; the number of possible diseases is therefore many; the body has a natural reactivity to morbidity, conceptualised as a process of coction; the progress of this therapeutic response in individuals may be visibly monitored through inspection of the general habit of patients, and in particular through the condition and quality of their evacuations; this empirical evidence is the only guide the physician has to treatment - but this is a complex and delicate task, and doctors should not be regarded as infallible; medical intervention should be cautious, should not threaten the patient, and may not be necessary at all if a healthy resolution is indicated; the aim of therapy is to assist the body's own curative mechanism when it appears to be failing (i.e. use of the similar remedy); and patient and physician are engaged in a co-operative and complementary therapeutic endeavour.

Harris Coulter suggests the use of the terms 'Rationalist' and 'Empirical' to describe the contrasting (allopathic-homoeopathic) approaches of the Hippocratic theorists. He explains as follows: 'Therapeutic theories in all their variety are attempts to make sense out of the healer's experience with the patient', and:

The great medical thinkers have all sought a rule or rules permitting correct interpretation of the primary data of experience. History shows that the search for interpretative rules can be conducted along two alterna-

tive lines. One is to emphasize the paramount significance of the sensory data. The other is to look for a
higher order of reality assumed to be lurking behind the
data of sense perception, treatment being guided by the
physician's assumptions about this reality ... A ...
customary pair of terms for this dichotomy has been
'empirical' and 'rationalist'.[61]

And, as the substantive elaboration of these perspectives
in terms of the Hippocratic texts cited above has shown:

The conflict between the Rationalist and Empirical
assumptions extends to every category of medical
knowledge and therapeutic practice, e.g. the interpretation of the symptom,˙ the relation between theory
and practice, the meaning of disease 'cause', the number
of possible diseases, the role of the physician vs that of
the physis [natural healing power of the body] etc.
...[62]

Thus Rationalist physicians, according to Coulter, would
interpret signs and symptoms as morbid sequelae; theory,
grounded in logic and ratiocinative processes, as guiding
practice; the number of diseases as limited; and the role of
the physician as that of dominating the disease and patient.
Empiricist physicians, on the other hand, would regard signs
and symptoms positively, as evidence of a curative process;
theory as originating in the observation of this phenomenon;
the number of diseases as many; and the role of the
physician as one of co-operation with the physis and its host.
Within the Empirical tradition, Coulter continues, diagnosis and therapy are intimately linked in an observational
process. In Rationalism, however, the link is forged through
resort to theory in the auxillary sciences. Aristotelian logic
provided the doctrine of contraries. Later, the Iatrochemists
and Iatromechanists of the seventeenth century turned to
chemistry and hydraulics (disease as acid-alkali inbalance, or
as a product of blockages in the hydraulic system operated
by the pumping heart); later still, bacteriology was to
perform the same role. The problem, Coulter argues, in the
Rationalist tradition has always been the transition from
diagnosis to therapy - a problem which the Empiricists, by
starting with the curative process manifested by the body,
have never had to grapple.[63]

NOTES

1. The quote is taken from L.J. Boyd, A Study of the
Simile in Medicine (Boericke and Tafel, Philadelphia, 1936) p.
9. There is no complete translation of the Hippocratic Corpus

available in English: <u>Of the Places in Man</u> does not figure in
the collections currently available. Of these see e.g. J.
Chadwick and W.N. Mann, <u>The Medical Works of Hippocrates</u>
(Blackwell, Oxford, 1950). G.E.R. Lloyd's introduction to the
Pelican edition (Harmondsworth, 1978) provides a useful
commentary on the texts, and draws together invaluable
information on medical practitioners in Greek society.

2. H.L. Coulter, <u>Divided Legacy, A History of the</u>
<u>Schism in Medical Thought</u>, 3 vols. (Wehawken Book
Company, Washington, 1973-7).
3. Anon., 'The Nature of Man' in G.E.R. Lloyd (ed.),
<u>Hippocratic Writings</u>, Translated by J. Chadwick and W.N.
Mann (Pelican, Harmondsworth, 1978) pp. 260-71. All subsequent references to Hippocratic texts refer to this
collection.
4. Ibid., p. 261.
5. Ibid., p. 262.
6. Ibid.
7. Ibid.
8. Ibid.
9. Ibid., p. 263.
10. Ibid., p. 264.
11. Ibid., p. 265.
12. Ibid.
13. Ibid.
14. Ibid., p. 271.
15. Ibid., p. 266.
16. Anon., 'The Sacred Disease' in G.E.R. Lloyd
(ed.), op.cit., pp. 237-51.
17. Ibid., p. 251.
18. Anon., 'Regimen IV' in G.E.R. Lloyd (ed.),
op.cit., pp. 252-9.
19. Ibid., p. 258.
20. Ibid., p. 259.
21. Anon., 'Airs, Waters, Places' in G.E.R. Lloyd
(ed.), op.cit., pp. 148-69.
22. Ibid., p. 153.
23. Anon., 'A Regimen for Health' in G.E.R. Lloyd
(ed.), op.cit., pp. 272-6.
24. Ibid., p. 273.
25. Ibid.
26. Ibid., p. 275.
27. Ibid., p. 272.
28. Ibid.
29. Anon., 'Aphorisms' in G.E.R. Lloyd (ed.), op.cit.,
pp. 206-36.
30. Ibid., p. 206.
31. Anon., 'Tradition in Medicine' in G.E.R. Lloyd
(ed.), op.cit., pp. 70-86.
32. Ibid., p. 75.
33. Both passages from ibid., pp. 77-8.

34. Ibid., p. 78.
35. Ibid.
36. Ibid., pp. 83-4.
37. Ibid., p. 78.
38. Ibid., p. 79.
39. Ibid., p. 78.
40. Ibid., pp. 78-9.
41. Ibid., p. 82.
42. Ibid., p. 80.
43. Ibid.
44. Anon., 'Epidemics I' in G.E.R. Lloyd (ed.), op. cit., pp. 87-112.
45. Ibid., p. 100.
46. Ibid., p. 93.
47. Ibid., p. 94.
48. Anon., 'Epidemics III' in G.E.R. Lloyd (ed.), op.cit., pp. 113-38.
49. Quotes from ibid., pp. 132-3.
50. Anon., 'Prognosis' in G.E.R. Lloyd (ed.), op.cit., pp. 170-85.
51. Ibid., p. 177.
52. Ibid.
53. Ibid., p. 176.
54. Anon., 'Aphorisms' in G.E.R. Lloyd (ed.), op.cit., p. 220.
55. Anon., 'Regimen in Acute Diseases' in G.E.R. Lloyd (ed.), op.cit., pp. 186-205.
56. Ibid., p. 204.
57. Anon., 'Aphorisms' in G.E.R. Lloyd (ed.), op.cit., p. 223.
58. Ibid., p. 208.
59. Ibid., p. 209.
60. Ibid., p. 212.
61. H.L. Coulter, op.cit., vol. I, pp. viii-ix.
62. See the discussion, ibid., pp. xiv-xvii. Original italics.
63. See the discussion, ibid., pp. xvii-xviii.

Chapter Three

THE DOMINANCE OF RATIONALISM -
SOME SOCIOLOGICAL REFLECTIONS

Volumes I and II of Coulter's argument are concerned to show
the oscillation between the Rationalist and Empirical
perspectives in medical thought from Hippocrates to the
nineteenth century. Following the legacy of Greek medicine,
the leading representatives of the former school included
figures such as Galen (129-199?); the iatrochemists Sylvius
(1616-72) and Willis (1622-75); the iatromechanists Boerhaave
(1668-1738) and Hoffman (1660-1742); the iatromathematician
Cheyne (1671-1743); von Haller (1708-77); Cullen (1710-90)
and Brown (1735-88) of Edinburgh; Bernard (1813-78) and
Magendie (1783-1855) of the Paris school; and Virchow (1821-
1902). Significant philosophical influences came, at
appropriate points, from the work of Aristotle, Newton and
Descartes, with Harvey's demonstration of the circulation of
the blood and von Haller's experiments on muscular irritability
also providing key physiological insights for theoretical work.
The rival perspective in Greek therapeutics remained
subdued throughout the centuries long domination of medical
thought by Galen. The first serious Empirical challenge to the
Galenic system came, Coulter suggests, from Paracelsus
(1491-1541). Thereafter, the Empirical tradition was continued
by van Helmont (1578-1644); Sydenham (1624-89); Baglivi
(1668-1707) in Italy; Stahl (1660-1734) at Berlin; Bourdeu
(1722-76) at Montpellier; Hahnemann (1755-1843) in Germany;
and Cabanis (1757-1808), Pinel (1745-1826) and Laennec
(1781-1826) at Paris. Again, philosophical work was
important. Scepticism, according to Coulter, helped to
underpin the Empirical approach in Greek medicine after
Hippocrates, with Bacon's work (1561-1626) providing later
epistemological support.
Simply to present lists of prominent medical thinkers
representing each school is, of course, to do violence to the
individual subtlety of their views. Not every Rationalist
thinker would have subscribed whole-heartedly to all the
tenets which have been used to characterise Rationalism;
similarly, Empiricist thinkers would sometimes be less than

fully committed to every element attributed to the Empirical perspective. Nevertheless, Coulter's central point that the history of medicine '... takes the form of an oscillation back and forth between the Rationalist and Empirical poles of the spectrum',[1] with the former usually in ascendance, is clear enough.

Some final points are worth emphasising. The first concerns Hahnemann's concept of proving medicines on healthy subjects. Hahnemann, in fact, was not the first to suggest this technique, though he was the first to make systematic use of it.[2] And this was a decisive contribution to the Empirical tradition, because it allowed the therapeutic domain of medicines to be determined in advance of their use on sick individuals. By arguing that the symptoms which a substance produced in a healthy person were the guide to its remedial action, Hahnemann provided a criterion which would allow the expansion of the pharmacopoeia to proceed on a systematic rather than trial and error basis. Effectively, by seeing medicines as the diseases they would cure (whether this is correct is not at issue here), Hahnemann bridged the gap between diagnosis and remedy, and gave direction to an otherwise random empirical search for treatments. (In this sense, the extent to which allopathic medicine has relied on 'chance' discoveries for some of its most potent drugs – antibiotics, for example – can be seen as an indication of its failure to find a consistent solution to this problem.)

Secondly, although Coulter's thesis is an admirable antidote to the teleological tendencies of medical historians – tendencies which write medical history in terms of a unilineal and progressively enlightened intellectual development, beginning with Hippocrates and 'inevitably' culminating in the scientific revolution of the nineteenth century – his own analysis is vitiated by an associated problem: 'the great man theory' of the history of medicine.

What needs emphasising is that for centuries the medical care available to the majority of people was simply traditional folk medicine, handed down from mother to daughter, or practised by wise-women, and consisting of advice and remedies whose respectability was grounded in their cultural longevity. Often this knowledge would be of herbal medicines, perhaps admixtured with magic and various charms. Of this lay medicine little, of course, is known: its primary mode of inter-generational transmission was oral – necessarily, since literacy was confined to the educated elite. Occasionally, however, this traditional wisdom would be collected and published in the form of 'herbals' (Barbara Griggs book, Green Pharmacy, provides an interesting glimpse of this material.)[3] There is little doubt, however, that prior to the consolidation of the industrial revolution in Europe, the primary health care available to agrarian communities was largely lay health care - much of it domestically dispensed and very largely the province of women.

This does not compromise Coulter's thesis on its own terms. His 'object of thought', after all, is the schism in medical theory, and since the history of medical theory is the history of the literary output of educated thinkers, it is therefore inevitably a male and elitist history. But drawing attention to the great undercurrent of traditional or folk medicine does shed light on Coulter's use of the terms 'Empirical' and 'Rationalist' to characterise the theoretical schism in which he is interested.

It is clear from his discussion of these positions that both are ultimately rooted in different epistmological perspectives: Empiricism is built on a theory of knowledge that accords priority to the products of perception; Rationalism, on the other hand, from Plato to Descartes, doubts the reliability and validity of sense data, and turns instead to logic and ratiocination as the guarantor of knowledge claims. Both positions, as articulated by Coulter, are clearly theoretical structures or paradigms. However, while they have an obvious utility in drawing attention to different traditions in medical theorising, they are less able to encompass the different traditions in the practice of healing. To secure the latter objective, a tripartite conceptual structure is required. The terms comprising this vocabulary would be, firstly, 'vitalism-holism' (corresponding to Coulter's Empiricism, and referring to one tradition in masculine-elite medical theorising); secondly, 'mechanism-particularism' (corresponding to Rationalism, and to the other half of Coulter's theoretical schism); and thirdly, 'empiricism' (with a small 'e'), corresponding to folk and lay healing. That is to say, less coyly, to the care and healing services historically provided by women to family, friends and neighbours, with practice grounded in the largely oral transmission of an ad hoc herb lore rather than in elite epistemological argument.

Finally, it is necessary to ask why the mechanistic-particularistic tradition came to enjoy an institutionalised dominance among educated physicians in the post Hippocratic era. As already suggested in Chapter Two, the answer would not seem to lie in any special therapeutic superiority. Coulter makes the following observation:

> The acceptance of Rationalism was not determined by its value as a therapeutic instrument but because it enhanced the professional pride and prestige of the physician, made it easier for him to earn a living in the practice of medicine, and demarcated the physician from the layman.[4]

This socio-economic answer to the problem is certainly worth exploring.

32

In any therapeutic encounter, the physician is under pressure to demonstrate to the client that something is being done in return for the fee charged for treatment. In turn, this means that medication - preferably with a pronounced effect upon the patient - is favoured, and likely to be prescribed after consultation. Physicians, then, need to be seen as being engaged in an overt struggle against disease on their patient's behalf. This socio-economic imperative favours the adoption of a therapeutic outlook which advocates the aggressive elimination of disease from the body via the opposing remedy. Additionally, it is in the physician's economic interest to maximise the number of patients that can be treated in any given period. Thus it is an advantage if diagnosis is both rapid and authoritative. A theoretical structure which readily isolates specific causes and classes of disease as the proper subject of the therapeutic endeavour is therefore preferable. Something like a four humoural theory (or iatrochemicalism or iatromechanism) fulfills this requirement exceptionally well. Such an intellectual structure also has the benefit of a claim to esoteric and specialised knowledge - knowledge important to the self-esteem of the practitioner. Moreover, this helps to increase the social distance between physician and client, making the latter dependent on and subject to expert knowledge, and emphasising the disjuncture between lay and exclusive professional culture.

In contrast, a vitalistic-holistic approach encourages prolonged and careful observation of individual healing processes before medication is prescribed. Since such medication focuses on the encouragement of this process, a similar remedy will be used. Care must be taken, however, not to pervert the vitalistic response through excessive stimulation. Remedies will tend, therefore, to be gentle and supportive, rather than aggressive and reactive. Often, it may be judged that no remedy is required at all. Additionally, the focus of the therapeutic performance - careful systematic observation of the physis at work - means that claims to specialised knowledge regarding the internal nature and cause of disease receive less emphasis. To the extent that diagnosis and treatment are grounded in the observation and interpretation of signs and symptoms - data available to both patient and physician - the importance of particular and esoteric knowledge (exclusive to the physician) is reduced, and the social distance between doctor and client correspondingly closed.

At every level, then, the economic, social and psychological implications of therapy based on vitalism-holism would appear to have had less potential to increase the income, prestige and authority of physicians than its mechanistic-particularistic counterpart. A Rationalist approach, Coulter argues, has always been a more attractive proposition for practising physicians - and this, he suggests, accounts for the historical dominance of the allopathic perspective in the post-Hippocratic medical 'profession'.

Coulter's explanation is sociologically attractive. It is worth pointing out, however, that he gives scant historical data about the actual socio-economic conditions relating to physician employment in Greek society. This is unfortunate as far as his explanation for the dominance of Rationalism is concerned - but the deficiency is not irredeemable.[5] We know, for example, that the technical status of medicine in Ancient Greece was a precarious one. Medical practitioners' training usually took the form of an informal apprenticeship with an established doctor (the greater the physician's reputation the better), but ended without formal certification. In this sense, Greek physicians were on a par with any lay-person who claimed to be able to heal the sick, with mid-wives, herbalists, drug sellers, and with quacks and charlatans. Trained doctors thus often found themselves in the position of having to defend medicine as a genuine science, which required skill and training, and which merited privileged status vis-à-vis rival lay practitioners. Such defences of medicine are clear in a number of Hippocratic texts: The Sacred Disease, Regimen in Acute Diseases, Tradition in Medicine, and most especially in The Science of Medicine. A constant need, then, (at bottom an economic one) to demarcate scientific medicine from lay practice suggests the attractiveness of adopting the more elaborate and abstract conceptual apparatus of Rationalism.

The social status of physicians was also low. Anyone who depended on earned income for economic survival was regarded as inferior by the aristocratic consciousness of Greek society - and, what is worse, it is fairly clear that doctors had also gained a reputation for avariciousness. Rationalism could do little to ameliorate the problem of status inferiority, but the fact that Greek doctors were itinerant, as Airs, Waters, Places makes clear, and depended on the fees of the clients they won and did their best to retain, is significant. Economic survival depended on reputation as a practitioner, and the emphasis in the texts on diagnosis, and especially prognosis, demonstrates the concern of physicians to win the confidence of patients. Hence the interest of doctors in refraining from treating hopeless cases: as the author of Prognosis states, 'By realising and announcing beforehand which patients were going to die, the physician would absolve himself from any blame'.[6] Again, then, the economic interests of rapid diagnosis, of prognosis, of gaining the confidence of patients by the use of apparently expert knowledge, and of maximising the number of clients who could be seen during a stay in any one locality, would seem to favour the adoption of Rationalism over Empiricism.

Coulter's socio-economic explanation of Rationalism's dominance does therefore seem attractive in view of the known exigencies of medical practice in Greek society. Moreover, the problems of demarcating medicine from lay practice, of defending its scientific status and credentials, and of earning an economic livelihood from treating the sick, are ones which doctors would continue to face in subsequent eras.

Coulter, however, ignores one particularly important issue. It needs to be emphasised again that educated physicians in Greek society, and thereafter, were male. If Sherry Ortner's claim[7] of a fundamental social dichotomy of 'nature' and 'culture' can be pressed, where women are reproductively associated with nature, and men with culture, then the fact of gender becomes significant in the explanation of Rationalism's historical dominance in medicine.

Ortner argues that whereas culture tends to be given positive social evaluation (social survival ultimately depends on the ability to control and exploit the natural environment through cultural products and processes), nature is correspondingly evaluated in negative terms. To the extent that women are perceived to be closer to nature than men, on the basis of cycles of menstruation, pregnancy, parturition, lactation, child rearing and menopause, so masculinity is associated with culture, and regarded as superior to feminity. The argument helps to account for the universal subordination of women to men, and of the general social estimation of the inferiority of the work of women, whatever form that may actually take, to the roles and tasks undertaken by their male counterparts. Here, however, Ortner's position is important in that in so far as the Empirical tradition in medical theorising subordinates itself to nature, it becomes clear that it is one at risk of negative social evaluation - especially by a body of male physicians. The cultural orientation of Rationalism is, once again, the more attractive proposition.

There is a second and related issue here. The nature-culture distinction helps in understanding the preference of an existing body of male physicians for Rationalism, but the fact of masculinity itself - its socio-psychological construction as a gender type - is also important. To the extent that the acquisition of masculine identity turns on the rejection and suppression of the nurturing, expressive, caring and supportive qualities historically associated with the roles of women, and is instead contingent on the cultivation of qualities of independence, control, objectivity and emotional neutrality, so male physicians will tend to endorse a Rationalist orientation in medical theory. If a broad historical generalisation may be permitted: a good deal turns on the fact that women mother and men (regrettably) do not, i.e. women's work is person centred, and that of men object centred. And Rationalism in medicine does, as a matter of fact, treat the human body as object, as something to be directed, manipulated and controlled. Empiricism, on the other hand, is person centred, and as such (at the risk of over-statement) is antithetical to the social practice of masculinity, and therefore to the practice of medicine by men. Whatever the strengths and weaknesses of these explanations, it remains the case that Rationalism has been the dominant tradition in professional thought and practice in the Western world. For Coulter, this is a '... tragedy of medical history...' since it has meant that:

> Allegiance is preferred to abstract principles, and the correctness of their application can be decided only by the corporate body itself. In this way the physician is shielded from society and cannot be called to account for his errors.[8]

In fact, Coulter rather forgets his own evidence in this final sentence: volume three of Divided Legacy is actually a demonstration of the way in which public rejection of violent allopathic practice in nineteenth century America, and patronage of homoeopaths in particular, led to the competitive reform of orthodox practice. A major theme of succeeding chapters will be to examine this process in more detail, with particular reference to the relationship between homoeopathy and regular medicine in Britain.

NOTES

1. H.L. Coulter, Divided Legacy, A History of the Schism in Medical Thought, 3 vols. (Wehawken Book Company, Washington, 1973-7) vol. I, p. xxxi.
2. See the discussion in L.J. Boyd, A Study of the Simile in Medicine (Boericke and Tafel, Philadelphia, 1936), pp. 104-6.
3. B. Griggs, Green Pharmacy (Jill Norman and Hobhouse, London, 1982).
4. H.L. Coulter, op.cit., vol. I, p. 323. His discussion, pp. 322-33, develops the points in the quotation.
5. Information in the discussion which follows is based on the editorial remarks in G.E.R. Lloyd (ed.), Hippocratic Writings (Pelican, Harmondsworth, 1978), pp. 12-21.
6. Anon., 'Prognosis' in G.E.R. Lloyd (ed.), op.cit., p. 170.
7. S.B. Ortner, 'Is Female to Male as Nature is to Culture?' in M.Z. Rosaldo and L. Lamphere (eds.), Women, Culture and Society (Stanford University Press, Stanford, 1974), pp. 67-87.
8. H.L. Coulter, op.cit., vol. I, p. 333.

Part II

MEDICINE IN THE NINETEENTH CENTURY:
OCCUPATIONAL STRUCTURE, THEORY AND PRACTICE

Chapter Four

THEMES AND ISSUES

The nineteenth century witnessed a momentous transformation of medicine - a transformation which revolutionised the understanding of disease, the nature of therapeutics, and the organisation of the profession. Even in the 1830s, however - the period during which homoeopathy first emerged in Britain - most of these changes still lay in the future. Much of medical practice was still influenced by monocausal theories of disease suggested by previous theoreticians such as Hermann Boerhaave, Friedrick Hoffman, Albert von Haller, William Cullen and John Brown, which variously ascribed pathological conditions of all kinds to the disordered functions of hypothesised mechanical, hydraulic, chemical or 'irritable' body systems. The most significant developments in medicine, however, came not through further theoretical work of this kind, but from a heightened interest in anatomical and physiological investigation, the development of more precise descriptions of particular diseases, and the correlation of morbid signs with the data revealed by post-mortem examination. These developments, already characteristic of Paris medicine, were aided by the growth of a hospital system which had increased the opportunities for clinical and pathological inquiry. The work of the 'great men of Guys', among which the names of Richard Bright (1789-1858), Thomas Addison (1793-1860) and Thomas Hodgkin (1798-1866) stand out in particular, were symbolic of these important trends in British medicine. But if these more practical concerns had displaced impetuous theorising from the centre of the medical stage, the effect of such systems lingered on - most particularly in the form of the violent, or heroic, therapy which they had helped to legitimise.

One change already underway in the early decades of the century was the gradual erosion of the tripartite structure of the profession. Traditionally physician, surgeon and apothecary had been distinct estates, each with their separate occupational rights and spheres of practice. With a burgeoning urban population, however, the emergence of the general practitioner began to undermine these divisions. Certain issues had served to unite ordinary medical practitioners more strongly than increasingly anachronistic concerns of status purity: one in particular was the competition from unqualified practitioners or quacks. Homoeopathy was in a peculiar position here. Orthodox doctors were for the most part convinced that it was absurd, and so like quackery - yet, incomprehensibly, it was taken up by their peers and colleagues. Moreover, homoeopathy constituted a major critique of received medical wisdom. If homoeopathy was right, allopathy had been wrong in the past and was still wrong. Indeed, if Hahnemann was correct, it was allopathy that was absurd. Thus the emergence of homoeopathy within the ranks of the profession constituted not only an economic threat to the livelihoods of regular practitioners in proportion to its popularity, but also an intellectual threat to the knowledge on which claims to professional esteem were to be increasingly based. This helps to explain the vehement reaction against homoeopathy within the ranks of the profession itself.

What follows is an attempt to put this reaction in context. Chapter Five presents an overview of the evolving profession of medicine in the nineteenth century, focusing on structural changes, and the major issues, disputes and reforms with which medical practitioners were concerned; Chapter Six emphasises the theoretical gulf between homoeopathy and regular medicine by comparing Hahnemann's system with the work of Sir Thomas Watson, who wrote what has been called 'The most important English treatise on the practice of medicine in the first half of the nineteenth century ...',[1] and Chapter Seven examines the nature of orthodox treatment that was typically prescribed for patients around the period of homoeopathy's introduction to Britain. This points up the practical disjunction between allopathic and homoepathic therapeutics at the time, and in so doing suggests reasons for the latter's popularity.

NOTES

1. F.H. Garrison, History of Medicine, 2nd. edition (W.B. Saunders Company, Philadelphia and London, 1917), p. 434.

Chapter Five

THE PROFESSION - ORGANISATION, STATUS AND CHANGE

Before the passage of the Medical Act of 1858, the organizational structure of the medical profession was in a state of near chaos. There were nineteen different licensing bodies in the United Kingdom by the early nineteenth century, and the rules governing their recognition were a tangle of conflicting rights and powers. Medical men practised with university degrees, various forms of medical licences, sometimes a combination of these, and sometimes with none at all. Medical training varied from classical university education and the study of Greek and Latin medical texts on the one hand, to broom-and-apron apprenticeship in an apothecary's shop, on the other - and sometimes involved no recognizable education at all. Quacks, 'empirics', and drug pedlars practised freely with no legal sanctions against them, while a physician in London could be disciplined by his College for preparing and selling a prescription to his patient.

The key to understanding the structure of the early nineteenth century medical profession is to be found in a commonplace of medical history: the separation of medical men into three orders - physicians, surgeons, and apothecaries. These three orders took corporate form in the Royal College of Physicians [RCP], the Royal College of Surgeons [RCS], and the Society of Apothecaries [SA], and they defined the social structure of the profession and, in theory at least, the division of medical labour.[1]

Of the three medical estates, the physicians were the most prestigious. This had more to do with the esteem attached to their social graces and skills than with their medical expertise. As university graduates, physicians had mixed with social elites, and had had an elite education. Not all physicians, however, belonged to the Royal College. Those practising in the provinces could become Extra Licentiates, but this was not compulsory. Only in London was firmer control attempted. Here, physicians enjoyed a monopoly on the practice of 'physic' (internal medicine) and, formally at least, had to be affiliated to the College as Licentiates or Fellows.

Full access to the benefits and privileges of College membership, such as exemption from jury service and taxation, and enjoyment of voting rights in College elections, was allowed only to the minority of Fellows - and Fellowship itself was largely restricted to those with an Oxbridge degree and a London practice. Additionally, Fellows could not practise surgery or make up and dispense medicines: this was the work of the lower orders of the medical hierarchy - respectively, the surgeons and apothecaries. Licentiates, however, while enjoying fewer of the privileges of College membership, were correspondingly less restricted in occupational terms. Licentiates were freer to engage in general practice.

The elite status of physicians among medical practitioners was matched by their numerical scarcity. Of the 14,700 practitioners in England in 1850, less than five per cent reported some kind of affiliation with the RCP, and the overwhelming majority of these were practising in London.[2] This compares with some 8,000 who held a licence from the RCS.[3]

Surgeons were essentially craftworkers - skilled manual operatives trained by apprenticeship. Predictably, they were regarded as the social inferiors of university educated physicians. In 1843, with the designation of the RCS as an English, rather than a specifically London corporation, a new membership rank - that of Fellow - was created. Candidates assumed the rank either by election or examination. Some 200 had acquired this distinction by mid-century.[4] Fellows were not required to have a London practice, but this was necessary if access was to be gained to the real centre of power, the ruling council of the College itself. Council members were also required to be solely engaged in surgery. In this respect, council members represented the surgeon elite, for many members of the College - which did not anyway enjoy a monopoly of surgical practice - prescribed and dispensed drugs as well. Indeed, as the century progressed, surgeons increasingly added a second qualification, from the SA, to their MRCS, a process which consolidated the emergence of the general practitioner.

If the status of surgeons was largely determined by the craft connotations of their work, then that of the apothecaries was the product of their connection with trade. Trained by apprenticeship, apothecaries had originally been responsible for the compounding and sale of drugs, but had increasingly found themselves being called on to provide medical advice and diagnostic services for their customers. In short, they were really practising generally well before the nineteenth century. This situation was formally ratified in 1815 with the passing of the Apothecaries' Act, which not only allowed the SA to examine candidates for medical practice, but also required all those who prescribed and dispensed medicines in England and Wales to acquire the Society's Licentiate. Between 1815-34, some 6,000 candidates were successful, more than half of whom also held the MRCS.[5] Again, trade distinctions were only maintained by the elites of the SA, who were forbidden either to cut or prescribe, and who enjoyed the privilege of exclusive rights of practice within the City of London.

In sum, although the medical corporations were to remain a feature of medical life throughout the century, the occupational distinctions which they had originally been developed to maintain and protect became increasingly irrelevant to the majority of their members. This process was already underway at the beginning of the nineteenth century, and although it was to be some time before it received formal recognition (in effect, it began in 1815), it was certainly the case that demarcation had already become a matter of concern really only for the corporation elites. Indeed, the emergence of the general practitioner was testimony to the implicit fact that the majority of practitioners had more in common with each other than with distant, elitist and tradition bound London Colleges.

Partly this was a product of the changing role of the hospital in the education of medical practitioners. London experienced a dramatic growth of hospital facilities during this period. By 1850, the capital boasted eleven major general institutions. The newer hospitals were supported by charitable donations from the wealthy, whose largesse gave them the right to nominate patients, and access to important posts on the governing bodies of the institutions themselves. Despite this lay control, hospital posts were highly prized by doctors - they provided an introduction to the affluent philanthropists who supported the institution, and whose social milieux was a source of potential clients in the attempt to establish a flourishing practice.

More significantly, the expansion of hospitals provided opportunities for physicians and surgeons to acquire extensive experience. Many more cases could be seen in the wards in a day than private consultation could possibly yield. Hospitals, too, changed the relationship between doctors and patients. Since a criterion of admission was inability to pay for private treatment, fees present and future were generally not a primary consideration as far as the interaction of medical staff with patients was concerned. This meant that attention could be focused more clearly on diseases instead of persons. Observation, comparison, suspension of judgement, and post-mortem data were therefore available in a way which was proscribed by the exigencies of practice based on individual, private consultation, where cultivating the social loyalty of clients was often as important as treating their medical problems.

In turn, opportunities for more precise and perceptive description of various diseases, the correlation of these findings with information provided by post-mortem investigation, and the elaboration of anatomical and physiological knowledge generally, led to a new recognition of the inadequacy of mere verbal 'history taking', and to the importance of the physical examination of the patient in diagnosis. Here, the growing use of the stethoscope was a major innovation (recognition of the importance of the pulse rate and of body temperature was of longer standing - though effective thermometers for medical use were not available until after 1850).

In the early years of the nineteenth century, the hospitals had played only an informal and relatively minor role in medical education. Students and apprentices would attend to see members of staff at work, but on a fairly ad hoc basis - the focus of their training was either at the university or in the practice to which they had been articled. But the realisation of the importance of clinical experience - made possible by the very growth of hospitals themselves - produced rapid changes. By the 1840s, apprenticeship was on the wane; private anatomy and other schools had developed to equip students with advances in medical knowledge; and then hospital staffs themselves began to organise formal in situ lecture courses and to supervise students as they developed the skills of physical examination. In short, the focus of medical education shifted to the hospitals - hospitals became medical schools. Indeed, the control of education by medical staff represented the first assertion of independence by doctors from lay authority in the hospitals - an independence which would grow stronger and wider as the century drew to a close.

These developments had important effects. Firstly, it meant that medical students shared an increasingly homogenous educational experience and background, which tended to further erode the old corporate divisions. Secondly, it led to the emergence of consultants, i.e. those who held hospital appointments and thus supervised medical education. Thirdly, by the middle of the century, it had emphasised a new disjunction in the organisation of medicine, a disjunction between the general practitioner and the elite of the Royal Colleges - for consultants were now leaders in a double sense, in control not merely of medical education, but also of the Royal Colleges whose Fellowship was usually a prerequisite for the more important hospital appointments.

The emergence of hospitals as centres of medical education gave further impetus to the process of gradual erosion of corporate divisions among medical practitioners. As noted, some physicians were already practising generally (especially those outside London); most apothecaries not only dispensed but also did some surgical work (such as dentistry and bleeding); while many surgeons also engaged in physic. At the grass roots level of the profession, the informal emergence of general practice had thus rendered corporate divisions largely irrelevant. Consequently, to the new general practitioners, the ancient and conservative Royal Colleges and Societies, which had been built on the preservation of occupational and status distinctions, seemed increasingly irrelevant too. The feeling was reciprocal. For the most part, the elites of the profession - the London based consultants/ Fellows - remained insensitive to the interests and problems of the predominantly rural and provincially based general practitioners.

This attitude had the effect of stimulating the rank and file to form its own associations. It was one of these, the Association of Apothecaries and Surgeon Apothecaries formed in 1812, which succeeded in securing the Act of 1815. The Act fell some way short of the original progressive intention of establishing a new licensing body to regulate general practice, largely because of opposition from the old corporations, but by requiring all those who prescribed and dispensed medicines to take the Licentiate examinations of the Society - itself a qualification which gave formal recognition to the fact that apothecaries where practising physic - the role of surgeon and apothecary were effectively fused. Surgeons who had been dispensing drugs now had to take the LSA examinations; and though those holding the LSA were not formally required to obtain a qualification from the RCS in order to practise surgery, many in fact did. The Apothecaries' Act, then, though failing to achieve any major overhaul of medical licensing, nevertheless had the effect for many of transforming an informal status - general practitioner - into a formal one. Surgeons who had practised generally had now to hold qualifications from more than one corporation.

The years after 1815 saw a proliferation of local and provincial medical societies. Established to represent and protect the interests of those in general practice, especially from the competition of quacks and unlicensed practitioners (no threat, of course, to the London elite), the most important of these was undoubtedly the Provincial Medical and Surgical Association (PMSA). Founded in Worcester in 1832, the Association rapidly assumed status as the national voice of the general practitioner. Realising that any kind of medical reform or legislative action would be impossible without the support of the London corporations, the PMSA's approach tended towards conciliation rather than denunciation.

Others felt that the London Colleges were not worthy of such respect. Here, the name of Thomas Wakley, an East End practitioner and founder and editor of The Lancet, stood out above all others. Possessed of a literary style which owed little to the niceties of nineteenth century professional discourse (he once described the London medical elite as consisting of '... craftly, intriguing, corrupt, avaricious, cowardly, plundering, rapacious, soul-betraying, dirty-minded BATS'),[6] Wakley gave radical, if not always entirely representative expression, to the general concerns of rank and file practitioners: the need to protect the qualified from unlicensed competition, the need for democratic reforms within the organisation of medicine as an occupation and a more substantive role for GPs in its politics, and anger at the discrepancy between the often impecunious position of many ordinary doctors and the wealth of the London elite.

In 1856, the PMSA - embracing many of the local and other provincial societies - became the British Medical Association (BMA). Two years later, its struggle for medical reform finally found expression in the passing of the Medical Act of 1858. In fact, from 1840 numerous medical bills had been introduced into parliament. All but the sixteenth had failed, usually on the grounds that they were either unacceptably radical for the Colleges, or too cautious for the rank and file. Indeed, the 1858 Act succeeded only because it represented a just acceptable compromise to the parties concerned. For many GPs (and especially for Wakley) it did not go nearly far enough.

The most important feature of the Act was the creation of a General Council of Medical Education and Registration (GMC), with responsibility for the supervision of medical education, and the registration and annual publication of the names of all qualified practitioners. On the debit side, however, the Act left much of the original structure and organisation of medicine intact. Since there was no provision for general practitioner representation on the GMC, it was dominated by the corporation elites, whose individual Colleges continued their licensing functions. Effectively, the creation of the GMC meant that those already in charge of medical education were now legally required to supervise their own performance. The unification of the profession by the creation of the GMC was thus in name only, since it actually permitted the continuation of corporate exclusiveness.

In sum, to their control of the Colleges and domination of the London hospitals, the medical elites had now also added control of the GMC, which consolidated their advantage vis-à-vis the GP. Moreover, the reformers also keenly felt the failure to secure in the Act any legal protection for doctors from the competition of unqualified practitioners. The furthest parliament was prepared to go was to bar those not entitled to medical registration from government employment. Undoubtedly, the influence of laissez-faire philosophy played its part in this decision, since it suggested that rational individuals must be free to exercise informed choice in the purchase of goods and services. Monopoly infringed this right, as well as that of potential producers to offer goods and services to consumers. It is worth reflecting, however, that parliament might have been inclined to listen with greater sympathy to general practitioner demands for protection from the unqualified if it had been convinced either that the latter constituted a serious health hazard to the public or that medicine's materia medica was more effective than more or less innocuous quack nostrums. And there were really insufficient grounds, at the time, for accepting either hypothesis. Besides, government tax on patent remedies was an important source of revenue. This meant that quackery was implicitly seen, in official terms, as a source of health care for the public. Indeed, medical practitioners themselves tended to advance their claims against the unqualified more in terms of protection from economic competition than the superiority of their methods.

Yet if medicine in the first half of the nineteenth century was still awaiting fundamental scientific and therapeutic breakthroughs, the ground was being prepared by the developments in anatomy, physiology and pathology made possible by the emergence of hospitals in expanding urban centres. In turn, these developments began to be reflected in medical education. Courses at university, as well as the training required for MRCS and LSA qualifications, tended to increase in length and complexity in order to accommodate advances made in the basic branches of medical knowledge - and, where appropriate, in recognition of the emergence of general practice. Apprenticeship became less important and less time was spent with individual tutors. Instead, the hospital increasingly emerged as the focal point of medical education. By the 1850s the private medical schools, which had first flourished by providing the various lecture courses required for certification, had all disappeared.

One of the traditional claims to the occupational superiority of the physician had been a classical university education - especially that provided at Oxbridge - which imparted the social characteristics valued by a status conscious society. The possession of such attributes was for long to remain at least as important (and in many cases probably more so) to a successful career than technical competence - itself something that could only be achieved in what was, after all, publicly recognised as a very imperfect art. These particularistic criteria, plus the activation of nepotistic obligations and the influence of powerful friends, remained important in obtaining access to prized hospital and College appointments (the former, significantly, being made by the lay governing bodies), and in the cultivation and retention of a clientele able to support a flourishing practice. And for a large part of the century, many practitioners seemed not to have reacted with reluctant acquiescence to lay evaluation of their merit on social rather than technical criteria. On the contrary, they tended to use the same values in the assessment of their colleagues, a situation which only gradually yielded to the more universalistic judgements made possible by the elaboration, later in the century, of a scientific and technical basis for medical practice.

Leaving aside the fashionable elite, however, who in total constituted probably only about one per cent of all medical practitioners,[7] the general status of medicine vis-à-vis the other professions was low - predictable enough, given its strong association with trade and craft practices. Peterson's admirable discussion of The Medical Profession in Mid-Victorian London (see note 1 below) documents the point well. It is also a view which finds its way into the nineteenth century novel. Though such illustrative material should be treated with due caution, a few examples may be usefully recorded.

George Eliot's Middlemarch is rich in such material. Mrs Cadwallader, for example, is driven to compare Casaubon, the fossil bridegroom of the young Dorothea, to a dose of medicine, 'nasty to take and sure to disagree'. And Lady Chettom, in commenting on the superior family connections of the country practitioner Lydgate, remarks:

> One does not expect it in a practitioner of that kind. For my own part, I like a medical man more on a footing with my servants; they are often all the cleverer. I assure you I found poor Hicks's judgement unfailing; I never knew him wrong. He was coarse and butcherlike, but he knew my constitution.[8]

Anthony Trollope provides a second example. In The Vicar of Bullhampton he ascribes the following opinion to Miss Marrable:

> She would not absolutely say that a physician was not a gentleman, or even a surgeon; but she would not allow to physic the same absolute privilege which, in her eyes, belonged to the law and the church.[9]

And Matthew Arnold, in a literary criticism of Keats's romantic correspondence, added the barb that his prose was like that of a 'surgeon's apprentice' (he had been), it being 'underbred and ignoble, as of a youth ill brought up'.[10] Similar illustrations can be found in the work of Charles Dickens, particularly The Pickwick Papers.

The low status of medicine as a profession was also reflected in - and indeed was partly a product of - the inferior social origins of the majority of its members. Even among the elite - Fellows of the RCP - the extent of family connection with the aristocracy and landed gentry was small, and that normal prerequisite of good social standing, a public school education, an exception. Neither did the professional middle classes perceive medicine as a career of first choice for their children: the law, church or army were preferred. Even the children of professional people who took up medicine tended not to be allowed the benefit of an education at public school.[11] It was a vicious circle. The low prestige of medicine as a career meant that it attracted relatively few recruits from the children of status conscious families; the profession was thus largely constituted from among those lacking the valued cultural polish imparted by public schools, and this helped to confirm the impression that a medical career would involve downward social mobility for the children of professional people.[12]

This general deficit of cultural capital among medical practitioners was keenly felt, a fact which the various licensing bodies attempted to rectify by instituting preliminary examinations, designed to ensure a minimum standard of general - i.e. liberal/classical - education for candidates prior to their registration. Only in the 1880s did these examinations assume a more scientific content. Compared to other professions, however, the great majority of medical practitioners were 'uncultured'. Only among the College elites was a classical education, in the form of an arts as well as a university medical degree, to be found - though again, even here the possession of both seems to have been the exception rather than the rule.[13]

By far the most common product of medical training was a career in general practice. This would require some four to five years of education and would cost, in total, between £185 to £300 [14] in the provinces - a figure well within the reach of the lower middle class, especially if there was already some family connection with medicine. With the preliminary examination passed, and having registered with one of the Colleges (and, after 1858, with the GMC), the student would commence the academic and practical training offered by a chosen hospital medical school. Typically, students would aim to leave with both the MRCS and LSA, i.e. qualifications in surgery as well as in medicine - though only one was actually required for registration. (After 1861, the LSA tended to be replaced by the new Licentiate from the RCP.) Obtaining qualifications for general practice, however, was one thing. Establishing a successful practice was an altogether different proposition. Nowhere was the necessity of conforming to the values of lay society in achieving this aim more apparent. As Peterson observes, 'No one felt this dependency in the social judgement of patients more acutely than the young man starting out in practice'.[15]

Emulation of the manners, morals, habits and opinions of respectable society was so important to the economic success of general practice because clients and public remained justifiably sceptical about the therapeutic value of the knowledge to which medical certification was a testimony. This meant, firstly, that the profession had no sound defence against competition from quacks and empirics and secondly, that social credentials become correspondingly more important, both in terms of distancing the profession from unlicensed practitioners, and as an index in terms of which public judgements about the distribution of patronage among medical practitioners themselves could be made. The newly licensed practitioner, then, in attempting to establish a career:

... was confronted with a lay public whose recognition of the value of qualified practice was less than wholehearted. Many, perhaps most, people frequently relied on home remedies or patent medicines purchased at the local chemist's shop. People of all classes resorted to the unlicensed ministration of the herbalist, bonesetter, homoeopathist, or midwife. A general practitioner at a dinner party might blush to hear his gentlemanly host scoff at the doctor-patient relationship as a case of 'the blind leading the blind' and a course of treatment as 'a course of groping in the dark'. Medical opinion on matters of public health was sometimes ignored, sometimes not even sought. Employers of medical men treated them as employees, rather than as experts.[16]

Besides, for those without the option of an established family practice to join, starting a career was also expensive. The central problem was to cultivate and retain a clientele. This would take time for a new practice, and could prove impossible where a town already had several practitioners. Savings would certainly be necessary as a means of support until economic viability had been secured. The early years would also require financial outlay in order to develop that outward appearance of sobriety and gentility without which customers could not be attracted. A suitable residence, suits, carriage, houses, servants and a wife (given the social mores of the time, women patients, as well as their husbands, deemed this only proper) were all important. Money was also required to purchase drugs and equipment. No less vital was time to socialise and entertain. Clients who preferred to pay by means of an annual bill could not be turned away - but added to the drain on hard pressed resources. Many newly qualified practitioners, of course, could not afford all these indulgences. About £100 was probably the absolute minimum required in the first year just to survive.[17]

Less risky was the decision to purchase either a
partnership or a single-handed practice. These were
advertised in the pages of medical journals, and solo practices
would be priced according to the annual income which they
customarily generated. Though the purchase of an existing
practice helped to overcome the problem of attracting clients
they were by no means cheap. A good practice, i.e. one
which was non-dispensing and had a middle class clientele
(higher fees could be charged to wealthier customers), might
cost over £1000.[18] Others, in which the doctor made up
medicines and dispensed, and which were situated in poor
and/or densely populated working class areas, were less
attractive. Here fees were lower, the work harder and often -
particularly with frequent obstetric work - time consuming.
Prices might be as low as £100.[19]

In the absence of family connections, then, beginning a
career in general practice was a difficult, expensive and
competitive business. Few have given better literary testimony
to this than that most acute observer of rural and provincial
life, Anthony Trollope, who, particularly in Chapter Three of
Dr Thorne - published in 1858 - painted a most illuminating
picture of the professional rivalries and social exigencies
involved. And if the early years in particular were likely to
be impecunious, even established general practices rarely
yielded a comfortable income. About £700 per annum was
probably required in the 1870s to sustain the material appearance of respectability, but it is conceivable that most practitioners earnt about half this figure. Though fee schedules
provide only an imperfect guide to average earnings - since
fees charged would vary according to services required and
the financial resources of the client - ten calls per day at an
average of 2/6d per call would not have been that unusual.
Over a year, however, this would yield - even assuming a six
day week - only some £390.[20] No practitioner, then, could
really succeed without appropriate social credentials: often
these were lacking to begin with, and impecuniousness might
frustrate subsequent attempts to acquire the material trap-
pings of a respectable household.

Not surprisingly, general practitioners often sought to
supplement their income by part-time employment in a government or other private post. Should a career in general
practice fail, or could not even be initiated, such employment
would have to be full-time. There were expanding opportunities in this respect. The Victorian years saw a proliferation of government appointments - such as Public
Vaccinator, Prison Medical Officer and Poor Law Medical
Officer - as well as posts in private institutions (e.g. in
public schools or orphanages, in various kinds of asylum or
charitable or even commercial and entrepreneurial organisations, in provident dispensaries and in the sick clubs of
workers' associations).

Appointments of this nature, if increasingly available, were neither lucrative nor professionally rewarding. Generally, salaries were very low and in most cases the appointment was made by lay authorities and remained subject to lay control. The post of Poor Law Medical Officer was a classic illustration of these tendencies. Part-time, a doctor could earn as little as £5 to £10 per annum in the 1840s.[21] Appointed by lay administrators, and subject to their annual reappointment, the everyday work of the doctor was also under lay control in the form of the Relieving Officer, who was responsible for deciding which pauper applicants should receive treatment. Until the 1840s doctors were obliged to bid or tender for Poor Law appointments. With the emphasis on economy rather than ability, the lowest bid usually secured the position. The fact that doctors were prepared to accept such meagre remuneration is illustrative of the competitiveness of medical careers in the nineteenth century.

In London especially, this competition was fierce, with one practitioner for every 750 people – approximately twice the national average (in 1861, this was about 1:1400; by 1891, it had risen to 1:1500). Competition tended to depress medical incomes generally, as well as reinforcing the association between trade and physic. Peterson notes:

> Whether in [private practice], public employment, salaried posts, sick clubs, or dispensaries, medical men shared the fate of being subject to, ruled by, and dependent on their lay employers. Such lay dominance was possible because of the overcrowding of the profession and the consequent competition among medical men for practice wherever it could be found.[22]

It was also a situation which followed naturally from the low public regard for medical knowledge itself. The formation of general practitioner associations – such as the BMA, the Poor Law Medical Officers' Association (1868), and the Association of Medical Officers of Health (1856) – showed that despite the competitive nature of their existence, doctors could co-operate in the pursuit of collective interests, but ultimately such action could only produce an improvement in their economic and social position, and greater autonomy in work, when medical skills, qualifications and expertise ceased to be regarded as less important than the social bearing of practitioners themselves. And in turn, this transformation depended on developments in the theory and practice of medicine and surgery which would lend the dignity and authority of science to the training and work of the profession. By demarcating the practice of the professional from that of the quack, these developments would provide a more secure basis on which claims to occupational status and self-regulation could be pressed.

The decline of lay control over medical work which began to occur in roughly the last quarter of the nineteenth century was among the first of the practical effects of the scientific revolution in medicine on the occupational position of doctors. Significantly, at the apex of the profession, appointments in the teaching hospitals began to be based more on peer assessment of people's record of research, their contribution to the development of medical knowledge, and on their clinical or surgical skill, and rather less on their possession of exclusive social attributes. Claims, too, were successfully pressed for bringing auxillary medical staff, such as nurses, under the control of hospital physicians and surgeons. If, it was argued, patient care demanded the exercise of soundly based specialised knowledge, the work of all those involved in patient care should be directed by the trained expert:

> The system of gubernatorial control [in hospitals] died slowly, but the demands of the hospitals for skilled staff, the growing certainty among laymen that training was prerequisite for medical judgement, and medical men's assertion of authority based on medical knowledge - all these opened the door to professional power in the hospitals.[23]

Fundamental changes, then, occurred in the organisation of medicine in the nineteenth century: the tripartite structure of physician, surgeon and apothecary collapsed with the emergence and formal recognition of the general practitioner; hospitals emerged as centres of medical education; the elite of the profession consolidated its control over education, licensing and the Royal Colleges; and general practitioners, failing to find support and representation from the leaders of the profession, began to form their own associations. General practice, however, was no route to wealth or social esteem. Unprotected from unlicensed competition, it was highly competitive; earnings were low and reflected the lack of prestige with which medicine was regarded by society. Largely of undistinguished social origin themselves, medical practitioners - whether in private practice, government employment or in hospitals - were subject to lay authority; and success, if it was to be had at all, lay not so much in expertise, as in the emulation of the habits, manners, morals and general life-style of genteel society. On the possession, acquisition or absence of characteristics such as these were practitioners judged by employers, by clients, and, indeed, by colleagues.

Yet the emergence of the hospital also provided the material foundation for the scientific advances destined to occur later in the century. Patients were now physically examined, and many diseases more precisely recognised from the opportunity for post-mortem examination. Eighteenth century theorising, though lingeringly influential, was more

or less abandoned. Therapeutics, however, remained violent
for many years. Though the work of men like Pasteur and
Koch was later to revolutionise the understanding of disease,
and certain developments in immunisation bore tentative fruit
(e.g. for anthrax, rabies, cholera, typhoid), even by the
end of the century the range of safe and generally effective
drugs was small.
The important new drugs of the scientific revolution
were those used in anaesthesia. Microbes may have been
singled out as a necessary (if not sufficient) condition for the
appearance of some infective diseases (in fact, between 1874
and 1894 the bacteria responsible for gonorrhoea, typhoid,
pneumonia, erysipelas, diphtheria, tetanus, meningitis and
the plague had all been identified), and though this general
understanding helped to make surgery and childbirth safer,
there was as yet no 'magic bullet' which would save those
already suffering from life threatening infections. Nevertheless, bacteriology represented the culmination of scientific
developments in nineteenth century medicine. Working in a
discipline which had thus gained, towards the end of the
century, from the authority of scientific achievement, medical
practitioners had a firmer basis on which to lay claim to, and
achieve, greater professional prestige and occupational
autonomy.
When homoeopathy first appeared in Britain, most of
these important developments lay in the future. Not surprisingly, homoeopathy's subsequent career was to be affected by
them. Indeed, as will be seen, homoeopathy managed to effect
important changes in conventional practice in its own right.
Clearly, however, the medical terrain in which homoeopathy flourished was one which would invite its condemnation
by medical practitioners. At the same time, it was a terrain
which, through competitive exigency and client power,
encouraged the adoption of homoeopathy by certain practitioners. The profession was overcrowded and largely dis-
valued. A practitioner who 'broke rank', achieving status and
prosperity through the practice of a special system of
medicine, represented not only an intellectual, social and
professional threat to a medical community struggling for
social recognition, but also a direct economic threat to its
individual members. Naturally, too, practitioners were liable
to react strongly to colleagues who implied that the conventional wisdom of the profession merited not merely low
prestige, but in fact no prestige at all. In effect, this was
exactly how the bulk of the profession interpreted the
homoeopathic critique - though it ought to be said that few
homoeopaths, either in Britain, Europe or America, really
argued such an extreme position. Clarification of the theoretical points at issue between the two schools, however, is
best achieved by comparing Hahnemann's own work with that

of a leading teacher, practitioner and writer of the orthodox medical world in the 1830s - Sir Thomas Watson.

NOTES

1. M.J. Peterson, The Medical Profession in Mid-Victorian London (University of California Press, Berkeley, 1978) pp. 5-6. Chapter Five owes much to Peterson's excellent discussion. Other useful texts here are J. Berlant, Profession and Monopoly (University of California Press, Berkeley and Los Angeles, 1975); N. Parry and J. Parry, The Rise of the Medical Profession (Croom Helm, London, 1976); C. Newman, The Evolution of Medical Education in the Nineteenth Century (Oxford University Press, London, 1957); and F.N.L. Poynter (ed.), The Evolution of Medical Education in Britain (Pitman, London, 1966).
2. M.J. Peterson, op.cit., p. 8.
3. Ibid., p. 10.
4. Ibid.
5. Ibid., p. 11.
6. Quoted by M.J. Peterson, op.cit., p. 26.
7. Ibid., p. 137.
8. Quoted by F.H. Garrison, History of Medicine, 2nd edition (W.B. Saunders Company, Philadelphia and London, 1917) p. 754.
9. Quoted in A.M. Carr-Saunders and P.A. Wilson, The Professions (Clarendon Press, Oxford, 1933) p. 295.
10. Quoted in M.J. Peterson, op.cit., p. 342 (note 2 to chapter 5).
11. For a more detailed statistical documentation of these points, see the discussion indicated at note 12 below.
12. See the discussion, ibid., chapter 2, especially Table 3, p. 54; and chapter 5, especially Table 9, p. 198.
13. Ibid., Tables 1 and 2, pp. 50-1.
14. Ibid., pp. 74-5.
15. Ibid., p. 91.
16. Ibid., p. 90.
17. Ibid., p. 97.
18. Ibid., p. 99.
19. Ibid.
20. See the discussion, ibid., pp. 206-24.
21. Ibid., p. 111.
22. Ibid., p. 116.
23. Ibid., p. 188.

Chapter Six

HAHNEMANN AND WATSON - CONTRADICTION AND
DISJUNCTION IN MEDICAL THOUGHT

In selecting texts with which to compare the Organon, it is
actually of more value to choose material published when
homoeopathy was establishing itself as a significant force in
British medicine, than from work current during the 1790s,
when Hahnemann was developing the homoeopathic system.[1]
This helps to highlight the differences between the two
approaches which would have been perceived by medical
practitioners in the middle of the nineteenth century.

The clearest exposition of the principles and nature of
regular practice for this period is probably found in the work
of Sir Thomas Watson, whose Lectures on the Principles and
Practice of Physic were first published in 1843.[2] Watson,
formerly a Fellow of St. John's College Cambridge, was
physician to the Middlesex Hospital, and also a Fellow of the
Royal College. The lectures which comprise the publication of
1843 were first delivered at King's College London in 1836-7,
and were repeated, more or less unchanged, for several years
afterwards. First serialised in the Medical Gazette before
appearing in book form, the lectures acquired a high
reputation - not by virtue of any innovatory content which
they possessed, but rather because of the elegant clarity with
which the author pursued a formal statement of the discipline
for medical students. Indeed, as the preface to volume one
makes clear, Watson's main hope was that the collected
lectures '... may prove useful as a textbook for students'.[3]
His hopes were more than fulfilled: 'For more than a quarter
of century, this work continued to pass through many
editions and enjoyed a well deserved popularity ...'.[4] For
present purposes, Watson's work is therefore an ideal selection. It was popular, it influenced several generations of
medical students, and it represents a clear and distinct
statement of contemporary theory and practice.

On every important issue, however, Watson and
Hahnemann assume diametrically opposed positions.[5] These
disjunctions in medical theory help to explain the strength of
the ensuing allopathic reaction to the homoeopathic movement.

ON THE NATURE OF THE HUMAN ORGANISM

Scattered throughout Watson's lectures are numerous state-
ments which reveal a concept of the human organism as a
complex piece of machinery. Some of the more isolated
examples could be interpreted as metaphorical devices, whose
appearance and utility in a pedagogic context might easily be
anticipated. Thus in discussing the pathological changes to
which the human system is subject, Watson remarks:

> You cannot fail to perceive the injurious effects which
> many of these changes in the various solids are calcu-
> lated to produce upon the movements and working of the
> living machine; how some of them must impede or
> derange its natural action; some stop that action
> altogether.[6]

Yet other instances clearly indicate that the mechanistic
analogy is meant literally. The human organism is not merely
like a machine; it is not even the case that, for medical
purposes, it might be usefully considered as a machine - it is
a machine:

> The most cursory examination of the animal economy
> suffices to show that it is made up, not merely of
> separate parts, but of several distinct systems. There is
> one set of organs for the mechanical circulation of the
> blood; there is an apparatus expressly designed for the
> repeated exposure of the blood to the air; a system for
> regulating the movements and feelings of the body;
> another for receiving, preparing, and appropriating its
> nourishment; another for the elaboration of matters that
> are useful or essential to its functions; another for
> carrying off its impurities, and for removing its
> superfluous or effete materials; and another for the
> continuance of the species.[7]

And even more strongly:

> Observe the ample provision that is made, in the con-
> struction of the body, for carrying on and maintaining
> [the circulation of the blood]. First, there is an
> extensive hydraulic apparatus distributed throughout the
> frame, and consisting of the heart and other blood
> vessels. Next, there is a large pneumatic machine,
> forming a considerable part of the whole body, and
> composed of the lungs, and the case in which they are
> lodged. Lastly, the power by which this machine is to be
> worked and regulated is vested in the nervous system.
> Each of these systems must continue in action, or the
> circulation will stop, and life will come to an end.[8]

Watson's mechanistic perspective has profound implications for nosology, pathology and therapeutics. If the body
is a machine, then sickness is a mechanistic disorder. Human
'machines' being essentially identical, they are liable to
common and recurring malfunctions of their constituent parts.
This lays the basis for the identification of classes of disease
as the proper subject of the therapeutic endeavour. Mechan-
istically, there can be no individuality of sickness. The
physician's first task is to name the disease – and then to
treat it by aiming to remove or oppose the mechanically based
disorder characteristic of a particular class of morbidity.

Hahnemann, on the other hand, argues for a vitalistic
appreciation:

> In the healthy condition of Man, the spiritual vital force
> (autocracy), the dynamis that animates the material body
> (organism) rules completely, and retains all the parts of
> the organism in admirable, harmonious, vital operation,
> as regards both sensation and functions ...
>
> The material organism, without the vital force, is capable
> of no sensation, no function, no self-preservation ...
> The material organism derives all sensation and performs
> all the functions of life solely by means of the immaterial
> being (the vital force) which animates the material
> organism in health and in disease.[9]

Summarising, then: for Watson, organic life is dependent
on hydraulic and pneumatic mechanical systems, activated by
power supplied through the nervous system; for Hahnemann,
individuals can only be understood in terms of a vital force
which '... rules completely and retains all the parts of the
organism in admirable, harmonious, vital operation ...'.
Disease is thus a vitalistic problem, affecting and involving
both the physical and mental disposition of the individual.
Treatment therefore needs to focus on the whole person,
whose idiosyncratic response to illness rules out the possibility of elaborating standardised categories of disease. Moreover, since the vital force is responsible for the equilibrium
of health, the signs and symptoms of illness can be viewed as
the expression of its attempt to restore normality. The task
of the physician should therefore be to assist this process.

The difference between a mechanistic and vitalistic
appreciation of the human organism is fundamental to an
understanding of homoeopathy's dispute with medical
orthodoxy in the nineteenth century, for it is in the contrast
between these initial premises that all succeeding points of
disagreement are ultimately rooted. This will become clearer
as the discussion proceeds.

ON DISEASE

If, for Watson, the body is to be understood as an inter-
connection of mechanical systems, then it follows that disease
should originate from adverse structural changes and/or
functional impediments. This is precisely the perspective
which Watson employs:

> There are various ways, capable of intelligent descrip-
> tion, in which the different parts of the body may be
> altered by disease.
>
> The solid parts may be altered in bulk; in form; in
> consistence; in their intimate texture, i.e. in the
> qualities and arrangement of their component particles;
> and in situation.
>
> The fluid parts may also be altered in quantity; in
> quality; and in place.[10]

Watson elaborates as follows:

> [Solids] may be simply altered in bulk without any
> change of texture; and that in two ways. They may
> become larger than natural, or smaller than natural. In
> the one case the change is called hypertrophy, in the
> other, atrophy.[11]

And:

> Hypertrophy ... is believed to depend upon more active
> nutrition of the part. More materials are laid down in the
> part by the blood, and assimilated, than are received
> back from the part into the blood to be taken out of the
> body.[12]

The mechanistic perspective is again revealed in Watson's
discussion of the relationship of hypertrophy to disease:

> Thus we have it in the hollow contractile organs, the
> office of which is to propel fluids:- in the heart, when
> the progress of blood suffers from some mechanical
> disorder: in the bladder when the urine and in the
> intestinal canal when its contents are somehow hindered
> in their natural course; or when, from some stimulus or
> irritation, these parts respectively are urged for a long
> time together to excessive, or too frequent action.[13]

Atrophy, on the other hand, occurs when 'Building
materials are not provided by the blood, or are provided
inadequately'.[14] And when atrophy:

... is morbid in its nature, [it] may be the consequence
of inaction, of compression, of chronic inflammation, and
of various diseases; but in all cases the deficit of
nutrition which constitutes the atrophy seems to be
resolvable into a diminished supply of blood through the
arteries.[15]

Changes in bulk often involved changes in form: for
example, 'You will have one or two of the chambers of the
heart greatly enlarged, while the others remain of their
natural size'.[16]
A third set of morbid changes occurs when organs
become too hard (induration) or too soft: 'Induration of an
organ may happen ... in consequence of inordinate fullness of
its blood vessels'.[17] Or:

... from the expression of its fluid, and compression of
its solid parts. We see this extremely well in the lung,
when it has been thrust and flattened against the
vertebral column by fluid effused into the pleura.[18]

But more frequently:

... induration depends upon the presence, in the
internal texture of parts, in the little spaces left
between their component tissues, of fluid or solid
matters which are not found in the healthy state. Bony
or earthy particles are sometimes laid down, and the
part thus changed is said to be ossified ... [Such
changes are] especially common in the coats of the
arteries ...[19]

Tumours and tubercular nodules were also instances of
induration, since they involved '... the deposition or growth
of irregular masses of matter within the body, differing
remarkably from any of the solids or fluids that enter into its
healthy composition'.[20]
While some structures of the body may be immune to
induration, however, 'There is scarcely any tissue of the
living body in which softening may not take place ... brain
... cellular tissue ... muscles ... mucous membranes ...
even the bones ...'.[21] Inflammation was usually the culprit:

Every part, I believe, that is inflamed undergoes, in the
first instance, a diminution of its consistence. This
appears to be almost the necessary consequence of the
stagnation of the blood, the effusion of serosity, and the
suspension of healthy nutrition.[22]

Finally, tissues may undergo transformation of their
intimate texture. Watson mentions that tissues may become

fatty, or fibrous, or like cartilage;[23] and the altered
position of solid parts was of morbid potential when, for
example:

> In the chest, a whole lung may be displaced, ... by the
> blood, or serum, or air effused into the cavity of the
> pleura ... And in the abdomen and pelvis, the various
> forms of hernia may be adduced as involving very
> dangerous changes in the place and relative position of
> parts.[24]

Watson's discussion of the alteration in the quantity,
quality and situation of body fluids proceeds along similar
lines. Though he recognises the existence of fluids other than
blood in the body, Watson is most interested in blood itself.
The central task here was to:

> ... inquire what morbid changes the blood itself is liable
> to undergo.

> The blood, then, is subject, first to remarkable vari-
> ations in its quantity, both in respect of the whole
> system [general plethora or congestion], and in respect
> to particular organs and tissues [local plethora or con-
> gestion].

> Closely connected with these differences of quantity is
> the variety which is observable in regard to the propor-
> tions between the several proximate constituents of the
> blood ... blood drawn from a vein is thinner, manifestly
> more watery, less rich in fibrin and in colouring matter,
> than blood of the standard quality.

Again

> ... the blood is liable to great change in its chemical
> composition, and, therefore, in its physical quality. This
> appears to be the case in sea scurvy, and in the
> analogous disease called purpura [bruising from sub-
> cutaneous haemorrhages] and it is doubtless so in many
> other complaints.[25]

Congestion, we are told, is responsible for major categories of disease:

> If we comprehend rightly this subject of plethora or
> congestion, we shall be prepared to understand some
> most important morbid states, of which it seems to be in
> many, if not in all cases, the earliest approach. Inflam-
> mation, haemorrhage, dropsy, all acknowledge and imply
> a previous condition of congestion.[26]

Logically, general plethora implies local plethora of every organ and tissue. A general deficiency, however, does not necessarily mean an absence of local congestion. 'Far from it. Local determinations of blood are very common in persons in whom the mass of that fluid ... has been considerably diminished by disease, or by haemorrhage'.[27]

Watson goes on to distinguish three kinds of congestion: active, associated with '... increased velocity of blood in the arteries ...';[28] mechanical, due to '... any mechanical obstacle in the veins';[29] and passive, where blood accumulates in the capillaries.[30]

For Watson - and he was merely reiterating a medical commonplace of the period - understanding the forms and implications of plethora was almost the physicians's equivalent of the philosopher's stone. To know the qualitative and quantitative capriciousness of blood was, in truth, to lay 'the foundation for the better understanding of those three great classes of disease - Inflammations, Haemorrhage, and Dropsies'.[31]

Before turning to the contrasting perspective found in Hahnemann's writing it is worth emphasising two points. Firstly, Watson's analysis of pathology is seen to be firmly rooted in a material and mechanistic view of the human organism. Disease becomes a malfunction of the parts and systems of the human machine. Secondly, disease is seen as an internal problem. Symptoms only represent its external appearance. The physician must become expert at using symptoms in order to interpret the hidden nature of the real problem - but the signs and symptoms are not the disease itself. It will be necessary to return to this issue later, but it must be made explicit here in order to highlight the alternative perspective taken in the Organon.

In discussing the nature of illness, Hahnemann writes:

The unprejudiced observer takes note of nothing except the changes in the health of the body and of the mind ... which can be perceived externally by means of the senses. He notices only the deviations from the former healthy state of the new diseased individual, which are felt by the patient himself, remarked by those around him and observed by the physician. All these perceptible signs represent the disease in its whole extent, that is together they form the true and only conceivable portrait of the disease ...

Removal of all the symptoms of the disease and of the entire collection of the perceptible phenomena of the disease leaves nothing besides health. The unhealthy alteration in the interior is eradicated ... It is only the vital force, deranged to such an abnormal state, that can furnish the organism with its disagreeable sen-

sations, and incline it to the irregular processes which
we call disease. As a power invisible in itself, and only
recognizable by its effects on the organism, its unhealthy derangement only makes itself known by the
manifestations of disease in the sensations and functions
of those parts of the organism exposed to the senses of
the observer and the physician; that is by disease
symptoms, and in no other way can it make itself known
... The consideration of disease as being a thing
separate from the living whole, that is from the organism
and its animating vital force, could only be imagined by
minds of materialist stamp.[32]

Comparing this account with Watson's analysis of the
types and forms of human morbidity, certain key areas of
disagreement are revealed. Firstly for Hahnemann, disease is
not purely organically based nor mechanically caused. Essentially it is a derangement of the animating vital force of the
human organism. Secondly, the effect of disease on the vital
force is only apparent to the physician in terms of the signs
and symptoms which it produces in the individual. Indeed,
that is all that disease consists in, and when the symptoms
are removed, health is restored. Thirdly, since disease
consists solely in the symptoms generated by a deranged vital
force, and since the vital force is all pervasive, mental as
well as physical symptoms are important. Disease is always
disease of the whole organism.

ON NOSOLOGY

In the Lectures Watson's remarks on the classification of
disease are fairly brief. His writing suggests him to have
been a man of practical persuasion, concerned more with
activities in the ward and at the bedside, and with emphasising the importance of this clinical experience to his
students, than with the more academic areas of medical
inquiry. Watson thus gives nosology fairly short shrift.[33]
     For the purpose of his own discourse, Watson adopts an
eclectic position. His main principle is to classify diseases in
terms of '... the anatomy of regions - the place and situation
of organs ...'[34] affected, though he occasionally makes use
of alternative rationales, such as the body system or body
tissue involved. Classifying diseases in terms of symptoms,
however, is rejected. Watson states that he is not going to
'... attempt to construct a nosological system by grouping
together certain sets of symptoms, and calling each set, in its
collective form, a disease'.[35] This option is unsatisfactory,
since symptoms merely represent the appearance, not the
reality, of disease.

More important for Watson than nosology is the precise and accurate diagnosis of diseased conditions. For this:

... defines and fixes the objects about which observation is to be exercised, and experience collected. When we can once identify a given diseased condition, we obtain the privilege of watching the behaviour of that diseased condition, again and again, under the operation of therapeutic measures; and from that time the increase of our knowledge concerning the appropriate management of that particular disease becomes progressive and sure.[36]

This observation goes to the heart of the matter. The mechanical similarity of people's bodies, and mechanical interpretation of disease, underpins a materialist nosology which focuses on unchanging disease entities whose appropriate therapeutic management can be refined through the accumulation of clinical experience. Skill in the interpretation of symptoms is certainly necessary for accurate diagnosis - but it is the diagnosis which counts for Watson. Quite how diseases are classified after they have been accurately identified is a subsidiary problem - and one which, even if satisfactorily solved, has no obvious therapeutic pay off.

Hahnemann's approach is quite different. It has already been indicated that, homoeopathically, there is nothing more to disease than the symptoms themselves. The physician needs to know, in great detail, precisely what symptoms the individual experiences:

The patient details the history of his sufferings. Those about him tell of what they have heard him complain, how he has behaved and what they have noticed in him. The physician sees, hears and remarks by all his other senses what there is of an altered and unusual character about the patient. He writes down accurately all that the patient and his friends have told him in the very expressions used by them ... The physician begins a fresh line with every new circumstance mentioned by the patient or his friends. Thus the symptoms are arranged separately one below the other ... When the narrator has finished what he would say of his own accord, the physician then reverts to each particular symptom and elicits more precise information. At what period did the symptom occur? Did the symptom occur before taking the medicine he had hitherto been using? Whilst taking the medicine? Or only some days after leaving off the medicine? What kind of pain? What exact sensation? Where was the precise spot? Did the pain occur in fits? By itself? At various times? Or was the pain continuous?

How long did it last? At what time of day or night? In what position of the body was it worse or ceased entirely? What was the exact nature of this or that event or circumstance described in plain words?[37]

The resulting symptom picture of the patient would thus be individualistic. For Hahnemann, then, nosological exercises were largely fruitless, since each instance of disease was unique:[38]

The physician must regard the pure picture of every prevailing disease as if it were something new and unknown and investigate it thoroughly for itself, if he desires to practise medicine in a real and radical manner. The physician must never substitute conjecture for actual observation, never taking for granted that the case of disease before him is already wholly or partially known. He must examine the illness in all its phases, because a careful examination will show that every prevailing disease is in many respects a phenomenon of a unique character ...[39]

ON THE CAUSES OF DISEASE

Watson divides the causes of disease into three classes: predisposing, exciting and proximate. A predisposing cause is defined as '... anything whatever which has had such a previous influence upon the body as to have put it in a condition of greater susceptibility to the exciting cause of the particular disease'.[40] Thus a family might have a constitutional predisposition toward consumption (predisposing cause), while exposure to a cold damp climate (exciting cause) might result in the actual appearance of the disease. Clearly, however:

It is sometimes difficult, or impossible to say of a given cause whether it ought to be ranked among the exciting or among the predisposing causes: whether it has prepared the system for being affected by some other agent, or whether it has itself produced the disease ...[41]

Among those predisposing (or exciting) causes cited by Watson are extremes of heat or cold, dampness or dryness, different electrical conditions in the atmosphere, differences of pressure, a deficiency of light, poor diet or overeating, excessive drinking, certain occupations (e.g. coal-mining), lack of exercise, overwork, anxiety, too much or too little sleep, and air when '... loaded with impurities ... contagious ... and noxious gases'.[42]

65

The sensible physician, of course, will advocate the removal, where possible, of any identified cause. Hahnemann agrees: 'Every intelligent physician will first remove any manifest or maintaining cause of disease'.[43]
The real disagreement between the two writers turns on the concept of the proximate cause. For Watson, this is '... nothing less than the disease itself - the actual condition of the body, from which the whole train of morbid phenomena essentially flows'.[44] Actually, he does not consider the concept of 'proximate cause' a very helpful one. On the contrary, he suggests that it is confusing, and prefers instead to talk of 'diseases' instead of 'proximate causes'. The dispute, then, turns on the concept of disease itself - a subject already addressed. Whereas Watson regards disease as an internal functional or structural disorder, Hahnemann argues:

> The dominant school of medicine affects to possess a supernatural insight into the inner nature of things and so renders it impossible for man to know disease. It is in consequence impossible for the dominant school to cure disease. That which needs to be cured in illness is not in fact shrouded in mysterious obscurity. Illness is the sum of its symptoms.[45]

ON SYMPTOMS

Sufficient ground has already been laid to enable remarks here to be brief. Watson argues that '... although diseases are not constituted by symptoms, they are, in the living body, disclosed by symptoms',[46] and that the physician should '... always strive ... to penetrate beyond the symptoms to the disease of which they are significant ...'.[47]
Hahnemann, on the other hand, insists that the distinction between 'internal disease' and 'perceptible symptoms (or signs)' is a false one. Arguing that 'The sole and infallible oracle of the healing art is pure experience',[48] it follows that the only pathological reality on which physicians can reliably focus is that which is constituted from data immediately perceptible to themselves or their patients. Thus 'There is nothing that needs to be removed from a disease in order to achieve a state of health, apart from the totality of the signs and symptoms of that disease.'[49]
Watson and Hahnemann are not only in disagreement about the relationship between disease and symptoms. They also adopt different stances with respect to the morbidity of signs and symptoms themselves. For Watson, signs and/or symptoms clearly are, in general, morbid. A pathological

condition produces pathological signs and symptoms: as he says, a '... whole train of morbid phenomena ...' flows from the disease. (There were, however, some exceptions to this rule - for example, those signs which indicated, or were felt to indicate, that a lesion was healing.) Hahnemann, though, makes a more positive interpretation. While symptoms indicate that a derangement of the vital force has occurred, they also indicate the way in which the vital force is reacting to the disease. Hence the more positive appreciation of symptoms in the homoeopathic system - and the rationale for the similar remedy.

ON TREATMENT

Inflammation, for Watson and his contemporaries, was almost always involved in disease. Indicating the treatment of this condition provides an excellent opportunity to examine the rationale of the contrary remedy, and to appreciate the scope of its application.

Approvingly, Watson quotes Dr Alison's view that there is:

... no kind of diseased action of which any part of the living body is susceptible, which is not connected, sooner or later, with increased afflux of blood towards that part, either as its cause or its effect; and the immediate object of all our most powerful remedies is to act on these irregularities of the circulation.[50]

Watson agrees: pain, swelling, redness and heat - all signs or symptoms of inflammation - depend upon '... the increased influx of blood into the part'.[51] All treatment of inflammatory conditions thus focused on relieving pressure from an excess of blood and in undoing, if appropriate, the internal adhesion of parts which inflammation was felt to produce.

The first step in achieving these objectives was the imposition of the 'antiphlogistic regimen', which involved the '... avoidance of every stimulus that can be avoided, whether external or internal'.[52] The patient was to be protected from all forms of mental or physical agitation or stimulus; inflamed parts, where accessible, were to be immobilised; diet was to be bland, excluding animal foods and strong drink, and the patient was to remain in bed in a quiet, moderately lit and temperate room. The rationale for these precautions was to avoid raising the heart beat, as this determined the force with which blood was pumped into the inflamed organ.

These initial measures attended to, the physician's next task was to relieve pressure by venesection. 'Of all the direct remedies', Watson observes, 'of inflammation, the abstraction of blood ... is by much the most effectual and important.'[53] Following venesection:

The evacuation next in importance ... is purging ... two points are gained by it. The stomach and intestines are freed from accumulated faeces, or other matters which, by their bulk or acrimony, might prove irritating, and at the same time depletion is carried on by means of the serous discharge which is produced from that large extent of mucous membrane.[54]

Mercury was one of the medicines which had a purgative effect. But its use in combating inflammation was valued for other reasons. As Watson puts it, mercury is '... a very powerful agent in controlling ... adhesive inflammation; such as glues the parts together, and spoils the texture of organs',[55] since it has '... a loosening effect upon certain textures; it works by pulling down parts of the building'.[56]

Other medicines with a role in the anti-inflammation regimen were antimony (antimonial tartrate - the tartar-emetic) which '... subdues the action of the heart and arteries',[57] as well as procuring further depletion through its emetic effect; digitalis (Digitalis purpurea, Foxglove) - but Watson is less enthusiastic about this remedy, since the precise dose required to achieve a reduction (!) in heart rate was difficult to estimate; and opium, which '... soothes ... nervous irritability'.[58]

Cold baths or ice bags might be employed to reduce pain or heat. Warm poultices might also be used, though this was not a similar remedy, since the rationale was to encourage blood to 'determine to the surface'[59] from an engorged organ. Finally, counter-irritation of the skin was employed: 'It probably operates', Watson argues, 'by attracting blood into the neighbouring parts, and in the same degree diverting it from the inflamed part.'[60]

Each of the above remedies is justified in terms of the principle of opposition: remedies are useful to the extent to which they oppose the cause of the disease in question. Significantly too, the remedies - perhaps with the minor exception of cold applications - are not aimed directly at the signs or symptoms of the disease (swelling, redness, pain, tenderness, heat, etc.), but at the internal phenomenon held to be responsible for their appearance, i.e. plethora, peccant material, and the internal adhesion of parts.

Hahnemann, however, was strongly opposed to the kind of practices which informed the allopathic treatment of inflammation and other disorders. This opposition was grounded in a number of convictions. First, disease was held to consist of nothing more than the peculiar symptoms experienced by individual patients. This meant that a category such as 'inflammatory disease' was rendered meaningless: the symptoms of someone with a sore finger would be very different from those of someone with sore tonsils. It also meant that remedies should be selected by reference to symptoms, and not to any hypothesised internal cause. Secondly, Hahnemann was convinced that allopathic remedies did not cure. The large doses used might produce temporary relief - but would, in so doing, add a further medicinal or iatrogenic disease to the original:

> Allopathic treatment, without ever being able to remove and cure the original (dissimilar) chronic disease, only develops new artificial diseases beside it. As daily experience shows, this practice renders the patient much worse and more incurable than before.[61]

Moreover:

> The ordinary physician imagines he can get over the difficulties of antipathic treatment by giving a stronger dose of the remedy at each renewed aggravation of the illness. By this method an equally transient suppression of disease is effected and then there is still greater necessity for giving every-increasing quantities of the palliative. There ensues either more serious disease or frequently danger to life, and then to death itself.[62]

The third and most important basis of Hahnemann's rejection of allopathic treatment is that the principle of opposition itself is wrong:

> Had physicians been capable of reflecting upon the sad results of antipathic treatment they would have long since discovered the grand truth that the true radical healing art must be found in the exact opposite of such an antipathic treatment of the symptoms of disease. The homoeopathic employment of medicines according to similarity of symptoms will effect a permanent and perfect cure, if at the same time the most minute doses are exhibited instead of the large doses of the ordinary physician.[63]

As was made clear in Chapter One, Hahnemann's own experiments with quinine had suggested that substances capable of producing certain sets of symptoms in healthy persons will relieve those symptoms in sickness. His typical response to disbelievers was to invite them to try the principle for themselves. That it worked, he argued, was more important than why it worked. Nevertheless, Hahnemann - drawing on Hunter's idea that two diseases rarely concur, and hence that an artificial disease will tend to cure by a

process of displacement - did attempt to construct a theoretical explanation of the principle of similarity.
His first contention is that all medicines are capable of producing illness:

> ... it is very evident that medicines could never cure diseases if they did not possess the power of altering man's state of health ... their curative power must be due solely to this power they possess of altering man's state of health.[64]

The second premise concerns the interaction of diseases within the body. Hahnemann argues that if two dissimilar diseases meet together in the human organism, the stronger will oust the weaker, or if of equal strength, the original disease will repel the newcomer:

> If two dissimilar diseases meeting together in the human being are of equal strength, or still more if the older one is the stronger, the new disease will be repelled by the older one ...

And:

> When a new dissimilar disease is stronger than the original illness, the original illness will be kept back and suspended by the accession of the stronger disease ...[65]

However, if the dissimilar diseases occupy different parts of the body (an inconsistent point for Hahnemann to make), then a multiple or complex diseased state ensues: 'The two diseases join together and the patient is thereby rendered more diseased.'[66]
Herein lies the rationale for the rejection of allopathic treatment, for the contrary remedy, like all medicines, produces a disease, but one which is different from the malady. Hence depending on the relative strength or situation of the two diseases (medicinal plus original illness), any of three things may happen: the original illness repels the medicinal illness; the medicinal illness takes the place of the original illness (during which some temporary alleviation of symptoms would be expected); or the two diseases occupy different parts of the body to form a compound problem. In any event, the patient is not helped and could well be made worse.
However, if two similar diseases meet, the stronger of the two ousts the weaker, and at the same time stimulates the vital force to more energetic reaction, which eventually overcomes the substituted illness. Since this latter is artificially

designed to be of shorter duration anyway, the vital force is rapidly successful in its attempt to restore health:

> A somewhat stronger, similar, artificial disease is brought into contact with, and as it were pushed into the place of the weaker, similar, natural disease. [Hence the possible initial aggravation of symptoms produced by the primary action of the medicine.] The vital force is instinctively compelled to direct an increased amount of energy against this artificial disease. On account of the shorter duration of the action of the medicinal agent that now affects the organism, the vital force soon overcomes the artificial illness. As in the first instance the organism was relieved from the natural disease, so it is finally freed from the substituted artificial medicinal one, and hence is enabled again to carry on in health.[67]

Hahnemann's discussion does not really bear close examination. His explanation of the action of a homoeopathic remedy actually makes reference to vitalism redundant. If the stronger artificial similar disease displaces the weaker original illness, and is said to have an action of short duration, then it will apparently disappear of its own accord, irrespective of any vitalistic or other physiological response. Nevertheless, his judgement that allopathic drugs of the period created disease and debility in their own right, exacerbated existing conditions, and rarely cured, was a telling enough point.

POSOLOGY

> There are practitioners ... who affirm that digitalis may be given, after due depletion, and in acute inflammation, in very large, and I should say startling doses, with the very best effects - doses which range from half a drachm to half an ounce, and even six drachms of the official tincture.[68]

Watson opines that this was excessive - but the heavy prescription of drugs was commonplace, and Watson himself, though on the cautious side of an extravagent spectrum in this respect, was quite prepared to use large doses where relatively smaller ones had failed to produce any immediate impression. He describes a case where '... a child of twenty-eight months took in nine days 350 grains of calomel [a mercurial medicine] ...; and in six of these days 136 grains of jalap [a purgative] ...' but notes that '... large doses of this kind are never to be given, until the inefficiency of smaller ones has been ascertained'.[69]

Examples of the contemporary attitude toward the quantity of drugs required to deal with illnesses are littered through the literature of the period. One such case is that described by John Elliotson, physician to St Thomas's Hospital, in a clinical lecture of 1832 reprinted in The Lancet.[70] The patient had severe neuralgia (or 'tic douloureux') of the finger. Feeling, like Watson, that large doses are not necessary if 'a small one will answer', Elliotson added:

> But I deem it quite as absurd to give small doses when you know that they will not answer ... When a disease is very violent indeed, of course you must bring up your forces in a commensurate manner. No one would think of sending a regiment of soldiers to remove an old apple women; but no one would send two policemen to storm a castle.

Since the neuralgia was indeed violent, Elliotson proceeded to marshall his assault with appropriate vigour. The treatment decided upon was carbonate of iron, and began with 'half an ounce three times a day; and when he had taken that for five days without any benefit whatever, he took the same quantity every four hours'. In addition, '... a quarter of a grain of muriate of morphia ...' was given, as well as bathing the finger in a solution of 'cyanuret of potassium'. This was found ineffective, and was replaced by ether, to cool the finger. The dosage of morphia was increased to a grain every night, and the iron '... to the quantity of an ounce, and it was given every four hours'. To the carbonate of iron was then added sulphate or iron, first in five grains every three hours, and then in ten and fifteen grain doses. After three months, the iron was discontinued, the patient no better.

Strychnine was the next choice, being gradually increased from one twelfth of a grain to three fifths of a grain three times a day; meanwhile the dosage of morphia had risen to two and a half grains per night. The iron was reintroduced: 'He began with half an ounce three times a day, which was increased to an ounce, and then to four times a day', and the morphia was increased 'to three grains twice a day'. Strychnine had produced no improvement, and was replaced by arsenic. This was increased to nine minims three times a day, and was accompanied by hydrocyanic acid to prevent the nausea created by the arsenic. The dose of arsenic was then raised to 'twenty minims three times a day'. (Elliotson adds that the patient 'now began to look thin again', and 'did not look so well as before'). Arsenic was at length discontinued, and to ensure that the patient could sleep, the morphia had meanwhile been raised to 'eight grains twice a day'. Unfortunately, the patient now 'looked as ill as he did when he first came in', and 'wished to go out of the hospital for a fortnight for a change.'

Elliotson's attitude here clearly reveals the prevailing
allopathic concept of disease as a powerful enemy, which
needed to be met with violent, strenuous and indeed heroic
measures. (It also reveals the physician's desire to demonstrate to the patient that effort is not spared on his or her
behalf, with the physiological effect of powerful medicines
becoming the overt measure of conscientious service.)
For Hahnemann, however, this approach was either
ineffective, or dangerous - or both. Asserting that 'The
highest ideal of cure is rapid, gentle, and permanent restoration of health or the removal and annihilation of the disease
in its whole extent, in the shortest, most reliable and most
harmless way',[71] Hahnemann argued that 'uncommonly small
doses of medicine are sufficient by the similarity of their
symptoms, to overpower and remove similar and natural
disease',[72] and that 'it is highly desirable that the dose is
reduced to the degree of minuteness appropriate for a gentle,
remedial effect.'[73]
The doctrine of the minimum dose is intimately connected
with Hahnemann's theory of the power and action of
medicines, and of how their energy can be tapped. A
summary of his ideas on this matter is given immediately
below. Before broaching this issue, however, it is also worth
drawing attention to Hahnemann's insistence that: 'It is never
permissible to administer more than one medicinal substance at
a time.'[74] Again, this contrasts with the prevailing
allopathic view that remedies could be used in combination.
Often a combination of remedies was to be found in a single
medicine. 'Addison's pill' (after Thomas Addison), for
example, contained calomel, digitalis and squills (a
diuretic).[75]

ON THE ACTION OF MEDICINES

A mechanistic conception of the human organism leads into a
mechanistic appreciation of pathology, and inevitably to the
search for remedies whose activity is explicable in terms of
their capacity to exert mechanical effects. Sufficient has been
seen of Watson's work to require little elaboration of the
point: abstraction of blood empties engorged organs or
tissues; purging expels irritating matter and pressurising
fluid via the bowels; emetics clear the stomach of peccant
material; counter-irritation attracts blood from one area of the
body to another; opium calms an irritated nervous system;
digitalis reduces hydraulic pressure by depressing the
pumping rate of the heart, as does antimony; and mercury
works (in inflammation) by either 'causing blood to be
distributed in larger quantity than common upon several
surfaces at the same time', thus reducing 'excessive
congestion or accumulation in any one organ',[76] or by

'stopping, controlling or altogether preventing the effusion of coagulable lymph; of bridling adhesive inflamination.'[77]

Hahnemann's explanation of the action of medicines is quite different. If disease is a product of the derangement of the invisible, incorporeal, animating vital force, then it follows that medicines, if they are to be effective, must be capable of exerting a spiritual effect. In Hahnemann's words 'The power of medicines to heal depends upon the quality of influence which their energy can bring to bear upon the vital force.'[78] Hahnemann stated that to release this energy:

> The homoeopathic system of medicine develops for its special use a mechanical action upon the smallest particles of the substance by means of rubbing and shaking with an inert substance, so as to cause separation of those particles. A remarkable change occurs in the quality of the substance. The power to heal is released, so that even a totally inert substance can come to influence the vital force. The process is succussion or trituration and the change produced in the substance is called potentizing. These three phenomona were not known before my time.[79]

Preparing the first (centesimal, IC) potency of botanical or animal derived remedies involved making a 'mother tincture' of plant or animal extract and alcohol, adding one part of this to 99 parts of an inert medium - alcohol again, or an alcohol and distilled water mixture - and succussing (shaking) the resulting solution. Where medicines were prepared from solids, one part of the substance was added to 99 parts of milk sugar, and rubbed (triturated) together. The second centesimal potency (2C) was made by taking one part of the first, and succussing or triturating it once more with 99 parts of the appropriate substrate. Higher potencies were produced simply by repeating the procedure, the resulting remedies being labelled either according to the centesimal (C) or, if one-to-ten ratios had been used in preparation, the decimal (X) range. The medicine itself could be administered to the patient in a number of ways. Usually, a drop in water, or tiny pills of milk sugar moistened with the potency were employed.

For Hahnemann, 'High dilutions of the medicinal substances prepared in this manner potentize their properties to an incredible extent.'[80] Moreover, since most physicians were ignorant of this phenomenon, they 'cannot believe in what they regard as being the magical powers of homoeopathic remedies. In truth, potentizing a substance which has hidden medicinal properties ... spiritualizes that material substance.'[81]

Once Hahnemann had asserted that disease was a spiritual or immaterial phenomenon, he really had little option but to proceed to a metaphysical posology, since he was then faced with a therapeutic version of the Cartesian dilemma: how could (medicinal) matter affect (the morbid) mental/ spiritual realm? While Descartes had resorted, with desperate inconsistency, to the pineal gland as the organ where the transaction between the two realms was effected, Hahnemann's solution, though logically more coherent, was conceptually and technically much bolder - spiritualise matter. To put it bluntly: if the problem was a pharmacological attack on immaterial disease, the solution was to dematerialise the medicine through potentisation.

This bequeathed enduring problems to the homoeopathic movement. First, was there a limit beyond which potentisation should not proceed? Hahnemann himself suggested the thirtieth centesimal dilution as the upper limit [82], but since beyond the twelfth it was known that it was unlikely that any of the original medicine was left in the remedy, this was neither logical nor defensible - and certainly many homoeopaths ignored it. Second, to the problem of remedy selection, Hahnemann's peculiar posology added for practising homoeopaths the problem of choosing the correct potency. This was to lead to the eventual split in the movement between those who favoured 'high power' and 'low power' remedies. Thirdly, it opened the door to ridicule from materialist science, seemed to condemn homoeopathy to the status of placebo therapy as far as regular practitioners were concerned, and saddled subsequent generations of homoeopaths with a problem equivalent to squaring the circle: how to produce a satisfactory explanation, in terms of conventional science, of the clinical efficacy of high potencies, which unless solved would close the doors of medical legitimacy in perpetuum.

Whatever one's view of the potency issue, homoeopathic remedies prepared according to Hahnemann's method, compared to allopathic drugs of the same period were, at the very least, undoubtedly extremely gentle - and totally safe.

The remaining problems - which remedy to use in a particular case of illness - was solved through the principle of similarity, i.e. the matching of a patient's symptoms with the results of drug proving on healthy volunteers. Hahnemann advised that these latter should also be based on potentised remedies: 'It is best to investigate the medicinal powers of substances by giving the experimenter a daily dose of four to six very small globules of the thirtieth potency.'[83]

Unfortunately, these principles were also compromised by problems of consistency with the other elements of the homoeopathic system. On the one hand, Hahnemann had also argued, in defence of the potentised dose, that it worked because of the greatly heightened sensitivity of the diseased body to medicinal illness. But if this was correct, it did not make sense to prove drugs on healthy people in potentised make sense to prove drugs on healthy people in potentised form. Rather, Hahnemann should have held to his original practice of proving medicines in allopathic dosage. Finally, if provers responded to medicinal illness in an individualistic way - and according to the principle of idiosyncrasy of disease they would - it is hard to see how useable drug pictures could logically be produced. Each prover would present unique symptoms which would never precisely match those of any patient. Hence if the principle of individuality was correct, the precisely matching remedy was not logically available; if the matching remedy was found, then the principle of individuality was wrong.

ON THE DEVELOPMENT OF A PHARMACOPOEIA

Whatever its implications for other elements of the homoeo-pathic system, the principle of proving medicines did provide a basis on which the development of a pharmacopoeia could be undertaken. Effectively, it suggested a way of identifying the therapeutic domain of a drug in advance of testing its effec-tiveness against particular disease states. At bottom, this was grounded in the notion of 'seeing' medicines as the diseases they would cure. Here homoeopathy had a decisive advantage over orthodox medicine, which had to rely on empirical results, and on trial and error. As Watson observed:

> That rhubarb will purge, and opium lull to sleep ... are truths which experience alone could suggest, and successive trials alone confirm. They are purely empirical truths. No one could guess them beforehand. No skill in the discrimination of disease has even a tendency to teach them ... diagnosis does not, of itself, afford us any direct information as to the cure of diseases ...[84]

Not so for Hahnemann: homoeopathically, diagnosis identified the appropriate remedy from among the record of drug provings. Whatever it happened to be in any particular instance, the patient could rest assured that it at least would do no harm. Of the medicine advocated and taught by Watson, the same could not be said.

NOTES

1. For example W. Cullen, First Lines of the Practice of Physic, 4 vols. (Bell and Bradfute, Edinburg, 1796). This is a posthumous edition: Cullen had died in 1790. The First Lines were originally written between 1766-84, and were for years 'authoritative on medical practice', F.H. Garrison,

History of Medicine, 2nd edition (W.B. Saunders Company, Philadelphia and London, 1917) p. 358.
2. T. Watson, Lectures on the Principles and Practice of Physic, 2 vols. (John W. Parker, London, 1843).
3. Ibid., vol. 1, preface.
4. F.H. Garrison, op.cit., p. 434.
5. H.L. Coulter adopts a similar procedure of comparison in order to bring out the points of conflict between regular and Hahnemannian medicine, but refers to authors relevant to the American context. See Divided Legacy, A History of the Schism in Medical Thought, 3 vols. (Wehawken Book Company, Washington, 1973-7) especially vol. III, chapter 1.
6. T. Watson, op.cit., vol. 1, p. 42.
7. Ibid., pp. 4-5
8. Ibid., pp. 59-60.
9. E. Hamlyn (ed.), The Healing Art of Homoeopathy, The Organon of Samuel Hahnemann (Beaconsfield Publishers Ltd., Beaconsfield, 1979) pp. 15-16.
10. T. Watson, op.cit., vol. 1, p. 17. Original emphasis.
11. Ibid., p. 17. Original emphasis.
12. Ibid., p. 18.
13. Ibid.
14. Ibid., pp. 24-5.
15. Ibid., p. 26.
16. Ibid.
17. Ibid., p.27.
18. Ibid. Original emphasis.
19. Ibid., p. 28.
20. Ibid., p. 29.
21. Ibid., pp. 30-1.
22. Ibid., p. 31.
23. Ibid., pp. 36-7.
24. Ibid., p. 41.
25. Ibid., p. 46. Original emphasis.
26. Ibid., p. 47.
27. Ibid., pp. 49-50. Original emphasis.
28. Ibid., p.55.
29. Ibid.
30. Ibid.
31. Ibid., p. 58. Original emphasis.
32. E. Hamlyn (ed.), op.cit., pp. 14-17.
33. In contrast with earlier writers, such as William Cullen, who was sufficiently enthused by the subject to distinguish as many as 34 different varieties of chronic rheumatism. See F.H. Garrison, op.cit., p. 358.
34. T. Watson, op.cit., vol. I, pp. 4-5.
35. Ibid.
36. Ibid., pp. 112-13.
37. E. Hamlyn (ed.), op.cit., pp. 37-8.

38. This did not mean that Hahnemann refused to recognise conditions such as smallpox, measles, cholera etc. - merely that any patient's experience of these diseases would be slightly different from that of any other, and that therefore different treatment may be necessary.
39. Ibid., p.41.
40. T. Watson, op.cit., vol. I, pp. 75-6.
41. Ibid., p. 76.
42. Ibid., pp. 77-8.
43. E. Hamlyn (ed.), op.cit., p. 15.
44. T. Watson, op.cit., vol. I, pp. 75-6.
45. E. Hamlyn (ed.), op.cit., pp. 17-18.
46. T. Watson, op.cit., vol. I, p. 5. Original emphasis.
47. Ibid., p. 116.
48. E. Hamlyn (ed.), op.cit., p. 19.
49. Ibid., p. 19.
50. T. Watson, op.cit., vol. I, p.47.
51. Ibid., p. 144. Original emphasis.
52. Ibid., p. 212.
53. Ibid., p. 213. Original emphasis.
54. Ibid., p. 227. Original emphasis.
55. Ibid., p. 228.
56. Ibid., p. 230.
57. Ibid., p. 234.
58. Ibid., p. 237. Opium - from the poppy, Papaver somniferum
59. Ibid., p. 239.
60. Ibid., pp. 239-40.
61. E. Hamlyn (ed.), op.cit., p. 27.
62. Ibid., p. 28.
63. Ibid., p. 29.
64. Ibid., p. 18.
65. Both passages from ibid., pp. 22-3.
66. Ibid., p. 24.
67. Ibid., pp. 20-1. Hahnemann had previously conceptualised this process of vital reaction as the 'biphasic action' of drugs where 'Most medicines have more than one action; the first a direct action, which gradually changes into the second (which I call the indirect secondary action). The latter is generally a state opposite of the former'. See S. Hahnemann, 'Essay on a New Principle for Ascertaining the Curative Power of Drugs' in S. Hahnemann, The Lesser Writings of Samuel Hahnemann. Collected and translated by R.E. Dudgeon MD (W. Headland, London, 1851) p. 312. Original emphasis.
68. T. Watson, op.cit., vol. I, p. 236. The reader may find a table of the metric equivalents of Apothecaries' weights useful:

1 scruple (20 grains) = 1.29598 grammes
1 drachm (3 scruples) = 3.88794 grammes
1 ounce (8 drachms) = 31.10348 grammes
(The Apothecaries' ounce is the Troy ounce of 480
Avoirdupois grains)
69. Ibid., p. 432.
70. John Elliotson, 'Clinical Lecture', The Lancet, vol.
I (1832-3) pp. 323-5. All quotes illustrating Elliotson's discussion of the case are to be found in the pages indicated
above.
71. E. Hamlyn (ed.), op.cit., p. 13. My emphasis.
72. Ibid., p. 31. My emphasis.
73. Ibid., p. 91. My emphasis.
74. Ibid., p. 90.
75. F.H. Garrison, op.cit., p. 431.
76. T. Watson, op.cit., vol. I., pp. 228-9. Original
emphasis.
77. Ibid., p. 230. Original emphasis.
78. E. Hamlyn (ed.), op.cit., p. 16.
79. Ibid., pp. 89-90.
80. Ibid., p. 51.
81. Ibid., p. 90.
82. See H.L. Coulter, op.cit., vol. III, p. 57. In 1829,
Hahnemann observed that 'There must be an end to the
thing, it cannot go on to infinity. By laying it down as a
rule that all homoeopathic remedies be attenuated and
dynamised up to X (thirtieth dilution) we have a uniform
mode of procedure ...' Anon, 'The Ethics of Mongrelism', The
British Journal of Homoeopathy, vol. XXXIX (1881) p. 271.
Hahnemann's notation is confusing, but here X is the thirtieth
dilution.
83. E. Hamlyn (ed.), op.cit., p. 51.
84. T. Watson, op.cit., vol. I, pp. 112-13. Original
emphasis.

Chapter Seven

HEROIC THERAPY IN ACTION

'Bless me, you are surely not mad enough to think of
leaving your patients without anybody to attend them',
remonstrated Mr. Pickwick in a very serious tone.
'Why not?' asked Bob in reply. 'I shall save by it, you
know. None of them ever pay. Besides', said Bob,
lowering his voice to a confidential whisper, 'they will be
all the better for it; for being nearly out of drugs just
now, I should have been obliged to give them calomel all
round, and it would have been certain to have disagreed
with some of them. So it's all for the best!'

Charles Dickens, The Pickwick Papers

'Things have arrived at such a pitch that they cannot be
worse.'

Sir John Forbes, Homoeopathy,
Allopathy and 'Young Physic'

Homeopathy was an elaborate theoretical system which,
on every important therapeutic issue, constituted a radical
rejection of received medical wisdom. As theory differed, so
did practice. Where allopathic medicine strove to produce
violent reactions in the patient, matching the power of disease
with that of the remedy, homoeopathy was informed by the
idea of helping the body to heal itself. This was its great
strength, for even if homoeopathic medicines were therapeutically inert, homoeopathy was to teach the vital lesson
that people could get well without the punishment of heroic
treatment - and, indeed, could get well more completely and
more quickly, for the absence of violent therapy meant the
absence of iatrogenic complications.

The public perhaps came to appreciate this fact rather
more quickly than most regular doctors. This encouraged the
emergence of more homoeopathic practitioners: in turn, client
patronage of homoeopaths eventually persuaded regular prac-

titioners to moderate their own prescribing habits, for doctors who continued to practise heroically ran the risk of losing their clientele, either to homoeopaths directly, or to colleagues who had already adopted less aggressive methods, and thus their economic livelihood. Effectively, the public - by voting, or threatening to vote with its feet - was to intervene in and support a critique of medical practice which the regular profession itself had been loth to develop.

To have played a role in securing the abandonment of heroic therapy is one of homoepathy's most important legacies. That such a change was long overdue, the following discussion, which focuses on the prevailing norms and habits of medical practice, makes clear. Indeed, the attractiveness of homoeopathy as a therapeutic option to clients can hardly be rendered intelligible without establishing, in a more precise and concrete way, the nature of the allopathic alternative. This is not to be historically naïve: the privilege of temporal distance undoubtedly makes the typical modes of regular practice seem more tortuous than they would have appeared to those for whom such methods were an expected aspect of medical treatment. At the same time, however, the appearance of homoeopathy provided a bench-mark in terms of which their value as therapeutic agents could be assessed. Against this standard, orthodox medicine was mostly found wanting. Material from Watson's lectures, and from issues of The Lancet in the early 1830s, is sufficient to emphasise the degree of radical interventionism that had been attained by the profession in its approach to therapeutics.

In his advice on venesection Watson remarks that 'a sufficiently large orifice should be made in the vein; and sometimes it may be right to open a vein in both arms: and the patient should be bled in the upright position.'[1] The aim was to produce a rapid and dramatic effect upon the system. Enough blood should be taken to produce syncope or deliquium (i.e. to make the patient faint). Here Watson refers to Dr Marshall Hall's insistence that 'a patient under the influence of mere inflammation will bear to lose a far greater quantity of blood without becoming faint, than he could bear in health ... The amount of bleeding necessary to occasion syncope will be in proportion to the exigency of the case.'[2] With this convenient rule of thumb the physician could thus proceed to extract blood until syncope occurred, in the knowledge that when this event was procured sufficient blood had been removed to match the severity of the patient's condition. Moreover, bleeding could also be used as a diagnostic tool: it followed that if the patient did not bear bleeding well, and syncope occurred rapidly, then the chances were that the disease in question was not an inflammatory one.[3] 'To bleed or not to bleed' does not appear to have been a pertinent medical question. And one bleeding was usually regarded as insufficient, since 'if at the first blood-letting much blood flowed before any tendency to syncope manifested itself - an early repetition of that remedy will probably be required ...'.[4] Watson continues:

> I am almost afraid to tell you how much blood I <u>have</u> seen taken at one bleeding ... I once stood by, and saw, not without trembling - although I was quite free from responsibility in the matter - a vein in the arm kept open until seventy-two ounces (four pints and a half) of blood had issued from it.[5]

Students, however, were reassured that:

> It is very seldom that such large bleedings are required: you will generally find that five-and-twenty or thirty ounces, taken properly, will be sufficient to accomplish the purpose of the measure. Sometimes one such bleeding will extinguish, as it were, the inflammation; sometimes two or three, or half a dozen, may be necessary ...[6]

Watson advises that it is not recommended practice to open arteries, instead of veins (clearly, then, some doctors did) since it is sometimes difficult to stop the blood's 'egress when we wish to do so ...'.[7] Nevertheless 'Some persons are fond of opening the temporal artery when the inflammatory disease is situated in or about the head ...',[8] despite the 'after consequences which are far from being pleasant'.[9] Neither was it advisable to open the jugular vein in cranial inflammation. Though some practitioners adopted this practice with children ('where veins in the arm are small),[10] it always carried the danger of admitting air, which could lead to death. This 'frightful accident', Watson notes, 'has occurred in operations performed in this country'.[11]

While general bleeding remedied general plethora, local bleeding helped to relieve local symptoms. The two were invariably used in conjunction, each being a complement of the other (though where local plethora obtained in cases of general depletion, local treatment only would be used). The topical abstraction of blood was procured either by the use of leeches, or by scarification and 'cupping'. The scarifier was an instrument which made a series of small incisions in the skin. Over each incision, a cupping glass was placed in which a partial vacuum had been created by heat. The resulting imbalance of pressure forced the surrounding tissue into the glass, simultaneously squeezing out blood. Watson advises:

> With respect to the relative merits and disadvantages of cupping and leeches, as topical remedies for local inflammation; it may be said in favour of cupping, that the precise quantity of blood taken away is more accurately

determined in that manner, and the operation is sooner
over, and is less fatiguing, than the suction of leeches.
But on the other hand, the leeches seldom bungle in the
operation; while the surgeon often does. It requires a
good deal of practice to become handy and dextrous in
the application of the glasses - to avoid torturing and
burning the patient ... You may apply leeches also to
parts where the cupping glass could scarcely be
used.[12]

Watson preferred local bleeding to take place near the
site of the inflammation itself. He noted, however, that some
physicians bleed topically on the principle of 'revulsion', i.e.
the abstraction of blood at some distance from the inflamed
part, on the grounds that by so doing the flow of blood was
diverted from the affected organ. Thus 'they would put
leeches, for instance, on the insteps, to relieve an inflamed
throat'.[13] And 'in inflammation of the liver or intestines,
the French are in the habit of applying leeches in great
numbers to the verge of the anus'.[14] Watson was prepared
to agree that this was no doubt a 'good and useful practice',
but reflects that 'in this country we should find it difficult to
persuade many of our patients to have leeches planted'[15] in
such a sensitive area.
    Besides bleeding, active purging was thought to be of
great service in many conditions.[16] It helped to eliminate
irritating, inflammatory material from the bowels and stomach,
as well as reducing the fluid content of the body. Antimonial
tartrate was one favourite. Diuretics and enemas were freely
employed. And laxatives - such as oil of turpentine (from the
resin of coniferous trees), croton oil (croton tiglium),
calomel, scammony (Convolvulus scammonia), jalap (Ipomoea
purga), and senna (the 'black dose') were exhibited in
extravagent dose.
    Apart from its emetic quality, antimony was also prized
as a remedy which subdued '... the action of the heart and
arteries...'[17], and so could be used where further venesection was thought unwise. It was believed to be especially
useful in inflammation of the mucous membrane of the air
passages. Watson writes that when 'you give such a patient
repeated doses of antimony; he becomes sick, vomits ... feels
nausea; his pulse becomes less forcible, his face grows pale,
and he can breathe again'.[18] Antimony also sometimes acted
violently on the bowels.[19] Its emetic action, however, was
more generally valued: it could cut short attacks of
tonsillitis, intermittent fever, and even, Watson reports, help
in the initial sequelae of apoplexy.[20]
    One young patient, suffering from hydrocephalus - an
obvious candidate for diuretic treatment - was given a
medicine containing 'five grains of fresh squills: this was to
be one dose; and it was to be repeated every eight hours

... The patient took this dose three times a day for nearly three weeks ... It operated profusely by the kidneys ...'[21] Purging nearly always accompanied blood-letting, and the purging advised was usually <u>hard</u>.[22] In inflammation of the encephalon, for example:

> There is a great tendency to obstinate constipation in most cases; and this must be overcome, and free and frequent evacuations from the bowels obtained: five grains of calomel and fifteen of jalap should be followed in three or four hours by a strong black dose; and after that I should give, in such cases, three or four grains of calomel every four hours, and repeat the black dose at least every morning...[23]

In apoplexy, clysters were advised: 'Strong purgative and stimulating enemata must be thrown into the rectum: half an ounce, or six drachms, of turpentine, suspended by the help of the yolk of an egg, in gruel or warm water'.[24] In tetanus, however, the enema preferred was tobacco (<u>Nicotiana tabacum</u>), 'thrown up into the rectum: either the smoke of its burning leaves, or ... an infusion of them in water'.[25] (Regarding tobacco clysters Watson added, conscientiously, that 'you ought to know that, when injected in other emergencies ... mortal syncope has followed'[26]). Hysteria – reductively explained by Watson in terms of menstrual disorders[27] – was also a candidate for enemata: 'Signal good may ... be effected by ... the turpentine injection ... or ice cold water thrown into the rectum will often bring the fit to a speedy termination.'[28]

The anti-inflammatory regimen was by no means completed after depletion and purgation. 'Next to blood-letting, as a <u>remedy</u>, and of vastly superior value upon whole, to purgation, in serious inflammations of various kinds is <u>mercury</u>'[29]. Its efficacy was held to stem from its 'loosening effect upon certain textures',[30] an important consideration in cases of adhesive inflammation. The administration of mercury, Watson noted, was typically accompanied by 'increased watery evacuations from the intestines; or by an increased discharge of bile; or by an increased flow of saliva...',[31] and though these were felt to be positive signs that the curative action of mercury had taken hold:

> If you push this remedy ... other effects ensue: ... the gums become tender, and red, and swollen, and at length ulcerate; and in extreme cases, and in young children especially, the inflamed parts may perish: the cheeks, for example, sometimes slough internally. Not only the gums, but the throat and fauces grow red, and sore, and sloughy.[32]

Dr John Fosbroke, writing in The Lancet in 1831 felt,
even then, that his colleagues had been too zealous in the
exhibition of this destructive remedy:

> ... in every town in England, the number of consti-
> tutions ruined, and delicate persons murdered, of cases
> of general debility, of permanently enfeebled powers of
> stomach, of nervous irritability, of total destruction of
> muscular strength and mental energy, of morbid determi-
> nation of blood to the head and liver, and of increased
> susceptibility of all the impressions which cause inflam-
> mation, all produced by mercury, marks the wretched,
> indiscriminate, and empirical abuse of this powerful
> agent in common practice, when given to those upon
> whom it acts as a poison destructive of health and life
> from the first day it is taken. The French who come to
> this country, have a stronger feeling on this point than
> any other, from a notion that English practitioners give
> mercury for everything.[33]

Watson, though aware of the dangers, and of the difficulty of predicting which patients would prove particularly
sensitive to the effects of mercury, nevertheless considered it
an invaluable remedy:

> When we have to contend with acute inflammation, and
> desire to prevent or arrest the deposition of coagulable
> lymph, our object is, after such bleeding as may have
> been proper, to bring the system as speedily as possible
> under the specific influence of mercury.[34]

Two or three grains every four or six hours, he noted,
would usually suffice within 36 hours to produce the requisite
indications that this influence had been accomplished, i.e.
when 'The gums grow red and spongy...' and the patient
complains of '... a metallic taste, a taste like that of copper
in his mouth: and an unpleasant and very peculiar foetor ...
is smelt on the breath'.[35] These symptoms, Watson
observed, 'are enough: you need not in general look for any
more decided affection of the mouth, such as ulceration of the
gums, swelling of the glands beneath the jaw, and of the
tongue, and a profuse flow of saliva...'.[36]

Bringing the system under the influence of mercury
could, of course, be achieved more rapidly by increasing the
dosage (up to ten grains every two hours), and by combining
its administration with opium, to prevent the mercury running
off by the bowels. But different persons had varying degrees
of tolerance: in some, the remedy became unmanageable and
dangerous.[37] To illustrate the point, Watson cited the
example of a women who after only two grains of calomel,
salivated furiously 'in a few hours: and she died, at the end

of two years, worn out by the affects of the mercury, and having lost portions of the jaw bone by narcosis'.[38] Another example involved a man who found, after sleeping with his wife who had used a mercurial unguent on her neck for a skin disease, that 'his gums were tender for three or four days, and slight salivation took place'.[39] Watson noted that 'Cases similar to these occur now and then to most medical men: we cannot tell beforehand in whom such effects are to be looked for ...'[40]

For Watson, the iatrogenic effects of mercury - usually taken as either calomel or the 'blue pill' - were worth the risk. Nevertheless, he did recognise that '... so distressing sometimes are these effects ... upon the mouth...'[41] that he hastened to advise his students of ways of relieving this unfortunate but inevitable side-effect. Sore gums were a local inflammation, and so:

> ... apply eight or ten leeches beneath the edges of the jaw bones, and wrap a soft poultice round the neck, into which the orifices made by the leeches may bleed; and I can promise you that, in nine cases out of ten, you will receive the thanks of your patient for the great comfort this measure has afforded him.[42]

Both digitalis and opium were held to be of value in treating inflammatory conditions, the former through its effect on the circulation, the latter through its soothing effect on the nervous system. Again, however:

> ... if you give moderate doses of digitalis, its very peculiar effect upon the pulse comes on at very uncertain periods, and may be postponed until it is too late to be of any service. If, on the other hand, you give it in such quantity as speedily to affect the heart's action (which is what we want in acute and serious inflammation), then you are never sure against what may be called its poisonous effects: deadly faintness, frightful syncope, and even death itself. Most practitioners can tell of cases in which patients, who were taking full doses of digitalis, have suddenly expired; and when the remedy has appeared to have had more to do with the fatal event than the disease.[43]

As with digitalis, so with opium:

> ... this is a remedy which requires to be used, in inflammation, with great caution ... I certainly have known more than one person, labouring under extensive and severe bronchitis, so effectually quieted by a dose of the same medicine, that they never woke again. As a general rule I should say that you must be very careful

how you venture upon opium in inflammatory diseases that tend to produce death by <u>coma</u> or <u>apnoea</u>. [cessation of respiration] [44]

But:

> On the other hand, ... in cases where the tendency is towards death by <u>asthenia</u> [debility, loss of vital power] the use of opium, as a remedy for inflammation, is most serviceable. It has a capital effect often, after free bleeding, in cases of peritonitis, and of enteritis ... If there be any hope in such cases, it is to be found in the continued exhibition of opium in considerable doses.[45]

Counter-irritation was another weapon in the subjuguation (<u>sic</u>) of inflammation. A variety of dermatologically invasive techniques were used to create lesions which would attract blood away from the inflamed part or organ:

> Counter-irritation, by means of blisters [often raised by <u>cantharides</u> - the 'Spanish Fly', or Cantharides vesicatoria], irritating ointments, setons [threads drawn under the skin], issues [artificial ulcers], or moxas [burning vegetable matter placed on or near the skin] is often very beneficial. It probably operates by attracting blood into the neighbouring parts, and in the same degree diverting it from the inflamed part. ... To the chest, in thoracic inflammation, and to the belly in abdominal, blisters are not only perfectly safe, but of the greatest use...[46]

The fact that the pages of The Lancet during this period are littered with communications informing the readership of the efficacy of certain novel remedies or approaches in the management of particular conditions should not be allowed to obscure the fact that most practitioners relied on a few great 'sheet anchors' when it came to treating their patients. It was entirely logical. Most disease was inflammatory, and required anti-inflammatory remedies. Hence the regimen in the great majority of cases moved more or less systematically through venesection, leeches, cupping, purges, emetics, mercury, <u>digitalis</u>, opium, and blisters. Indeed, any practitioner <u>failing</u> to adopt these measures would have been regarded as professionally negligent.

One way of putting the near universal application of these remedies beyond any reasonable doubt would be to tabulate the 86 conditions discussed in both volumes of Watson's Lectures together with the treatments suggested for each. But this would probably serve to establish the point only by taxing the patience of the reader. It is perhaps better to bring the chapter to a close in a livelier way with some case histories taken from The Lancet. This helps to dispose of the lingering possibility that it was Watson's imagination, rather than the conventional materia medica, which was limited.

Forbes Winslow, surgeon, included the following case in his 1830 communication concerning cerebral disease:

> Susan [aged] 5 ... laboured under the following symptoms:- great languor, unwillingness to move her head ...; vision ... indistinct, the pulse quick, but feeble, the bowels irregular. The medical gentlemen, judging from the symptoms that inflammatory action was going on, applied eight leeches to the temples, and ordered her bowels to be emptied by a cathartic composed of calomel and jalap. The following day the child was worse, the leeches having failed to relieve the supposed inflammatory symptoms. On the second day four more leeches were applied to the temples, and a blister to the nape of the neck, notwithstanding which, the child gradually grew worse, and on the seventh day died.[47]

A case abstracted from the Edinburgh Medical and Surgical Journal of 1830, and reprinted in The Lancet, involved Janet Barclay, 28, who was suffering from amaurosis (i.e. a diseased optic nerve):

> The amaurosis, at its commencement in the right eye, was accompanied with deep seated pain in the eyeball, which, after a short time, disappeared, but recurred when the left eye became affected, and has continued more or less since ... Blisters have been applied to her temples and nape of neck, without effecting any improvement in the vision.

> The application of extract of belladonna [Atropa belladonna] to the eyebrows produced its usual effects. The system was affected slightly by mercury, and purgatives administered without any beneficial effect. Blisters were then applied to her temples, and one grain of strychnine [Strychnos nuxvomica] sprinkled on their surfaces. This application was continued till it occasioned vertigo, headache, tremours, etc.

The report ends with the rather optimistic statement that Janet 'was dismissed cured'.[48]

Francis Warren, 27, was admitted to the Westminster Hospital on 31 March 1830. Known to have laboured under syphilis in the past, he was diagnosed as suffering from debility and erysipelas: treatment included the tartar-emetic, ipecacuanha (Cephaelis ipecacuanha - also an emetic), calomel, ammonia acetate, jalap, fomentations (i.e. warming or medicated lotions), brandy, warm baths, and, at 10 pm on the 3rd, '... an injection of brandy, laudanum, and tinct. assafoetid [tincture of Narthex assafoetida] with gruel, was thrown up the rectum, but not retained.'[49] Further efforts were made on the patient's behalf, but to no avail. The patient expired at 7.00 am on the following day.

James Hale, 21, was more fortunate. Admitted to the Royal Western Ophthalmic Hospital on 1 April with 'gonnorhoeal ophthalmia' (conjunctivitis), he was discharged on the 27th, since by that time 'The slightest possible opacity remains where the ulcer of the cornea was, and that does not in the least interfere with his sight.' On admission, however, he had had 'three leeches applied ... but without any relief'. Jalap was included in his medication to clear the bowels; a mercurial unguent also appears to have been used (since the patient was reported as salivating by the 9th.) and:

A large quantity of the fresh made, or strongest, nitrate of silver ointment was applied to the eye by Mr Guthrie, and the lids then gently rubbed, so that it might be diffused equally over the conjunctiva. He was then cupped to the temple to twenty ounces, and ordered to foment the eye constantly.

April 2nd. The ointment caused considerable pain in the head and eye, which was, however, entirely removed by the cupping ...

3. ... The ointment repeated; to be well purged and cupped to twelve ounces in the evening.

4. ... Ointment applied, and twelve ounces of blood taken from the temple.

5. ... Better in every respect. The ointment and purgative medicines repeated.[50]

The improvement in vision, according to the report, seemed to continue.

A report of a meeting of the London Medical Society, held on 18 October, 1830, described a case related by one Dr Whiting:

The case ... was that of a middle aged lady ... whom he had attended in child bed. She bore two children and suffered a severe rigor; reaction came on, and a pain commenced in the region of the womb, which became very tender, and enlarged. What was to be done in such

89

a case as this? The variety of treatment recommended by practitioners was so great [sic], that he did not know what measures to resort; he thought it right, therefore, to read all the authors from whom he could expect to obtain information on the subject; accordingly he referred to Gooch, Hamilton, Armstrong, Gordon, Mackintosh and Campbell, and made up his mind that antiphlogistic measures would be most successful. Dr Gooch was the last writer on the subject, and he recommended that the patient should be bled to syncope; twelve hours, therefore, from the first attack, this (or nearly this) was done; leeches were then applied: she was purged from the first; three grains of calomel every three hours, with quarter or the eighth of a grain of tartrate of antimony, and one grain of opium. She recovered, but the progress was slow ...[51]

At the same meeting, a Mr Howell read a paper concerning his treatment of a case which, on post-mortem examination, had been identified as gangrene of the lung. The Lancet reported verbatim. Among the measures taken, Howell reports:

The bowels had been readily and actively purged ... I bled the patient moderately, and was particularly struck with the exhaustion the loss of a small quantity of blood seemed to produce ... On the 7th [of August, 1829] he complained of a recurrence of pain ... The pulse justifying me, I abstracted more blood from the arm, and applied a dozen leeches to the lower part of the right side of the abdomen...

By the 25th the pulmonary problem had become apparent, after which '... the patient rapidly declined, and died on the evening of the 3rd of September.'[52]

Dr Ellitoson, at St Thomas's Hospital on 18 October, 1830 - having lectured to his students on the diagnosis of pleurisy - then proceeded to outline his treatment of a particular case:

As to the cure, nothing can be more beautiful than the treatment of cases of acute inflammation. The body is more subject to inflammation than to any other disease, and no disease is more dangerous; while on the other hand there is no disease in which medicine can be employed more satisfactorily. If the diagnosis was perfectly clear in the present case, the treatment necessary to be pursued was equally so. I had the woman made to sit upright in bed, and ordered her to be bled, not to this quantity or that, but to fainting, and as soon as that was over, twenty leeches were applied over the seat of the pain, and after them a poultice. I ordered five grains of calomel, with three of opium to be given at the same time, and the calomel to be repeated every six hours afterwards.

The following morning, the patient had apparently improved, a fact which Elliotson used to demonstrate to his class the necessity for vigorous action by the physician.

I need hardly say to you, that in acute inflammation, the very best treatment that can be adopted is to procure a loss of blood from a vessel of some size; and further, that on the suddenness with which the bleeding is performed, its good effect materially depends ... i.e. the more decided will be the impression made upon the system.

To make sure his students got the message, Elliotson summed up by stating that 'you should go briskly to work, knock the disease on the head at once, and then follow the bleeding up immediately with the other necessary measures'. After all 'if, in this case, the leeches only had been applied, the disease might have gone on ... we might have pushed the disease about, but not have knocked it down'.[53]

Mr Lawrence, lecturing at St Bartholomew's Hospital in October 1830, had described his treatment of a patient with a protuberant naevus on her face. The Lancet reported his discussion of the case as follows:

... he passed in the first instance, a thick seton through the inferior part of the tumour; the seton was introduced by a large needle with a proportionate thread, in order to prevent the risk of haemorrhage ... ... he next sprinkled the seton with a little powdered nitrate of silver, and drew it into the opening; beyond pain and irritation, this produced little or no inflammatory effect. The nitrate of silver was again used more copiously, and a good deal of uneasiness was produced for twenty four hours ... The seton was then removed, and he introduced a stick of caustic potash into the opening and rubbed it in very freely ...[54]

Unfortunately, however, none of these measures had the hoped for effect, and Mr Lawrence eventually resorted to ligature and nitric acid.

The same Lancet report includes Mr Lawrence's handling of a hospital patient who suffered:

... a sudden and violent attack of apoplexy; the usual treatment was adopted, he was profusely bled, cupped, leeched, purged, and blistered, but with so little effect, that he (Mr Lawrence) abandoned all hopes of his

91

recovery; as a last experiment, however, he determined
on the employment of mercury in large doses, which was
pushed to salivation, and he eventually recovered
...[55]

Mr Lawrence's experience proving particularly instruc-
tive, it is worth drawing attention to his treatment of 'a
young woman named Robinson, who had been admitted to St.
Bartholomew's on the 19th of October', with a leg which had
become excessively swollen and painful:

A large bleeding was immediately directed and leeches to
be applied to the inflamed parts; the saturnine [lead]
lotion, and active purgative medicines were also
prescribed. Before the leeches were applied she was
accordingly bled to deliquium. Thirty leeches were afterwards put on ...[56]

- and that of George Booth, 38, in Henry Ward, who had
hepatitis and an abscess on the right hip: 'He was bled to
sixteen ounces. Had calomel and jalap, and a saline mixture,
with tartar-emetic and sulphate of magnesia, every sixth
hour. He was moreover cupped once, and had a blister to the
side.'[57]

John Alexander, MD, Medical Officer to the General
Dispensary for Children in Manchester, had ample opportunity
to witness cases of puerperal (childbirth) fever. He communicated the history of several of these to The Lancet. Case
three, which occurred in February 1829, involved one Mrs
Luke, who after giving birth to her tenth child with the aid
of a midwife, suffered from:

... a tense, painful, abdomen, and the other symptoms
of peritoneal inflammation. Dr Freckleton, Mr
Fawdington, and myself, visited this woman. The usual
remedies, bloodletting, blistering, enemata, cataplasms
[poultices], febrifuge [fever reducing] medicines, and
opiates, were employed. The disease subsided, and she
gradually regained her health.

Alexander, however, entertained doubts as to whether Mrs
Luke had really been suffering from the malady in question,
as the case had 'yielded to the common antiphologistic
treatment, which most practitioners, with but too great
reason, conceive inefficient in combating peurperal fever.'[58]

John Fosbroke, writing on the Pathology and Treatment
of Deafness, observed:

I have found the application of tartar-emetic ointment in
deafness with discharge, of signal service ... I was

asked by Dr Graham ... what difference there is
between the tartar-emetic ointment and a common blister.
There is a great deal of difference. It penetrates deeper
than Cantharides; and secretes not merely vesicular and
serous, but pustular and purulent, secretion. We want
manageable applications that will excite a purulent discharge. The tartar-emetic touches not merely the surface
of the cutis, but pierces the cellular tissue.

This was not all: 'In the second stage of local treatment, I
have been accustomed to excite the ear ... I have introduced
volatile ammonia and tobacco fumes ...'.[59]
At the Westminister Medical Society meeting of 19 April,
1831, the Chair was addressed on the subject of measles:

In reflecting, Sir, int he plan of treatment adopted in
the present cases, I cannot avoid referring to them as
remarkable instances of the good effect of bleeding. I
have no hesitation in affirming it as my opinion, that if
this young lady had been treated as some of my much
respected friends would have recommended, by stimulants and blisters, we should most certainly have lost
her.

The speaker went on to observe:

I have referred to blisters particularly, it having fallen
to my lot to witness three little patients suffering from
the terrific gangrenous bones consequent upon such
applications, which made a most powerful impression on
my mind; and where, Sir, can we have a stronger argument against their use than such an appearance?[60]

W.R. Whatton, A Manchester surgeon, had the by now
all too familiar recommendations on the treatment of pertussis
(whooping cough):

The bowels should be well and effectively opened with
calomel and jalap powder, and leeches should be applied
over the cartilages of the larynx, so as to remove the
congestion, or to the back of the neck, or between the
shoulders, if there be also much determination upwards.
These may be repeated from time to time, until the
breathing be effectually relieved. A mixture composed of
four grains of tartrate of antimony dissolved in six
ounces of water, and sweetened with some simple syrup,
is what I usually employ, regulating the dose according
to the age and strength of the child, and repeating it
often enough to procure vomiting after the fits of cough-
ing.[61]

John Elliotson, lecturing on the treatment of hydrophobia (rabies) at the University of London on 13 October, 1831, described a particular case where he:

... wished also to give one fair trial to the carbonate of iron, and therefore proposed administering an electuary composed of carbonate of iron and treacle ... both in the way of clyster and by the mouth. The mixture was very easily thrown into the intestines by means of Weiss's syringe, but though administered repeatedly, it was invariably discharged as soon as it had entered.[62]

A Lancet correspondent drew attention to Dr Williams's treatment of fever:

The grand remedy on which Dr Williams places the greatest reliance in fever, is the administration of enemas. Throughout the disease, an enema, consisting of a pint of barley water, and half an ounce of the syrup of poppies, is injected twice daily - in the morning and in the evening ...

Dr Williams also applies mustard poultices to the abdomen, and if there be evidence of the internal irritation being very great, especially if we have any reason to suspect that inflammation already exists there, thirty, forty, or fifty leeches ... should also be applied to the abdomen ... If the symptoms do not disappear on the first application of leeches to the abdomen, they must be reapplied, even to a third time.[63]

Dr Billing, speaking on diseases of the heart at the London Hospital on 14 January, 1832, indicated his treatment of a case of Enlargement of the Heart produced by Acute Rheumatism:

It is unnecessary to enter into the daily minutiae of the case, the treatment having been in many respects similar to the last [hypertrophy of the heart, with severe diarrhoea]; he has been bled from the arm and cupped over the heart; he has had the saline antimonial mixture with colchicum [Meadow saffron] and also been subjected to the influence of mercury and digitalis.[64]

The Lancet occasionally carried lectures from continental physicians. Dr Andral, discoursing on the treatment of epilepsy at the University of Paris, advised as follows:

In the interval between the attacks, we must be guided in our medicines principally by the indication which the occasional causes afford ...

These occasional causes ... are very diversified. Our therapeutic plans must accordingly be exceedingly various in different cases. Venesection, leeches, purgatives, and cutaneous irritation, have thus the cases to which they are separately or collectively suitable. The modes of cutaneous irritation are manifold. Blisters, setons, especially in the neck, moxae to the base of the skull, the cautery ... This latter application has even been recommended to the head itself. Cases are on record, however, in which the application of fire to the skull has been attended with the most dreadful inflammation, erysipelas, caries of the bones, and death itself. The application of the cautery to a limb seems more promising.[65]

Despite Watson's later reflection that patients would be unlikely to accept leeches applied around the anus, Elliotson appears to have had sufficient authority to make his advice stick. Describing a case of piles, again at the University of London (November 26th, 1832), Elliotson observed: 'The symptoms were a swelling around the anus, accompanied by great pain. It was presently cured by keeping him in the horizontal posture, the application of leeches, cold and alum water.'[66]

Yet, as Watson subsequently remarked, leeches did have the advantage of 'being able to refresh themselves from parts where cupping could not reach'. There was, indeed, no organ safe from their attention. One Edward Smith, aged 60, was admitted to St Bartholomew's Hospital, on 31 January, 1833, suffering from a penis which was: 'much increased in bulk, indurated, and curved downwards'. On the following day, he was seen by Mr Lawrence, who helpfully advised 'twelve leeches to be applied along the penis, which is also to be fomented'. On 4 February, the 'state of the parts [was] the same. The leeches were applied, and, he fancies, afforded him some relief. He continues the pills and fomentations. Bowels opened by the senna mixture'. The next report occurs on the 8th: 'The leeches have been repeated. He says, they did not "bite well"; that they got little blood from the part. No alteration in the condition of the penis, nor in the general health of the patient.' By the 11th., Edward Smith appeared to be '... in very depressed spirits, and complains of the affected part being rendered "sore" by so much handling.'[67]

The depressing litany of heroic therapy continues throughout the voluminous proceedings recorded in The Lancet issues of the period. Two final examples illustrate the lengths to which this would be pushed where the disease itself was (quite rightly) seen as particularly ferocious. Cholera was a source of much concern at the time; all kinds of treatments were tried, to little effect. Dr Latta, of Leith, communicated his practice of saline treatment: 'On the 27th of May, at seven pm., a middle aged female was brought to the hospital ... Unconscious of existence, she was laid on the mattress. I instantly opened a vein in the right arm, and threw in 132 ounces of saline fluid, keeping the temperature above 105 ...' By midnight, however, '... she was as low as ever; eighty ounces of saline injection again restored her ... ' But by four in the morning, the patient was again 'in spite of every remedy', sinking, 'so I was compelled again to have recourse to the only thing that produced any improvement and ... four pounds nine ounces were again injected ...' Throughout the following day, 'mercurials, tonics, stimulants, with effervescing draughts were administered ...'.[68] Unfortunately, however, these drastic measures were to no avail, and the patient died on 30 May.

Joseph Ayre MD, of Hull, on the other hand, recommended small but frequent doses of calomel:

> The exclusive object sought for, has been to restore the secretion of the liver, and the means employed for this purpose have been no less exclusive, and have wholly consisted of calomel and laudanum, given in small quantities and frequently repeated ... The average quantity of calomel which I have given [in total] has been about eighty grains, and the highest quantity 176 grains.[69]

Everything recorded here would have been anathema to Hahnemann, and to most of his followers: with the introduction of homeopathy into Britain, however, it also began to appear increasingly objectionable to the public and, ultimately, and as a consequence, to the orthodox profession itself. As Sir John Forbes was moved to remark, in an article otherwise highly critical of homoeopathy: 'Things [in regular practice] have arrived at such a pitch that they cannot be worse.'[70] But if the violence of regular treatment had created fertile soil for the popularisation of homoeopathy, and if, following the homoeopathic stimulus, conventional practitioners eventually learnt the lesson that expectant therapy was superior to medical violence, the regular profession nevertheless refused to investigate homoeopathy seriously, or to admit homoeopathic doctors as respectable colleagues. The following chapters trace the growth of homoeopathy, and these allopathic responses, in more detail.

NOTES

1. T. Watson, Lectures on the Principles and Practice of Physic, 2 vols. (John W. Parker, London, 1843) vol. I. p. 213.
2. Quoted in ibid., pp. 219-20.
3. See ibid., p. 220.
4. Ibid., p. 221.
5. Ibid. Original emphasis.
6. Ibid.
7. Ibid., p. 225.
8. Ibid.
9. Ibid.
10. Ibid.
11. Ibid., pp. 225-6.
12. Ibid., p. 222.
13. Ibid., p. 227.
14. Ibid.
15. Ibid.
16. See ibid.
17. Ibid., p. 234.
18. Ibid., p. 235
19. See ibid., pp. 235-6.
20. Ibid., pp. 790, 745, 525.
21. Ibid., p. 447. Original emphasis.
22. See ibid., p. 384.
23. Ibid.
24. Ibid., p. 524.
25. Ibid., p. 571.
26. Ibid.
27. See ibid., p. 671.
28. Ibid., pp. 680-1.
29. Ibid., p. 228, Original emphasis.
30. Ibid., p. 230
31. Ibid., pp. 228-9.
32. Ibid., p. 230.
33. John Fosbroke, 'Practical Observations on the Pathology and Treatment of Deafness', The Lancet, vol. II (1830-1) p. 70.
34. T. Watson, op.cit., vol. I. pp. 230-1.
35. Ibid.
36 Ibid.
37. See ibid., p. 231.
38. Ibid., p. 232.
39. Ibid.
40. Ibid.
41. Ibid., pp. 232-3.
42. Ibid.
43. Ibid., p. 276.
44. Ibid., p. 237. Original emphasis.

45. Ibid., p. 238. Original emphasis. In the context, 'asthenia' could be a misprint. Watson may have meant 'sthenic' diseases, i.e. those characterised by an excess of vital or nervous energy.
46. Ibid., pp. 239-40. Original emphasis.
47. Forbes Winslow, 'Observations on Symptoms Attributed to Cerebral Disease', The Lancet, vol. I (1830-1) p. 36.
48. Anon., 'The Edinburgh Medical and Surgical Journal', The Lancet, vol. I (1830-1) pp. 90-1.
49. Anon., 'Westminster Hospital', The Lancet, vol. I (1830-1) pp. 92-4. Laudanum is a liquid preparation of opium.
50. Anon., 'Royal Western Ophthalmic Hospital', The Lancet, vol. I (1830-1) pp. 94-5.
51. Anon., 'London Medical Society', The Lancet, vol. I (1830-1) p. 152.
52. All quotes from ibid., p. 154.
53. All quotes from Dr Elliotson 'Clinical Lecture', The Lancet, vol. I (1830-1) pp. 157-8.
54. Mr Lawrence, 'Clinical Lectures', The Lancet, vol. I (1830-1) pp. 162-3.
55. Ibid., p. 163.
56. All quotes from ibid., p. 164.
57. Ibid., p. 165.
58. See John Alexander, 'Cases of Puerperal Fever', The Lancet, vol. II (1830-1) p. 2 for both passages.
59. John Fosbroke, 'Practical Observations on the Pathology and Treatment of Deafness', The Lancet, vol. II (1830-1) pp. 58-9 for both passages. Original emphasis.
60. Anon., 'Westminister Medical Society', The Lancet, vol. II (1830-1) pp. 108-9 for both passages.
61. W.R. Whatton, 'Hooping Cough', The Lancet, vol. II (1830-1) p. 521.
62. John Elliotson, 'Clinical Lecture', The Lancet, vol. I (1831-2) p. 162. Original emphasis.
63. 'Achaz', 'The Nature and Treatment of Continued Fever', The Lancet, vol. I (1831-2) pp. 184-5.
64. Dr Billing, 'Clinical Lecture', The Lancet, vol. II (1831-2) p. 330.
65. M. Andral, 'Lectures on Medical Pathology', The Lancet, vol. II (1832-3) p. 103.
66. John Elliotson 'Clinical Lecture', The Lancet, vol. I (1832-3) p. 321.
67. Anon., 'Reports from St. Bartholomew's', The Lancet vol. I (1832-3) p. 671.
68. All quotes from T. Latta, 'Correspondence - Venous Injections in Cholera', The Lancet, vol. II (1831-2) pp. 371-2.
69. Joseph Ayre, 'On the Treatment of the Malignant Cholera', The Lancet, vol. II (1831-2) pp. 458-9. Original emphasis.

70. Sir John Forbes, Homoeopathy, Allopathy and 'Young Physic' (William Radde, New York, 1846) p. 52.

Part III

HOMOEOPATHY AND REGULAR MEDICINE:
THE DIALECTICS OF PROFESSIONAL REACTION, 1830-1900

Chapter Eight

THE MAJOR FEATURES OF THE DIALECTIC

Homoeopathy first began to attract intellectual attention in
Britain in the 1830s. Even by 1841, however, there were only
some 'ten practitioners ... in the three kingdoms ...'[1]
hardly enough to warrant any major reaction by the profession. Ten years later, things looked very different. The
number of regular practitioners adopting the system had been
increasing by 110 per cent every thirty months, so that by
1851, there were probably 'about 200 open and avowed
homoeopathists ...'.[2] This constituted a rate of increase
which was greeted with enthusiasm by homoeopaths. Looking
forward a further ten years to 1861, they felt that 'we may
confidently predict there will be at least a thousand -
perhaps double that number ...',[3] in which case homoeopaths would have constituted some ten per cent of all UK
practitioners. In the event, this prognosis proved very
optimistic, but it was one which, at the time, regular doctors
countenanced as a serious possibility. At the 1851 meeting of
the PMSA, Dr Williams noted, 'homoeopathy [is] rampant
through the land, deluding ... the powerful, the learned, the
rich, and, more than all, the poor in multitudes.'[4]
    The prospect of homoeopathy's rise and rise among
medical practitioners - especially in view of the acknowledged
overcrowding of the profession - seemed by no means
unrealistic. Indeed, the 1851 meeting of the PMSA was so
concerned that a series of measures, designed to ostracise
homoeopaths and all practitioners who consulted with them,
was passed with enthusiastic support. Something, doctors
agreed, clearly had to be done to defend regular practice,
and to halt the spread of homoeopathy within the profession.
As Dr Cormack observed, action was urgently required 'to
prevent this enemy from stealing a march upon us, and
destroying our citadel'.[5]
    In effect, the measures turned out to be dialectical.
Officially, homoeopathy was subjected to an intellectual
critique and its practitioners to professional ostracism;
unofficially, the regular profession began to abandon heroic

therapy, and to moderate the size and frequency of doses administered to patients. Regular practice became less aggressive, cures being left more 'to nature' - so called 'therapeutic nihilism' or 'expectant therapy'. In short, regular practice began to look more like homoeopathy. The regular profession, however, was loth to admit that the new fashion of expectant therapy had anything to do with homoeopathy, or concerns about professional income.

Therapeutic nihilism itself, though, was an inappropriate economic ethic for regular practitioners. Patients expected their physicians to do more than advise rest, good nursing and a sensible diet. Expectant therapy soon gave way, therefore, to the search for new medicines, i.e. new specifics which could be used with advantage in the treatment of individual diseases. To this end, the regular profession - usually without acknowledgement - began to experiment with the homoeopathic idea of proving medicines on healthy subjects in order to identify their physiological action. Homoeopaths had already generated a considerable literature on this topic: by the 1870s, allopathic texts were appearing which clearly owed a silent debt to such sources. Remedies introduced by homoeopaths were adopted by the regular profession; others were now being prescribed on homoeopathic indications.

The allopathic reaction, then, was one of official rejection of all things homoeopathic, and a covert assimilation of its remedies and lessons regarding dosage and drug proving. Of these dialectical responses, the latter was a far more effective check to the growth of homoeopathy within the profession than the former. Once the regular profession had abandoned the procedures which had made homoeopathy popular, the economic advantage of homoeopathic practice was considerably reduced, and no longer outweighed the difficulties of professional ostracism which its adoption involved. Indeed, with this change in therapeutic orientation secured, the continuation of official hostility was probably redundant, and perhaps even counter-productive. The stance of official ostracism, by inculcating public support for the 'underdog', might well have helped to keep homoeopathy in the public mind for longer than its therapeutic attractions vis-à-vis regular medicine merited. By the 1870s, a rapid slow-down in new recruits to homoeopathy among medical practitioners was apparent.

During these years homoeopathy itself had also changed. If regular practice had moved away from Watson in the direction of homoeopathy, homoeopaths had moved away from Hahnemann towards an eclectically orthodox position. Much of Hahnemann's original system was abandoned (though regular practitioners often criticised homoeopathy as if this had never happened), leaving only the principle of the simile. The infinitesimal dose became the small dose; prescription based on the totality of individual symptoms became prescription based on the affinity of a drug for a particular organ or tissue; the simile principle was demoted from universal to general applicability; allopathic measures were used where homoeopathy failed to give benefit; and - perhaps most importantly - homoeopaths were constrained, by the same forces which had led regular practitioners to abandon heroic practice, to adopt the new technologies (instrumentation and hygiene) and new drugs (especially the anaesthetics) developed by orthodox medicine. Homoeopaths could not, and did not, ignore the scientific revolution in medicine. To have done so would have been suicide - yet the growing reputation of orthodox medicine, particularly in surgery, and the assimilation of allopathic developments by homoeopaths themselves, also meant that homoeopathy appeared both less important and less distinctive to medical practitioners and their publics alike.

Homoeopathy probably suffered in particular from the heightened status and importance of surgery. Given the moratorium on consultations between homoeopaths and allopaths - even in non-medical cases - it was difficult, when necessary, for the former, as general practitioners, to obtain surgical advice or, as hospital staff, to obtain external assistance.

These developments and reactions are elaborated below. Chapter Nine deals with the early history of homoeopathy in Britain, Chapter Ten with the response of the regular profession, and Chapter Eleven with the effect of homoeopathy on regular medicine, and the changes in homoeopathic practice itself. Though this summarises the main focus of each section, some overlap of material is unavoidable. Extensive use of quotation best conveys the flavour of exchanges between homoeopaths and the orthodox profession and, inevitably, the participants saw many of the issues referred to above as being intimately connected. In particular, the early history of homoeopathy in Britain can hardly be discussed at all without signalling the more extreme allopathic response of later years.

NOTES

1. Anon., 'The Persecution of the Homoeopathists', The British Journal of Homoeopathy, vol. IX (1851) p. 612.
2. Ibid.
3. Ibid.
4. Anon, Homoeopathy - Report of the Speeches on Irregular Practice (John Churchill, London, 1851) p. 19. The speeches were delivered at the 19th anniversary meeting of the PMSA, held at Brighton, 13-14 August, 1851.
5. Ibid., p. 9.

Chapter Nine

THE EARLY YEARS - HOMOEOPATHY AND
BRITISH MEDICINE 1830-1846

The first mention of homoeopathy in an English medical
journal occurs in The Lancet of 1826-7. On the evening of
24 September Dr Clutterbuck, President of the London Medical
Society, was pleased to inform his audience that:

... he had a subject to mention, which he had no doubt
would excite considerable interest among the Members; it
was the account of a new medical doctrine which had
sprung up in the German Universities, and which
appeared to be extensively diffused throughout Germany
and some of the neighbouring countries. It originated
with a Dr HALNEMANN ... and was called HOMOOE-
PATHIA [1]

Dr Clutterbuck, however, had little else to say about the
matter other than that 'There was much ingenuity, and
probably some truth ...'[2] in it.
    Whether misprint or not, the incorrect spelling of
Hahnemann's name in the passage quoted above portended the
often wilful misunderstanding of homoeopathy by its regular
opponents in the nineteenth century. Indeed, it was left to a
layperson, Sir Daniel Sandford, Professor of Greek at the
University of Glasgow, to publish the first serious and
extended discussion of the Hahnemannian system in Britain.
In The Edinburgh Review of January 1830, Sandford called
for the homoeopathic doctrines to 'be made known to the
British public, and submitted to the keen and sagacious
criticism of our own medical school' [3] - both of which objectives he hoped his article would help to achieve. His call for
the first was more than fulfilled, for the second, dis-
appointed. Certainly criticism from the regular profession
flowed sufficient to fill a library, but its keenness often lay
more in enthusiasm for ridicule and vilification than the sober
and acute examination intended by Sandford.
    Sandford's own discussion of the homoeopathic system
was objective enough. The arguments for the similar remedy,

the explanation of its operation, and the concept of disease as
the totality of symptoms were all fairly presented, and given
a cautiously favourable reception. But incredulity was
reserved for the issue of dosage since, he drily remarked,
'if the decillionth part of a grain have any efficacy, an ounce
of medicine thrown into the Lake of Geneva would be
sufficient to physic all the Calvinists of Switzerland'.[4]
However fantastic potentisation appeared to be as a medical
principle, Sandford nevertheless felt that it should be judged
by the results it achieved with patients. He believed that
positive clinical evidence was available on this score, and
concluded that it represented 'the main stumbling block to the
antagonists of Homöopathie. Anything like an equal list of
well-established instances of failures would be the best
possible answer to Hahnemann's whole system. But these his
opponents do not adduce.'[5]

Though Sandford felt that there was something to be
said for homoeopathy, he was less than enthralled with:

...the style and character of Hahnemann. Perpetually
assuming his system and truth to be identical, he sets
up claims to infallibility that sound very suspicious to
Protestant ears. There is a tone of earnest and solemn
vanity, whenever he speaks of himself and his pretensions, which provokes not merely laughter, but
disquiet. Yet ... the worst of his sins against sense, as
well as taste, is the vulgar and unseemly abuse which he
is not slow nor sparing to heap upon all the votaries of
Aesculpias that belong not to the sacred band ...[6]

Whoever started the mud slinging in the first place, it
was destined to flow thick and fast as the century progressed. Sandford could afford to be dispassionate in his
assessment of homoeopathy: for him, it was an interesting
theory - one which had seemed to produce some promising
results but whose popularisation, should it occur, did not
pose any threat to his own status or livelihood. Once such an
outcome was taken seriously by general practitioners,
however, objective medical commentary on homoeopathy became
almost impossible. The economic self-interest of the profession
made the bellicose rejection of homoeopathy mandatory. As Dr
Cowan put it at the meeting of the PMSA in 1851, homoeopaths were mystics whose 'creed is at variance with all
rational experience, and subversive of all previously acquired
knowledge'. Any homoeopathic doctor, he continued, must
have 'lost the ballast of his reasoning faculties'.[7]

Though in the early 1830s the extremity of such reactions by the regular profession still lay in the future, they
were nevertheless prefigured in the career of the first significant homoeopathic practitioner in Britain, Dr Frederick
F.H. Quin (1799-1879).[8]

Quin had graduated, with the degree of MD, from the University of Edinburgh in 1820. He had already been noted by London's political and social elites as a person of promise, and was immediately invited by Lord Liverpool to fill the government position of physician to Napoleon, then incarcerated at St. Helena. Inconveniently however, the Emperor died before Quin could take up this prestigious appointment, whereupon he joined the entourage of the Duchess of Devonshire, as a personal physician on her travels through Italy. There he soon gained a reputation as an acute wit and gifted conversationalist among the nobility with whom he mixed. Following the Duchess's death in 1824, he was appointed physician to his friend Prince Leopold, afterwards King of the Belgians. It was during this period that Quin first came into contact with homoeopathy; a member of the Prince's household fell sick, and though Quin felt he could do no more, the patient recovered while receiving treatment from a homoeopath. Quin was sufficiently impressed to learn more about the principles which had been employed.

Shortly after this incident, he arrived in London with the Prince. Here Quin drew the attention of Dr Johnson, editor of the Medico-Chirurgical Review, to homoeopathy, and an article was requested for the journal. However, when Quin, still with the Prince, next returned to London, for 'the season' of 1827, and was actually treating patients homoeopathically, Dr Johnson did not repeat his appeal. If he was the first editor of a regular medical journal to have second thoughts about publishing homoeopathic material, he was certainly not to be the last. The practice became standard as the struggle between the two schools sharpened.

Before long, Quin left the Prince's household. Having studied for nearly two years with Hahnemann himself, Quin found the opportunity to put his learning into extensive action in 1831 against an epidemic of cholera in Moravia. This he did, apparently with success, despite catching the disease himself. In 1832 he returned to London and established himself in King Street, St. James's, as the first permanent homoeopathic practitioner in Britain.

Quin was a person of professional determination, wit, social grace, and aristocratic connection. These qualities did much to establish homoeopathy institutionally, and to popularise it among the highest grades of society: indeed, even before Quin had settled in London, homoeopathy had obtained its share of royal patronage - Dr Stapf, at the invitation of Queen Adelaide, and Dr Belluomini, had both practised, albeit briefly, at court.

Quin's repartee was legendary at London's dinner tables. Sir Charles Lococke, on once meeting Quin, observed that he had been treating one of Quin's patients. 'Indeed?', Quin replied. 'Yes, and cured him on your own method too', rejoined Lococke. 'What medicine did you give?', Quin asked. 'Nothing', came the gleeful reply. Quin, however, made a rapid recovery. 'Well, it is curious', he added, '... I have been treating a patient of yours too, and I used your method'. 'Well', Sir Charles responded, 'and what was the result?' Lococke had failed to see the trap, and Quin quietly sprung it: 'Dead', he replied.[9]

Lacking the credentials required for London practice from the RCP, Quin was always open to its exclusionary tactics. These were made clear in 1833, when he received the following note, dated 4 January:

> We, the censors of the Royal College of Physicians, London, having received information that you are practising physic within the City of London and seven miles of the same, do hereby admonish you to desist from so doing until you have been duly examined and licensed thereto under the common seal of the said college, otherwise it will be the duty of the said college to proceed against you for the recovery of the penalties thereby incurred ...[10]

Quin ignored these instructions. A second letter was then sent on 1 February, again requesting Quin 'to desist from practising physic',[11] and expressing surprise that no reply to the first communication had been forthcoming. Quin responded to both letters on 3 February, merely pointing out that he had felt that no reply was due to the first, and acknowledging receipt of the second. There the matter ended. The College did not proceed with its stated intentions. Probably Quin's social reputation and influential friends, and a fear of making him a martyr to a cause which, if ignored, would likely disappear, were sufficient to warn the College off.

But if Quin felt no more of the College's corporate wrath, he continued to face its social disapproval. He had been proposed for election as a member of the Athenaeum Club in London. His name, together with that of his nominator, was inscribed in the appropriate book for the inspection of members. When Dr Paris, then President of the RCP, noticed it he was heard to remark that the club had come to a sorry state if 'quacks and adventurers'[12] were to be proposed as members, and that he was sure no member other than the nominator would support the application. Mr Uwins, a friend of Quin's, did not share Paris's view, and made the point by adding his name to Quin's nomination, and by promising to advise his friend that Paris thought him rather less than a gentleman.

The following day, on which new members were to be elected, Paris - with the assistance of other College members

- did succeed in organising the defeat of Quin's nomination. But the matter did not rest there. On the morning after, Paris was attended by Lord Clarence Paget, an officer in the Guards, on behalf of his friend Quin, with the message that Paris must either provide a written apology for his language, or else justify it with pistols. It soon became obvious to Paris that if he declined to meet Quin, on the grounds that a mere homoeopath was not a fit opponent for the President of the RCP, he would have to fight Paget, who regarded this sentiment about his friend as a personal insult. Since Paris probably felt that 'physician heal thyself' was likely to be a task beyond even his skills after the likely effect of Paget's military aim on his anatomy, he submitted, and signed a retraction of his views, and an apology.

Quin, in fact, contributed little to the development of homoeopathy as a system of medicine, merely editing and translating some of Hahnemann's work. His written output was low for one who enjoyed a long career, but this was more than compensated for by his organisational work. Even in 1834, he was developing ideas on the constitution for a British Homoeopathic Society (BHS). In 1837, he called a meeting of London homoeopaths with the intention of founding this organisation, but had, at the time, to abandon the idea. A few years later, things were more successful. The BHS was formally established on Hahnemann's birthday (10 April) in 1844, when Mr Cameron, Dr Partridge and Dr Mayne met Quin at his house in Arlington Street. Quin was instated as its first president, a post which he held until his death. The first volume of the Society's journal - The British Journal of Homoeopathy - soon appeared (dated 1843), and the first Annual Assembly of the BHS took place in August 1846. In the early days, the Society was notorious for its strictness with members: fines were imposed for failing to deliver promised papers, and for leaving meetings before business had been concluded.

Quin's other major ambition was finally achieved, after a major fund raising drive, when the London Homoeopathic Hospital (LHH), founded at 32, Golden Square in October 1849, opened its doors to patients on 10 April of the following year. In 1859 the hospital moved, opening new premises in Great Ormond Street. As was usual at the time, the hospital was a charitable institution, supported by voluntary contributions. Those who subscribed to its maintenance were entitled to governor status, and had the right to nominate patients in proportion to the size of their annual donation. For admission, patients therefore required a letter of nomination from a governor or subscriber, as well as the approval of the Medical Board of the hospital, which operated on the principle that:

No person who is capable of paying for medical attendance ... shall be admissible; and no person shall be
admitted, or permitted to remain as an in-patient, who is
capable of receiving equal benefit as an out-patient, or
is merely requiring such rest and attention as a work
house can supply.[13]

Quin's popularity among the aristocracy, and elite
support for homoeopathy, was clear from the hospital's list of
benefactors. These first included the Duchess of Cambridge
(patroness), the Duke of Beaufort (vice-patron), the Marquis
of Anglesey (president), and the Archbishop of Dublin, the
Marquis of Worcester, the Earl of Essex, Viscount Sydney,
Lord Gray, Viscount Maldon and Lord Francis Gordon (as
vice-presidents).[14]

If Quin's major legacy was the medical organisation of
homoeopathy, and a tide of support among the well-born,
others had focused on winning goodwill among a wider
clientele, and on developing lay associations for the promotion
of the new school of medicine. The first of these appears to
have been a body known as the Homoeopathic Association
(HA), founded in 1836, and chaired by Lord Robert
Grosvenor. Apparently, sympathetic medical practitioners were
also invited to become honorary members.[15]

Around the same time - 1835 - Mr Leaf, a wealthy
entrepreneur and lay enthusiast, invited Dr Curie, a well-
known French homoeopath, to come to Britain. Quin, in fact,
soon came to regard the activities of Leaf and Curie as
unprofessional (see below), but Curie does seem to have been
almost as influential in ensuring the early growth of homoeo-
opathy in Britain as his better remembered antagonist.
Curie's work, however, through a painstaking devotion to
dispensary and hospital activities, helped to popularise
homoeopathy among social strata much lower than those
engaged by Quin.

Although The Homoeopathic Medical Directory of 1853[16]
lists two dispensaries established as early as 1832 - in
Chelsea and Bristol - the first fruits of Leaf and Curie's
efforts in this direction materialised in 1837, with a dispensary in Finsbury Circus. Five years later, in 1842, the
HA succeeded in raising sufficient funds for the establishment
of a hospital in Hanover Square, with Dr Curie as its leading
practitioner. (According to the 1853 Directory, another
hospital, the Manchester Homoeopathic Hospital and Dispensary, had been established in the same year, but the two
events do not seem to be connected[17]). With this major
objective achieved, the HA appears to have disbanded.

A successor soon emerged. The English Association of
Homoeopathy (EAH), sometimes referred to in the literature as
the English Homoeopathic Association, was formed in 1845,
with Dr Curie, and probably Leaf, among its members.[18]

Again, its object was to fund, support and publicise the development of homoeopathy, especially in the form of the Hanover Square Hospital. The EAH, however, soon ran foul of Quin, and bad blood began to emerge between the lay association, and the professionals in the BHS.[19] The latter disapproved of the way in which affairs at the Hanover Square Hospital were being conducted. The EAH felt decidedly aggrieved by this lack of appreciation of its efforts on behalf of homoeopathy, though the points made by the BHS appear to have hit home with sufficient members to have created an internal squabble within the EAH itself. In the end Mr Sampson and Mr Heurtly, respectively the originator and honorary secretary of the EAH resigned, since they were convinced that the best way forward for the new school was to work with, rather than antagonise, the BHS. Sampson and Heurtly circulated all EAH members with their reasons for leaving, and formed a new group, the British Homoeopathic Association (BHA), in 1847. The EAH, however, did not dissolve - according to The Directory, it was still extant in 1853.[20]

In resigning the two men had sought the advice and obtained the support of Quin. Quin was prepared to give this enthusiastically, provided that a number of conditions, which firmly established the seniority of the BHS in the future partnership, were met. There were six conditions in all. The first two stated that:

... no consideration could induce members of the BHS to have their names connected in any way with the Homoeopathic Institution in Hanover Square, which, by the manner in which the professional department had been directed, had done so much to compromise Homoeopathy, and to reflect discredit, in the estimation of the profession and the public, upon the Homoeopathic practitioners in England ... [and] ... That they would never, under any circumstances, consent to act in any public capacity with Dr Curie.[21]

Curie's cardinal sin, as far as Quin's strict sense of professional etiquette was concerned, was to have participated in the public exhibition of patients who had apparently been cured by homoeopathic treatment. Quin also made it clear that neither he nor the BHS would countenance the idea of furnishing the BHA with case histories for publication, for this would 'lower the profession'.[22]

With Quin's support, the BHA launched itself into fund raising for the establishment of the LHH. In a few years this had been achieved. It was, to quote the title of the last address to the BHA its 'Concluding Task', and the Association was disbanded on 22 August, 1849.[23] The continued existence of the EAH, however, still caused ripples of discontent.[24] The Hanover Square Hospital having closed, a successor - the Hahnemann Hospital - was instituted on 16 October, 1850 at 39, Bloomsbury Square. Leaf was among the vice-presidents and Dr Curie again on the staff. When disagreement on the constitution of the LHH occurred within the BHS - some people feeling that its officers should not solely be restricted to BHS candidates - those holding this view looked to the rival institution, and 'expressed their public protest by giving in their adhesion to the more liberal principle of the Hahnemann Hospital'.[25]

The increase in the number of homoeopathic dispensaries, societies, practitioners, and in the quantity of books, pamphlets, tracts and periodicals which were published continued throughout the early 1840s. Apart from the Chelsea, Bristol and Manchester dispensaries already mentioned, by 1846 four more had opened in London (North London, 1842; East London 1843; Islington 1845; and Pentonville, 1846); seven more in the provinces (Liverpool, 1841; Glastonbury, 1843; Northumberland and Newcastle, Brighton, Leeds and Cheltenham, 1844; and Leicester, 1845); one in Edinburgh (1841); and two in Ireland (the Dublin Homoeopathic Institution, 1844; and the Dispensary of the Irish Homoeopathic Society, 1845, which opened in the same year as the formation of the Society itself). Two other provincial societies were also probably formed in this period - the Cheltenham Homoeopathic Medical Society, and the Northern Homoeopathic Medical Association.[26] Such developments, of course, were partly the consequence of an increase in the number of homoeopathic doctors. As The British Journal of Homoeopathy observed in 1846: 'In taking a general survey of this country, we find the greatest change to be in the numbers of homoeopathic practitioners and their adherents. England is now thickly studded with them...'.[27]

Homoeopathic literature began to appear from the early 1830s onwards. The first texts to come off the press were a translation of the Organon by Charles H. Devrient (1833); A Practical Appeal to the Public through a Series of Letters, in Defence of the New System of Physic, by the Illustrious Hahnemann by John Borthwick Gilchrist (1833); two medical texts edited by Quin (1834); A Letter Addressed to the Medical Practitioners of Great Britain, on the Subject of Homoeopathy by the Reverend Thomas Everest (1834); Practical Observations on Homoeopathy by W. Broakes MRCS (1836); and A Practical View of Homoeopathy, being an Address to British Practitioners on the General Applicability and Superior Efficiency of the Homoeopathic Method in the Treatment of Diseases, with Cases by Stephen Simpson (1836).[28] This, however, was merely the beginning of a huge output. By 1853, the homoeopathic community in Britain had produced a total of 241 publications aimed variously at

the public, the regular profession, and like-minded practitioners.[29]

The tactic of making direct appeals to the public - a
feature of the early texts cited above - did not amuse the
regular profession. First, it smacked of advertising; second,
it publicised disunity in the profession on medical matters;
and third, it suggested that lay judgement of medical issues
was as competent as that of educated practitioners. When
similar material was also published by lay enthusiasts, such
as the Reverend Everest, orthodox practitioners felt that
insult was being added to injury.

Clerical support for homoeopathy probably stemmed from
Hahnemann's contention that illness was essentially a spiritual
condition, and that potentisation released a corresponding
energy in medicines. Presumably, too, the homoeopathic
pharmacopoeia, derived from plants, animals and minerals,
could be seen as evidence of divine beneficience: in creating
the natural world, God had compensated for disease by
furnishing the environment with resources which, if used
correctly, could cure the ills from which people suffered.
Everest, for example, described homoeopathy as 'the medicine
of love', and 'the medicine of harmony'; whereas '...
medicines in a brute, material state, having a totally different
action on the human organism, are perfectly useless, or
rather merely injurious'. Moreover 'the art of cure separated
from the holy principles of love has lost its way, and fallen
into foul company, and consorted with all unloveable things -
cathartics, moxa, The Lancet, emetics and blisters'.[30]

The volume of homoeopathic publication elicited a
matching response from the regular profession. The reviewers
of the publications by Gilchrist and Broakes set the tone for
future allopathic ripostes. Of Gilchrist, one reviewer wrote,
'Homoeopathy may have cured his bodily maladies, but it has
yet to "minister unto a mind diseased".'[31] Broakes received
similar treatment. For those who practisse homoeopathy, or
consent to be treated by the system, 'there is nothing left
for it, but to laugh the parties out of their self-conceits or if
the matter be of graver tendency, to charitably shut them up
in a madhouse'.[32]

Much early Lancet commentary proceeded in a similar
vein. Of a German homoeopath who 'sought to seduce the
Egyptian government by the specious advantages of his
system of medicinal economy', the journal noted with pleasure
that 'the imposter', having 'achieved some remarkable
failures', was so far discredited that 'covered with contempt
the envoy of the homoeopathists was forced to abandon
Egypt'.[33] Soon after, The Lancet reported the results of an
attempt to evaluate homoeopathy by a regular practitioner in
France. M. Andral tried the system with 140 hospital patients
'labouring under intermittent fever, syphilis, inflammatory
fever &c., ... but in no single case was a marked improve-

ment observed, and after a few days M. ANDRAL was compelled to have recourse to the ordinary remedies, under which his patients were rapidly cured'.[34]

Andral had done the profession a great service, the journal felt, for he had shown that 'homoeopathy was either a dream ... or merely a new agent in the hands of charlatans'.[35]

At this time, however, The Lancet had targets besides homoeopathy on its mind. Instead of trying to galvanise the Royal Colleges into the suppression of homoeopathy, which system the journal rather felt should be allowed to 'die a natural death' under the weight of its own absurdity, it was far more urgent to remove obstructions to the important issue of medical reform by petitioning parliament to 'purge the profession of the governing President' of the RCP.[36] These more urgent professional concerns created space in which occasional notes of cautious and qualified approval of the homoeopathic system could be made. Indeed, The Lancet went so far as to print a case history of the apparently successful homoeopathic treatment of haematemesis (vomiting of blood) by John Epps.[37] This was the first and last time such a concession was to be made. Not surprisingly, Epps's article immediately attracted a rebuttal. The recovery of the patient, Dr Mackin argued, was due to previous allopathic treatment.[38]

George G. Sigmund, whose lectures on Materia Medica and Therapeutics at the Windmill Street School of Medicine were reported in The Lancet, suggested that although 'the foundation upon which the superstructure of homoeopathy is raised' was 'altogether fallacious ... I, nevertheless, must proclaim my opinion that Hahnemann collected together a number of very singular facts, and that upon some points connected with the power of therapeutic agents upon the human body, he has much originality, and some truth to boast'.[39] Dr Symonds agreed with these sentiments, advising his class of students in October 1842 that they should 'not disdain [from] taking a hint now and then from heretical professors ... for in most of the heresies in medicine [he had in mind homoeopathy, hydropathy and probably Mesmerism] as in religion, there may be a portion of truth ...'.[40] Lancet editorials were even moved to acknowledge the fact that in some cases a more expectant approach was superior to active drugging: 'A world of mischief has been produced before now by long protracted doses of powerful medicines in chronic cases, many of which would, on the contrary, have been benefited by non-interference with medicine, or - which comes to the same thing - by homoeopathic treatment'.[41]

A few years later, however, when homoeopathy still showed no sign of disappearing from the medical scene, and when Dr Forbes (see below) drew out the full implications for regular medicine of these editorial points, he was lambasted for his pains. The increasing perception of the inroads made by homoeopaths on professional incomes had created a climate in which any case for the new school had to be received with hostility.

Despite the occasional appearance of these more positive overtures, the major thrust of Lancet response was still, in these early years, one of hostility or amusement. One writer sarcastically wondered whether 'the doctrines of homoeopathy extend to the fees as well as the medicines. Doctor Quin will not have perfected the library of homoeopathy until he has constructed a ready-reckoner of hundred thousandths and millionths of a guinea, half-a-crown, and eighteen-pence'.[42] Particular scorn was reserved for aristocratic enthusiasm for the new school: 'There seems to be a peculiar proneness in the English nobility to run after quackery ...',[43] the journal remarked, and went on to discuss the Queen's 'confidence in this absurd system'[44] in tones of despair. After all, as a woman, and as a member of the highest rank of society, her intelligence had to be doubly doubted:

> ... Her Majesty is till persevering in the homoeopathic system, and she supposes that she derived advantage from it. Nothing, however, can be more absurd ... Her brother ... sends her these invisible pills from Germany, and they are such atoms that a quill filled with them lasts her Majesty a couple of months. And, [scurrilously] Her Majesty has also an extraordinary bottle [of homoeopathic medication] which she smells whenever she wants a movement in her royal bowels, and my correspondent tells me that the effect of smelling this bottle is so immediate that her Majesty is obliged to leave the room at a moment's notice.[45]

If the rationality of homoeopathy's enthusiasts was to be doubted, so were their morals:

> The French Academy has not yet given its answer to the minister on the propriety of establishing an homoeopathic hospital. We have, however, just received an explanation of this strange demand, which is amusing enough. The 'young wife' ... to whom DR HAHNEMANN has just been married, turns out to be an old mistress of M. THIERS, the Minister of Public Instruction. Hence the proposed voyage of the old homoeopathist to Paris and hence the proposition of the minister.[46]

Other Lancet comments prefigured the arguments and issues that were to be made over and over again in the

second half of the century: supposed examples of homoeopathic cures were due to either previous allopathic treatment,
spontaneous remission, or poor diagnosis - where a self-
limiting condition was wrongly diagnosed as a serious
illness;[47] homoeopathy in serious illness endangered the life
of the patient, as in the deaths of Lady Denbigh (under
treatment by Dr Curie) and, later, her son;[48] where
homoeoopaths attempted to engage in normal professional
relationships with regular colleagues, they should be
snubbed;[49] and, when possible, homoeopaths should be
removed from official posts. The first example of this form of
action concerned the Poor Law Commissioners. Mr Newman,
surgeon to the Wells Union, had adopted the homoeopathic
system; the Commissioners applied to the RCP for their view
of the matter, and Newman was promptly removed from the
service.[50] Apparently, the RCP felt it unjust that the Poor
Law beneficiaries of Wells Union would not be in a position to
choose whether they would take homoeopathic treatment, or be
in a position to take legal action as compensation for the
dangers it presented if they were really ill. The fact that the
destitute had no choice about receiving regular treatment, or
about turning for economic relief to the Poor Law Commissioners, does not seem to have been an issue which much
bothered the College.

Meanwhile rivalry between the two schools, in the form
of a vigorous exchange of views between Drs Black and Wood,
had been gathering momentum in Edinburgh. Dr Black
published A Treatise on the Principles and Practice of
Homoeopathy in 1842; Dr Wood responded with Homoeopathy
Unmasked; a rebuttal to this appeared in 1843 - Defence of
Hahnemann and his Doctrines - to which Wood once again
replied with a Sequel to Homoeopathy Unmasked.[51]

Wood concentrated his searching examination on the
reliability of statistics concerning homoeopathic cures, on the
dubious validity of symptoms recorded by drug provers, and
on the absurdity of material effect from infinitesimal doses -
matters which were to recur time and again in subsequent
literature. These arguments, however, did not deter William
Henderson, Professor of Medicine and General Pathology at
the University of Edinburgh, from beginning to experiment
with homoeopathic remedies on hospital patients. Henderson's
subsequent conversion to the system was a major surprise to
the regular profession, and initiated a train of events which
had far-reaching consequences for nineteenth century
medicine.

After trying the system, Henderson went so far as to
declare:

I have no difficulty or hesitation in declaring, that the
result of the treatment in these cases, as a whole, has
been decidedly superior to what I have ever witnessed in

117

my previous experience; - of which I may be permitted to say, that it has been neither inconsiderable, nor, in so far as I have learned, different from that of others who enjoyed the same advantages.[52]

Henderson published his results as An Inquiry into the Homoeopathic Practice of Medicine, which appeared in 1845.[53] In fact, he had treated some 600 cases homoeopathically, but the Inquiry records only the treatment of 122 patients whose conditions were felt to offer a reasonable trial of the remedies employed. Thus Henderson excluded cases 'of a slight nature', as well as those in which the conditions had a history of 'repeated and spontaneous alterations of decline and increase', and where patients were not prepared to give the medicines 'a fair trial in point of view of time and attention'.[54]

Overall, Henderson was able to say that of the 122 cases recorded, improvement occurred, 'In 90 per cent ... after the employment of the remedies, and within such a time from their first administration, as to suggest the inference, that they were due to the remedies employed.'[55] Furthermore 'a very considerable number of the successful cases had been treated in the ordinary way, by respectable and intelligent practitioners ... without having experienced relief'.[56]

Henderson's results had apparently been replicated by others. Earlier in his discussion he had referred to Dr Fleischmann, of the Homoeopathic Hospital of Vienna, who had 'lately given to the public a statistical report of the diseases treated in that institution since its foundation in 1832; and among these we find no less than 300 cases of acute pneumonia, 105 of peritonitis, and 224 of pleurisy ...'.[57] The number of fatalities for each disease treated homoeopathically by Fleischmann was nineteen, five and three respectively - which compared with (allopathic) results achieved in the Edinburgh Infirmary over roughly the same period of eighty deaths in 222 cases of pneumonia, six out of 21 cases of peritonitis, and fourteen out of 111 cases of pleurisy. Proportionately, the mortality ratio of cases treated homoeopathically and allopathically was therefore: pneumonia, one death in 15.8 cases to one death in 2.8; peritonitis, one in 21 to one in 3.5; and pleurisy, one in 74.7 to one in 7.9.[58]

The statistics provided by Fleischmann - of which the above represent only a sample - were to become notorious. The regular profession typically alleged that he had massaged the figures by deliberately excluding serious cases from his hospital, or by wilful misdiagnosis. It is difficult to assess these charges at such historical distance, but there does appear to have been some persuasive evidence in their favour, as later and more detailed critiques of the statistics, such as those of Drs Routh, Gairdner, Braithwaite and Barr

Meadows, were to show.[59] Henderson's position at the time, however, was that even allowing for perfectly accurate diagnosis on the allopathic side, and a fifty per cent diagnostic error on Fleischmann's part 'there would remain, notwithstanding, an average mortality considerably less than in ordinary practice'[60] - a result which tended to accord with the experience provided by his own trials.

Of these latter, Henderson hoped that their description and publication would be enough to 'solicit, if not demand, on the part of the profession at large, a practical examination of the system to which they relate'.[61] The stance of the regular profession had been - and remained - one which asserted that if homoeopathy could be shown to invite incredulity at the theoretical level (and given the dogmatism and extremism of Hahnemann's later work, this was not too difficult), then practical trials were unnecessary. Henderson had little time for this attitude. The proof of the pudding had to be in the eating:

> There is no hypothesis in Homoeopathy that is of smallest consequence to the practice of it: the question now is, not whether it originated in a mere speculation, or in an induction of facts; but whether it be, as actually employed in the treatment of disease, a valuable acquisition to the practice of medicine...[62]

Henderson's use of the term 'acquisition' was important, as it signalled his eclectic therapeutic stance:

> If any are still so prejudiced against the ordinary practice, as to deny its possession of many palliative, and not a few, curative expedients, which render it, with all its imperfections, of eminent service to mankind, when administered with discrimination and ability, I must avow my hearty dissent from their opinion.[63]

Homoeopathic treatment then, for Henderson, could produce results generally superior to those achieved in regular practice, but that was no reason to jettison all of the latter in favour of the former. But the real question which Henderson's trials did not settle was whether homoeopathy could produce results that were superior to no treatment at all. On this point, he remarked of patients treated by himself: 'Doubtless some of the cases may have improved independently of the means employed ...'.[64] But this, he felt, would still have left 'many in which the effects may be fairly claimed by the remedies which were used'.[65] This was to overstate the case, of course. Without a control group, and double-blind insurance, no such conclusion could, in fact, 'be fairly claimed'. (In fact, the first rigorous test of the activity of homoeopathic medicines did not take place until

119

1880. Its results were not encouraging. The double-blind trial of aconite 30C in America, organised by homoeopaths in Milwaukee, failed to distinguish between potency and placebo.)[66]

This methodological issue was destined to have a major impact on the conduct of medicine - an ironic result for an issue that was never definitively settled by either side at the time. The regular profession probably preferred not to subject homoeopathic treatment to experimental evaluation because there was already sufficient evidence to suggest that many patients recovered at least as well, and perhaps better, under homoeopathy than with orthodox medication. If a properly controlled and conducted trial confirmed this result, heroic therapy would need to be abandoned, and the intellectual credibility of the profession - fragile at the best of times in the eyes of the public - damaged still further. Indeed, an offer from the Duke of Westminister to finance trials of homoeopathic remedies, in regular hospitals and under regular supervision, was later refused. Similar offers from the capitalist Henry Edmund Gurney, involving St. George's Hospital, and from Mr Clifton to the Northampton Infirmary, were also turned down.[67]

Homoeopaths, on the other hand, were probably wary of repeated and controlled comparison of their system with a nihilistic regimen on the grounds that the results could possibly add weight - if not, they felt, completely vindicate - allopathic criticisms.

As Henderson noted, allopaths certainly did claim that homoeopathy was equivalent to giving no medicine at all. But this was a double-edged accusation, for if homoeopathy produced cures only through 'the beneficient influences of time, repose or imagination ...'[68] - and allopaths could not deny that patients <u>were</u> cured under a homoeopathic regimen - then 'what is the <u>advantage</u> of the treatment usually esteemed so necessary and so potent?'[69] The practical experience of homoeopathic practitioners and their patients constituted, in effect, the experimental result which the regular profession was afraid to formalise. Henderson pointed out the dilemma perfectly:

> ... those who maintain that the results which have followed the employment of [homoeopathic] remedies are no more than the remedial efforts of nature are capable of yielding, cannot avoid the predicament of conceding, that the severe measures of the ordinary practice might have been dispensed with. The only course, in this state of the question, that is presented ... if [practitioners are] conscientiously desirous not unnecessarily to enfeeble [their] patients, is to lay aside the ordinary remedies.[70]

It was a powerful double bind: people recovered under homoeopathic treatment; if this was due to nature, then heroic therapy seemed to be redundant; if it was due to the homoeopathic remedies themselves, the profession could not reasonably refuse to adopt them. Either way, it seemed, regular practice was destined to change.

The Lancet greeted Henderson's work with unconcealed contempt. Its caustic review of the Inquiry, pointing out the apparent inconsistency of Henderson lecturing in pathology while practising a system of medicine which denied its importance, drew to a close with the observation that:

To the reputation of the University of Edinburgh the publication of such a work, and the instruction of such a Professor, must be injurious. Every intelligent student cannot but regard the chair of pathology, and the lectures delivered from it, with a feeling very much approaching to contempt.[71]

Yet Henderson's conclusions could not be so easily dismissed by the regular profession. Sir John Forbes was the first to accept their implications. In Homoeopathy, Allopathy and 'Young Physic' 'forced from us in 1846 somewhat suddenly and prematurely by the perusal of Dr Henderson's book'[72], Forbes argued that, first, homoeopathic remedies were medicinally inactive (oudenopathic); second, that it could not be denied that patients recovered under homoeopathy; and third, that the aggressive drugging and debilitation of regular practice was therefore unnecessary. As Henderson pointed out, once the first premise had been argued, and the second conceded, there could be no other conclusion. Forbes had arrived by logical constraint at the result predicted by Henderson.

Forbes's discussion of homoeopathy was dispassionate, [73] though not in the end sympathetic. As always, the sticking point was the principle of the infinitesimal dose, which he felt was '... an outrage to human reason'.[74] Forbes, in fact, entertained suspicions about Hahnemann's own account of the origins of the principle of reduced dosage. In elaborating these, he succeeded in developing a particularly telling criticism. Hahnemann, Forbes noted, had begun by using normal doses in proving and medication, subsequently reducing these on the basis that the heightened sensitivity of the body to medicinal illness during disease made only the most minute quantities of medicine necessary. But Forbes suggested an alternative interpretation:

The consideration of this reduction of the homoeopathic doses, from a sensible to an infinitesimal amount, suggests to the sceptical or suspicious mind another explanation of the cause much less favourable to

Hahnemann's views. It may be said, for instance, that while medicines were administered in sensible doses, on the Homoeopathic principle, sim*ilia similibus*, they were found not to act beneficially, because any effect they produced was, at best, not curative, and probably, was injurious by disturbing the curative effects of nature. When they were reduced to infinitesimal doses, they ceased to produce any effect on the system, and so came to seem beneficial by not interfering with the vis medicatrix [vitalistic power].[75]

Moreover, Hahnemann had also instructed provings to be conducted with attenuated remedies. Clearly, however, this was inconsistent with the view that the efficacy of the infinitesimal dose stemmed from the sensitivity of the diseased body: as already noted, either this principle was wrong, or the symptoms recorded by the healthy provers were invalid. Forbes was quick to emphasise the problem:

There seems also to be a contradiction in the facts, as well as the reasoning of Hahnemann in regard to this matter. He says it is from the sensitiveness of the affected part being exalted to an extraordinary pitch by the disease that the remedy operates in the infinitesimal dose. If this is the case, how does he explain the alleged facts, on which all his therapeutics is based, viz., the production of such a multitude of symptoms ... in the healthy body, as recorded in his 'Materia Medica Pura' and his 'Fragmenta'?[76]

Forbes developed other criticisms besides. Clearly, though, it was Hahnemann's recommendation of the infinitesimal dose which provided the most important basis for Forbes' rejection of homoeopathy. And there the matter might rest, he thought, as far as the profession was concerned, were it merely a theoretical issue. But homoeopathy's rapidly increasing popularity with the public had transformed it into one which could not be disposed of so readily:

... if [homoeopathy] came before us only as a theory, it would be unnecessary to waste more time in the discussion of its merits ... But homoeopathy comes before us in a much more imposing aspect ... ... it comes before us now, not in the garb of a supplicant, unknown and helpless, but as a conqueror, powerful, famous, and triumphant. The disciples of Hahnemann are spread over the whole civilized world. There is not a town of any considerable size in Germany, France, Italy, England or America, that does not boast of possessing one or more homoeopathic physicians, not a few of whom are men of high respectability and learning; many of them in large practice, and patronized especially by persons of high rank. New books on Homoeopathy issue in abundance from the press; and journals exclusively devoted to its cause are printed and widely circulated in Europe and America. Numerous hospitals and dispensaries for the treatment of the poor on the new system have been established, many of which publish records blazening its successes, not merely in warm phrases, but in the hard words and harder figures of statistical tables. The very fact of the publication of a third edition of such a large and expensive work as Dr Laurie's [Homoeopathic Domestic Medicine] proves how widely the practice is spread among the public generally.[77]

Theoretical critique, then, foundered on the two great facts that the public were increasingly prone to patronise homoeopaths, despite the advice of regular doctors, and that statistics provided by homoeopathic hospitals indicated practical therapeutic success, despite the fact that such results were said to be impossibly attributable to the use of homoeopathic remedies. For Forbes, this meant that:

If, as is maintained by its advocates, it is indeed true, that with its infinitesimal doses it cures diseases ... and cures them in a larger proportion than is done by ordinary treatment; it matters but little whether its theory is false or true. If it can prove to us, that it does what we have just stated ... we are prepared to admit, that this is a kind of evidence sufficient to overthrow all the arguments we can bring against it.[78]

Was such proof available? Ultimately not, Forbes felt. No statistics were available which compared the relative success of homoeopathic treatment to that achieved by no treatment at all.

Of Fleischmann's statistics, Forbes felt that although it was true that 'No candid physician, looking at the original report ... will hesitate to acknowledge that the results there set forth would have been considered by him as satisfactory, if they had occurred in his own practice',[79] and that such data substantiated 'this momentous fact, that all our ordinary curable diseases are cured, in fair proportion, under the homoeopathic method of treatment,'[80] it was nevertheless the case that:

... the sagacious physician will not fail to be struck by the fact, that the relative proportion of cures, and the relative mortality of the different diseases one to another, are precisely the same as he is accustomed to see in his own practice.[81]

In effect, Forbes indulged in some sleight of hand here. Aware of the problem that statistics tend to reflect the activities, aims and definitions of the people or agencies responsible for their collection, he is explicit that no precise conclusions could be drawn from a comparison of Fleishchmann's results with those routinely reported by allopathic hospitals. This was an entirely reasonable basis on which to avoid the otherwise unwelcome conclusion, which Forbes wished to avoid, that Fleischmann's treatment record was superior to that achieved in regular institutions. Unfortunately, however, it was also an entirely reasonable basis on which to reject the conclusion that the recovery rates under homoeopathic and allopathic treatment were the same. Besides, what practitioner would have had anything more than a rough idea of rates of cure for different diseases in his own practice? In the absence of precise records - which the ordinary general practitioner would have been unlikely to keep (and, significantly, Forbes does not introduce any data of this kind) - such judgements would be subject to an inevitable and unquantifiable margin or error. Forbes then, having first questioned the value of available statistical comparisons to rescue allopathy, had to retract his doubts in order to argue that the recovery rates were similar under the two systems. The motive for this argumentative flexibility was clear. It allowed Forbes to derive the inference that the similarity of recovery rates under homoeopathic and allopathic regimens must be due to the operation of a third factor, the power of nature (see especially his Of Nature and Art in the Cure of Disease, 1857).[82] The implications for regular practice were obvious. Forbes did not hesitate to draw them:

> But while we are thus exalting the powers of nature at the expense of homoeopathy, are we not, at the same time, laying bare the nakedness of our own cherished allopathy? If it is nature that cures in homoeopathy, and if homoeopathy (as we have admitted) does thus cure, in certain cases, as well as allopathy, do we not by this admission, inevitably expose ourselves defenceless to the shock of the tremendous inference - that the treatment of many diseases on the ordinary plan must, at the very best, be useless; while it inflicts on our own patients some serious evils that homoeopathy is free from, such as the swallowing of disagreeable and expensive drugs, and the frequently painful and almost always unpleasant effects produced by them during their operation?[83]

For Forbes, this was not an argument for embracing homoeopathy. Doctors, after all, ought to do something to justify their existence, and embracing a therapeutic system whose remedies had been declared therapeutically inert would have seemed to be the equivalent of professional genocide. It was, however, an argument for leaving more to nature in the cure of disease, and for abandoning aggressive and debilitating medication. Forbes summarised his conclusions as follows:

1. That in a large proportion of cases treated by allopathic physicians, the disease is cured by nature, and not by them.

2. That in a lesser, but still not a small proportion, the disease is cured by nature in spite of them; in other words, their interference opposing, instead of assisting the cure.

3. That, consequently, in a considerable proportion of diseases, it would fare as well, or better, with patients, in the actual condition of the medical art, as more generally practised, if all remedies, at least all active remedies, especially drugs, were abandoned.[84]

Furthermore:

Homoeopathy has brought more signally into the common daylight this lamentable condition of medicine where things have arrived at such a pitch, that they cannot be worse. They must mend or end. We believe they will mend ... we yet hope to see raised the standard of 'YOUNG PHYSIC'.[85]

Concerning the implementation of the 'the great REFORMATION' that was to be 'Young Physic', Forbes had twenty recommendations. The tenth of these urged doctors to:

... discountenance, as much as possible, and eschew the habitual use (without any sufficient reason) of certain powerful medicines in large doses, in a multitude of different diseases, a practice now generally prevalent and fraught with the most baneful consequences.[86]

This is one of the besetting sins of English practice ... Mercury, iodine, colchicum, antimony, also purgatives in general and blood-letting, are frightfully misused in this manner.[87]

The overall structure of Forbes's argument is inconsistent. In the comparison of statistics relating to the relative success of homoeopathic and allopathic treatment, Forbes at the same time wishes to avoid saying that the former is less effective, as this would compromise his thesis about the curative powers of nature, or that homoeopathy is more effective, as this would be too much for regular colleagues, or himself, to swallow. Hence he argues that both systems produce comparable results. This allows the introduction of the third variable, i.e. the curative powers of nature, which in turn lays the foundation for the argument against heroic therapy. But if this actually assists in 'opposing, instead of assisting the cure', Forbes should have conceded the point that on balance, patients treated homoeopathically (in his terms, oudenopathically) would fare better than patients treated in the regular manner. Probably Forbes was aware of the inconsistency, but tolerated it in order to avoid accentuating an argument that already looked (and, albeit temporarily, subsequently proved to be) indigestible as far as regular colleagues and readers were concerned.

Despite these inconsistencies, the main thrust of Forbes's argument identified certain facts whose implication for the practice of medicine were to prove irresistible: homoeopathy could not be dismissed by theoretical argument alone as it was already a powerful and popular force among the public, and since people recovered from inflammatory conditions under treatment that was mild and palatable instead of violent and noxious, aggressive medication should be abandoned. Clearly, practitioners who proved reluctant to learn this lesson - a lesson increasingly being absorbed by their clients - would be in for an impecunious future.

The initial reception of Forbes's ideas, though, was a hostile one. His criticism of homoeopathy was forgotten. Instead, he was attacked as a sympathiser, and as a heretic who had impugned the wisdom of an ancient and dignified profession. A Lancet editorial commented of Homoeopathy, Allopathy and 'Young Physic' that there was 'hardly an honest man in the profession, out of Dr Forbes' own circle, who would not reprobate [it] wholly and unreservedly'.[88] And of Forbes's argument for greater reliance on the recuperative powers of the human organism, the writer went on to observe that: 'We are not on this side ... We rather brand the sorceries of Dr Forbes as "Vandalisms, striving to place their heavy heal on the neck of genuine science".'[89] One correspondent went so far as to impugn Forbes's professional ability:

> Those who are faithless regarding the efficacy of medicines may have grounds for their infidelity in their own incapacity to prescribe correctly ... so long ... as we can influence the quality and quantity of the human fluids ... so long will it be wise to adhere to the orthodox methodus medendi, uninfluenced by the theories of the speculative ... or the heresy of Forbes.[90]

The regular profession was much disgruntled. Indeed, in protest 1400 doctors withdrew their subscriptions to The

British and Foreign Medical Review, the journal of which Forbes was editor. Soon after the issue of January 1846, where Homoeopathy, Allopathy and 'Young Physic' had first appeared in article form, the journal was forced to close.[91] Such reactions, however, could not be sustained for long. While official hostility to homoeopathy intensified, regular practice quietly accommodated itself to 'Young Physic'.

Forbes, of course, had opened himself to attack from two sides: if his appraisal of homoeopathy had not been sufficiently negative for the orthodox, it had been far too dismissive for the converted. Henderson was quick to reply: three months after Homoeopathy, Allopathy and 'Young Physic' had first appeared in the British and Foreign, Henderson published his rejoinder. The Letter to John Forbes[92] was an extensive critique of Forbes's argument that homoeopathy was oudenopathic.

Two main lines of argument were pursued. First, that given the large number of cases involved - between 1835-43, Fleishchmann's hospital had treated 6,551 patients - it was permissible to use these figures as a means of comparing the success of homoeopathy with the results achieved by orthodox treatment of a similarly large number of patients in regular hospitals. Errors of diagnosis and the like on either side, Henderson argued, were likely to be self-cancelling.[93] Comparison, therefore, actually did show that homoeopathy produced superior results - a conclusion which, in all consistency, Forbes himself should have conceded in the light of his remarks about the debilitating effect of regular therapy on the vis medicatrix naturae. Second, that the homoeopathy canonised by Hahnemann in the later editions of the Organon was not the way in which most homoeopaths actually practised. Thus to criticise the former was not necessarily to impugn the latter. Henderson was at pains to point out that he himself was not prepared to dismiss all regular therapy as valueless; and, moreover, that advances in pathology and medical technology were of vital importance in improving homoeopathic diagnosis and therefore remedy selection. Besides, homoeopathic doctors tended to favour the low dilutions, sometimes even using drops of the undiluted mother tincture. Again, contrary to Hahnemann, homoeopathic remedies were often used in combination with each other, or with regular treatments (such as enemas), and were given frequently, instead of at long intervals, as advised in the Organon.

Moreover, the theory that potentisation released a 'spiritual' power inhering in medicines was, in general, not taken seriously. Few, also, accepted Hahnemann's view of all chronic disease as the product of either of three inheritable cutaneous miasms. (This was the so-called 'psoric theory': it made relatively little impact in Britain in the nineteenth century and was anyway a late and really superfluous embel-

lishment of the homoeopathic position by Hahnemann. Discussion of this particular item is therefore omitted here.) Again, Henderson himself was clearly using the simile principle on pathological and nosological grounds, rather than in terms of a holistic symptom complex.
These changes, signalled by Henderson, were to be cemented and extended by later recruits. And in practice, homoeopaths would come to resemble their post-heroic regular colleagues - apart from their continued adherence to a distinctive criterion of remedy selection. The orthodox profession, however, having silently absorbed lessons from homoeopathy, continued to attack its practitioners as Hahnemannian fundamentalists. This helped to justify tactics of professional ostracism. By the 1850s, general practitioners were in no doubt that if the regular profession was to safeguard itself from further homoeopathic defections, such action was imperative.

NOTES

1. Anon., 'Report of the meeting of the London Medical Society', The Lancet, vol. XI (1826-7) p. 55.
2. Ibid.
3. Sir Daniel Sandford, 'Hahnemann's Homöopathie', The Edinburgh Review, vol. 50, No. C (1829-30) p. 505. In the Review, the article is anonymous - but it is clearly attributed to Sandford in the following text: R.E. Dudgeon, Hahnemann, the Founder of Scientific Therapeutics (E. Gould and Son, London, 1882) pp. 23-4.
4. Sir Daniel Sandford, op.cit., p. 518.
5. Ibid., pp. 522-3.
6. Ibid., p. 506.
7. Anon., Homoeopathy - Report of the Speeches on Irregular Practice (John Churchill, London, 1851) p. 25.
8. The details of Quin's career are taken from Thomas Lindsley Bradford, The Pioneers of Homoeopathy (Boericke and Tafel, Philadelphia, 1897) pp. 532-48.
9. The conversation is reported in ibid., pp. 537-8.
10. Ibid., p. 543.
11. Ibid.
12. Ibid., p. 547.
13. Anon., The Homoeopathic Directory of Great Britain and Ireland (Henry Turner and Co., London, 1867) pp. 74-5.
14. George Atkin (ed.), The British and Foreign Homoeopathic Medical Directory and Record (Aylott and Co., London, 1853) p. 36.
15. See Geo. M. Carfrae, 'Presidential Address for the Session 1889-90', Annals and Transactions of the British Homoeopathic Society and of The London Homoeopathic Hospital, vol. 12, no date, p. 190. The early history of the

various lay associations is difficult to piece together from the available records, and the account here should be read as a provisional chronological reconstruction rather than a definitive statement. The article on Dr Curie in Thomas Lindsley Bradford, op.cit., pp. 217-24 is useful.

16. George Atkin (ed.), op.cit., pp. 36-44, 70-5.
17. Ibid., pp. 70-5.
18. Ibid., pp. 44-52, and also Anon., Report of the Proceedings of the Second Annual Assembly of the British Homoeopathic Society, August 1847 (Arthur Hall and Co., London, 1847).
19. See the discussion in ... the Proceedings ... of the BHS, August 1847, op.cit., esp. p. 24.
20. George Atkin (ed.), op.cit., pp. 44-52.
21. ... the Proceedings ... of the BHS, August 1847, op.cit., p. 27.
22. Ibid., p. 29.
23. Ibid., and see also A.H.H. Moreton, 'The Homoeopathic Hospital and College', The British Journal of Homoeopathy, vol. VIII (1850), p. 139.
24. See A.H.H. Moreton, op.cit., and also Anon., 'Proposed Homoeopathic Hospital', The British Journal of Homoeopathy, vol. VIII (1850) p. 281; Anon., 'Homoeopathic Intelligence', The British Journal of Homoeopathy, vol. VIII (1850) pp. 411-13.
25. See Anon., 'Homoeopathic Intelligence', op.cit., p. 412.
26. George Atkin (ed.), op.cit., pp. 36-44, 70-5, 76-8.
27. Anon., 'Editorial Address', The British Journal of Homoeopathy, vol. IV (1846) p. 11.
28. Charles H. Devrient, The Homoeopathic Medical Doctrine, or "Organon of the Healing Art"; A New System of Physic. Translated from the German of S. Hahnemann (Simpson, Marshall, and Groombridge, London, 1833); John Borthwick Gilchrist, A Practical Appeal to the Public through a Series of Letters, in Defence of the New System of Physic, by the Illustrious Hahnemann (Parbury, Allen and Co., London, 1833); F.F. Quin (ed.) Fragmenta de Viribus Medicamentorum Positivis sive in Sano Copore Humano Observatis (S. Highley, London, 1834); F.F. Quin (ed.), Pharmacopoeia Homoeopathica (S. Highley, London, 1834); Thomas Everest, A Letter Addressed to the Medical Practitioners of Great Britain, on the Subject of Homoeopathy (Pickering, London, 1834); W. Broakes, Practical Observations on Homoeopathy (Wilson, London, 1836); Stephen Simpson, A Practical View of Homoeopathy, Being an Address to British Practitioners on the General Applicability and Superior Efficiency of the Homoeopathic Method in the Treatment of Diseases, with Cases (J. Baillière, London, 1836).
29. See George Atkin (ed.), op.cit., pp. 132-44.
30. Quoted by Dr Cormack in Homoeopathy - Report on

the Speeches on Irregular Practice (1851) op.cit., p. 15.
31. Anon., 'Review of Gilchrist's A Practical Appeal
...', The Athenaeum Journal of Literature, Science and Fine
Arts (J. Francis, London, 1833) p. 646.
32. Anon., 'Review of Broakes's 'Practical Observations
...', The Athenaeum Journal of Literature, Science and Fine
Arts (J. Francis, London, 1836) p. 170.
33. Anon., 'M. Clot's Account of his Medical and
Surgical Proceedings in Egypt', The Lancet, vol. I (1832-3)
p. 399.
34. Anon., 'Editorial Comment', The Lancet, vol. I
(1834-5) pp. 931-2.
35. Ibid., p. 931.
36. Anon., 'Editorial Comment'. The Lancet, vol. II
(1836-7) p. 134.
37. John Epps, 'Case of Haematemesis', The Lancet,
vol. I (1843-4) pp. 542-4.
38. Dr Mackin, 'The Homoeopathic Cure of Haematemesis', ibid., pp. 642-3.
39. George G. Sigmund, 'Lectures on Materia Medica
and Therapeutics', The Lancet, vol. II (1836-7) p. 75.
40. Dr Symonds, 'Some Truths in Medicine that may be
Allied to Heresies', The Lancet, vol. I (1842-3) p. 244.
41. Anon., 'Editorial Comment', The Lancet, vol. II
(1842-3), pp. 316-7. See also Anon., 'Editorial', The Lancet,
vol. I (1842-3) pp. 685-8 which makes the same point, esp.
pp. 686, 687.
42. Anon., 'Editorial Comment', The Lancet, vol. I
(1834-5) p. 932.
43. Ibid.
44. Anon., 'Intercepted Letter', The Lancet, vol. I
(1834-5) p. 359.
45. Ibid. Original emphasis.
46. Anon., 'Editorial Comment', The Lancet, vol. I
(1834-5) p. 828.
47. See Anon., 'An Homoeopathic Cure', The Lancet,
vol. II (1836-7) p. 32 for an early example.
48. See Anon., 'The Late Lady Denbigh', The Lancet,
vol. I (1842-3) pp. 584-5, and Anon., 'Benefits of
Homoeopathy', The Lancet, vol. II (1842-3) p. 328.
49. See Anon., 'Homoeopathy in Leeds', The Lancet,
vol. II (1844), p. 353, and Anon., 'Homoeopathy and the
Medical Profession', The Lancet, vol. I (1845) p. 24.
50. See Anon., 'The College of Physicians on Homoeopathy', The Lancet, vol. I (1843-4) pp. 270-1.
51. Francis Black, A Treatise on the Principles and
Practice of Homoeopathy (James Leath, London, 1842);
Alexander Wood, Homoeopathy Unmasked; Being an Exposure
of its Principal Absurdities and Contradictions; with an
Estimate of its Recorded Cures (John Menzies, Edinburgh,
1844); Anon., Defence of Hahnemann and his Doctrines:

Including an Exposure of Dr A. Wood's "Homoeopathy Un-masked" (London, Edinburgh, printed 1844); Alexander Wood, Sequel to Homoeopathy Unmasked: Being a Further Exposure of Hahnemann and his Doctrines, in a Reply to Recent Anonymous Pamphleteers (John Menzies, Edinburgh, 1844).
52. William Henderson, An Inquiry into the Homoeo-pathic Practice of Medicine (William Radde, New York, 1846) p. 32.
53. The date of the Radde edition is 1846, though the work appears to have been available in 1845. See J.D. Comrie, A History of Scottish Medicine, 2nd edition, 2 vols. (Baillière, Tindall and Cox, London, 1932) vol. II, p. 623.
54. William Henderson, op.cit., p. 35.
55. Ibid., p. 153.
56. Ibid., p. 154.
57. Ibid., p. 15.
58. Ibid. Appendix. This gives figures for the Edinburgh Infirmary, as well as those at other regular hospitals.
59. C.H.F. Routh, On the Fallacies of Homoeopathy and the Imperfect Statistical Inquiries on which the Results of that Practice are Estimated (H.K. Lewis, London, 1852); W.F. Gairdner, A Few Words on Homoeopathy and Homoeopathic Hospitals, Chiefly in Reply to Professor Henderson, Being a Sequel to the 'Edinburgh Essay' on Homoeopathy (Adam and Charles Black, Edinburgh, 1857). Gairdner notes that his 'Homoeopathic Hospital Statistics' was first published in The Medical Times and Gazette, 3 April (1852), and that it later became the 'Edinburgh Essay' referred to above. Henderson replied to Gairdner's paper: 'A Note on Dr W.T. Gairdner's Essay on Homoeopathy', The British Journal of Homoeopathy, vol. XV (1857) pp. 299-320, and Gairdner made a further rejoinder, afterwards published separately as A Few Words ... The remaining two texts mentioned are W. Braithwaite, A Temperate Examination of Homoeopathy No. 3; The Statistics of Homoeopathy, Examined and Compared with the Regular Practice of Medicine (Simpkin, Marshall and Co., London, 1860), and Barr Meadows, The Errors of Homoeopathy, 3rd edition (G. Hill, London, 1876). See especially the Appendix to this work.
60. William Henderson (1846) op.cit., p. 16.
61. Ibid., p. 31.
62. Ibid., p. 30.
63. Ibid.
64. Ibid., p. 154.
65. Ibid.
66. Anon., 'A Crucial Test of Homoeopathic Medicines', The British Medical Journal, vol. II (1880) p. 633.
67. See the letter from Major W.V. Morgan in J.H. Clarke (ed.), Odium Medicum and Homoeopathy, 'The Times' Correspondence (The Homoeopathic Publishing Co., London,

1888) p. 18; and also the letter from D. Wilson, 'The London Hospitals and Homoeopathy', The Lancet, vol. I (1860) p. 611; and Anon, 'A Homoeopathic Challenge', The British Medical Journal, vol. I (1865) p. 576.

68. William Henderson (1846) op.cit., p. 14.
69. Ibid., p. 16.
70. Ibid., pp. 16-17.
71. Anon., Review of An Inquiry into the Homoeopathic Practice of Medicine', The Lancet, vol. II (1845) pp. 352.
72. Sir John Forbes, Homoeopathy, Allopathy and 'Young Physic' (William Radde, New York, 1846) p. 3. Forbes notes that the book was originally published as an article in The British and Foreign Medical Review, No. XLI (Jan. 1846). All subsequent references are to the Radde edition.
73. See esp. ibid., p. 5.
74. Ibid., p. 17.
75. Ibid., pp. 7-8. Original emphasis.
76. Ibid., p. 8. Original italics.
77. Ibid., p. 21. Original emphasis. Laurie's book proved more popular than even Forbes would have believed. See J. Laurie, The Homoeopathic Domestic Medicine, 27th edition. Revised by R.S. Gutteridge (Leath and Ross, London, 1885).
78. Sir John Forbes, op.cit., p. 22. Original emphasis.
79. Ibid., p. 26.
80. Ibid.
81. Ibid., p. 27.
82. Sir John Forbes, Of Nature and Art in the Cure of Disease, 2nd edition (John Churchill, London, 1858).
83. Sir John Forbes, Homoeopathy, Allopathy and 'Young Physic', op.cit., p. 45.
84. Ibid., p. 47.
85. Ibid., pp. 47, 52.
86. Ibid., p. 53.
87. Ibid., p. 55.
88. Anon. Editorial, The Lancet, vol. II (1847) p. 499.
89. Ibid., p. 500.
90. J.H., 'The Forbes Heresy', The Lancet, vol. I (1847) p. 23.
91. See J.J. Drysdale, Modern Medicine and Homoeopathy (Henry Turner and Co., London, 1870) p. 5.
92. William Henderson, Letter to John Forbes on his Article Entitled "Homoeopathy, Allopathy, and 'Young Physic'" (William Radde, New York, 1846). The Letter was first published as 'Letter to John Forbes', The British Journal of Homoeopathy, vol. IV (1846) pp. 148-219.
93. The point is made in William Henderson, An Inquiry into the Homoeopathic Practice of Medicine, op.cit., pp. 14-15.

Chapter Ten

SPURNING THE FOOL - THE OSTRACISM OF
HOMOEOPATHY 1847-1900

Henderson had been one of the first, and one of the most
distinguished practitioners in Britain, to adopt homoeopathy.
The Lancet was outraged, calling for his resignation. The
profession, it felt, should not hesitate to react in the
strongest possible way when faced with betrayal by one of its
own elite. Henderson had already been persuaded to relinquish the post of Professor of Clinical Medicine by the
university authorities at Edinburgh. This was not enough for
The Lancet. Henderson, it was argued, had also forfeited the
right to hold the Chair of Pathology. An 1845 editorial fumed
that:

> Whilst, on the one hand, he draws fees from the
> student's pocket on the plea of teaching him that
> science, he tells us, in his recent work, that for all
> practical purposes it is of no utility.
>
> How men like Drs ALISON, CHRISTISON, SIMPSON,
> SYME, etc., get on with such a colleague we cannot
> conceive. One thing at least is certain, that unless
> speedy means be taken to expel the homoeopath, the
> University of Edinburgh may bid farewell to its medical
> school.[1]

In fact, one way in which these men did try to 'get on'
with their wayward colleague was by attempting to make
attendance at Henderson's pathology lectures non-compulsory
for students.[2] The power of enforcing resignation, however, lay not with the university authorities, but with the
Town Council. By 1847, the latter body had still made no
move to dismiss Henderson, and The Lancet's frustration had
sharpened proportionately:

> Is there no means of remedying the evil? If Dr
> HENDERSON has not honour or honesty enough to resign
> a chair after he has entirely abandoned the principles

upon which he was elected to fill it, cannot the rest of the University Faculty bestir themselves to make him do so? We have conversed with some of the most distinguished members of the University ... and they are strongly in favour of memorializing the Town Council, with a request that this body should call on Professor HENDERSON to resign ...[3]

If the homoeopathic proclivities of Henderson in distant Edinburgh merited concern, the prospect of a homoeopathic hospital in London itself was contemplated with astonished fury. The Lancet had noticed an advertisement for the post of Resident Medical Officer to the proposed institution, which had asked for testimonials of qualification as a member or licentiate of a British medical college or corporation. The editor commented:

We should like to know the real use of a testimonial would it be, in fact, a proof of anything excepting that the party applying for the situation was a renegade from his true and lawful profession? ... Why did not its concoctors act boldly in their dishonesty, and say at once, 'we offer seventy-five pounds per annum, with apartments, to any young man who will become a renegade for that amount and privilege and we insist upon a qualification, that the advertisement may give us some semblance of scientific conduct in the eyes of the public'.[4]

The increasing stridency of these attacks did not reflect a concocted moral panic by the regular profession. The grounds for concern were real enough. Homoeopathy continued to win converts among doctors and patients. By 1853, 178 doctors in Britain and Ireland had publicly declared their allegiance to the new school, six veterinary surgeons had done so, 57 dispensaries and three hospitals had been opened, and nine societies formed. In-patients and out-patients at hospitals and dispensaries had numbered in excess of 150,000 by 1852.[5] Fourteen years later, in 1867, the number of self-confessed homoeopaths had grown to 251, veterinary surgeons to twelve, and the number of hospitals (five) and dispensaries (59) to 64. Readership for homoeopathic literature was sufficient to sustain two quarterly journals and three monthly publications, and practitioners could give their adherence to any of four major medical societies. Extant books on homoeopathy numbered 198, tracts and pamphlets 192.[6] By the end of 1866, the LHH alone had received 59,138 in and out-patients.[7]
These figures considerably understate the extent to which homoeopathy had imprinted itself on medical and public

consciousness. To begin with, as sanctions by the regular profession against homoeopaths began to bite, it required more and more courage to risk named inclusion in The Homoeopathic Directory. The 1867 issue makes this clear:

> ... we would wish to remark that the following list does not include the names of every practitioner of homoeopathy in the British Isles. In some cases we have been requested not to publish the names of new converts who ... are not yet prepared to avow their belief openly. While we think these gentlemen are wrong in thus withholding their public testimony as to the truth of homoeopathy, we cannot severely censure a course which the illiberality of the Allopathists has forced upon these members of our common profession.[8]

Neither is it possible to gain a definitive picture of the number of regular practitioners who, although not considering themselves homoeopaths, began to use some of the better known homoeopathic remedies as specifics. Finally it is also clear that, like John Gordon of Pitlurg, an unknown number of (more or less scrupulous) laypersons were making a living from treating patients with homoeopathic remedies.[9]

On the patient side, it is equally difficult to quantify the number of homoeopathic consultations per year. Although some hospitals and dispensaries routinely reported the number of in and out-patients treated, the information is neither comprehensive nor regular for the period.[10] Moreover, data on the practice size of doctors themselves appears to be entirely absent. The situation is still further complicated: one of the attractions of homoeopathy was that its essentials could be distilled into repertories, designed to teach laypersons the skills of prescribing for their families. Often, too, medicine chests could be purchased, designed to accompany the advice given in these books. Almost certainly, women constituted the major consumers and users of such products. Quite how many people received homoeopathic treatment in this form is incalculable. The least that can be said is that these repertories were among the most popular and largest selling of all homoeopathic publications. The Directory of 1867 lists 25 texts which obviously fall into this category. Most of them had gone through more than one edition: Dr Curie's had reached its third, Dr Malen's its fourth, Dr Epps's its sixth, Dr Chepmell's its eighth, Guernsey and Thomas's its ninth, and Dr Laurie's two publications their nineteenth and twenty-fifth.[11]

The 1850s and 60s, then, were a period of optimism and confidence for homoeopaths. The number of practitioners was growing, new hospitals and dispensaries for the poor were opening, and the system enjoyed a wide spectrum of public confidence, clerical sympathy and aristocratic patronage. Of those able to pay for medical services, probably only the lower middle class had little contact with homoeopaths. Demand meant that their fees were high enough to be prohibitive.[12] Dr Russell, addressing the Second Congress of Homoeopathic Practitioners in London (23-24 July, 1851) was so convinced that homoeopathy had laid a firm 'hold of the practical English and American mind that nothing', he believed, 'can now check its steady and rapid advance'.[13]

Regular practitioners shared this prognosis. The absolute number of professed homoeopaths may never have actually been very large in Britain, but the regular profession was certainly alarmed at the rate of increase in its medical adherents, and the growing volume of popular support which the system had enjoyed since the 1840s. At the time, as Forbes had observed, it appeared to the orthodox that homoeopathy 'comes before us ... as a conquerer, powerful, famous and triumphant'. And by 1851, Dr Cormack was sure that the advance of homoeopathy in the profession had reached the point at which 'it is time for us to be stirring, lest these apostates, when actually sheltered by [the PMSA], damage its respectability, and ultimately endanger its very existence'.[14]

The terms which the regular profession used to legitimate its action against homoeopaths - the preservation of the integrity of medical science, the defence of professional honour in the face of charlatanry, and a high-minded concern for public welfare - were really the public form in which deeper occupational interests about the collective social advance of medical practitioners found expression. The success of 'professionalism' as a strategy of group mobility depended on control over medical personnel and institutions, over the content of practice itself, and over the remuneration merited by professional status. Homoeopathy struck at all three concerns, but most immediately at that of finance. To the extent that patients dosed themselves homoeopathically, or sought the services of homoeopaths, so the livelihoods of regular practitioners were threatened. The overcrowded nature of the profession exacerbated the situation. Certainly, the financial temptation to practise homoeopathically was considerable. Homoeopaths themselves were open enough about this. As Dudgeon remarked 'any practitioner who declared himself a follower of Hahnemann was sure of getting rapidly into large practice. The mere material inducements to avow oneself a homoeopathist were of the most tempting character.'[15] Occasionally, too, these financial sentiments surfaced in allopathic literature. As the editor of The London Medical Review remarked, 'I venture to say, there is scarcely a medical man in the kingdom who has not felt the influence of this "delusion" on his professional income' - a situation which, he felt, was bound to worsen since 'I fear that the "delusion" is rather increasing than otherwise'.[16]

At bottom this financial threat originated in the parlous condition of regular practice. Public confidence in medical practitioners was low, and would not improve until, as Dr Jenks candidly admitted 'An earnest and truthful endeavour [was made] to improve our professional knowledge'.[17] This improvement ultimately had to await the scientific revolution in medicine in the later decades of the century, and in the general imposition of more exacting educational standards. But one step forward which could have been taken immediately was for the profession to absorb the homoeopathic lessons which Forbes had spelt out in the 1840s. More than anything else, this would have stemmed the haemorrhage of converts to the system, both among doctors and patients. In fact, this is precisely what happened. The free market in medical services saw to that. While this was the most effective of responses to the homoeopathic challenge, it was also, however, a covert one. The public stance of the profession was to fight with the tactics of ostracism, exclusion, dismissal and defamation. The campaign started in 1851.

At its nineteenth annual meeting, held at Brighton (13-14 August), the PMSA decided to act against irregular practice. A committee, consisting of Drs Cormack, Tunstall and Ranking, was appointed to consider what action might be taken. It reported on the 14th with a series of resolutions, all of which were adopted. The most important of these were, first: that homoeopathy was absurd, and that no reputable medical practitioner could or should have anything to do with it; second: that homoeopaths stood guilty of heaping abuse on the regular profession; third: that therefore no member of the PMSA should entertain professional contact with homoeo-paths; fourth: that pure or eclectic homoeopaths, or prac-titioners who consulted with them, should cease to be members of the Association; and fifth: 'That a Committee of seven be appointed to frame laws in accordance with these resolutions, to be submitted to the next annual meeting ...'.[18]

The by-laws proposed by this committee were read before the Association at Oxford the following year. These required that candidates for admission to the PMSA must give a written statement that they were not practising homoe-opathy, and never intended to do so, and that any current member suspected of using the system or dealing pro-fessionally with those who did so should, in the absence of a satisfactory defence, be excluded from the Association, provided a two-thirds majority of those present supported the decision. These measures were also adopted.[19] At the 1858 meeting in Edinburgh, it was resolved to instruct the General Council of the BMA (which the PMSA had become in 1856) to incorporate these strictures into its established legal frame-work.[20] In 1861, at Canterbury, the BMA reaffirmed its general support for all these policies.[21]

The consultation ban - since loss of fees would be involved in refusing to meet homoeopaths - could only be motivated, so the profession told itself, by a well-developed sense of professional honour. Acutally, one of the principal supports of this policy, the ostracism of those who broke the ban, depended for its force on an equally well-developed sense of material security. The potential loss of income from referrals by, and consultations with, regular colleagues was much greater than that risked from refusing to meet homoeopaths. In short, the threat of economic terrorism was the BMA's favoured weapon in ensuring the solidarity of its members.

A huge volume of correspondence in The Lancet and The British Medical Journal was generated as a result of the BMA's action. Surgeons wrote inquiring whether consultation was permitted in non-medical cases; accusations of practising or consorting with homoeopathy were made, defences written, and editorial comment elicited; and local societies usually endorsed, and sometimes argued about, the policies of exclusion and non-consultation. Regular medical journals of the period are rich in such cases. Only a few examples of the many instances which occurred are possible here.

The overwhelming message from local medical societies, predictably, was as hostile to homoeopathy as that of their parent organisation. The South Midland Branch, for example, resolved on 21 May 1858 that no honourable man could consult with homoeopaths, and that anyone who did so 'forfeits the respect of his professional brethren, and his membership of this branch ...'.[22] The Liverpool Medical Institution, however, had for a time tolerated homoeopaths among its members. A stormy meeting on 28 January 1859, much to The Lancet's satisfaction, put an end to this anomaly. A resolution, carried by 96 votes to twenty, amended the existing laws specifically to exclude current and future renegades.[23] In Reading, the branch's 1858 resolutions banning consultation were unanimously reaffirmed on 20 July 1864, after 'one of the subscribers to this resolution had recently broken his pledge ...'.[24] Reading's Pathological Society took similar action. At its meeting on 13 April 1881, the Society resolved to condemn 'emphatically ... any consultation between practitioners of general medicine and reputed homoeopaths'.[25] Feelings were much the same in 1896. On 24 October the Lancashire and Cheshire Branch of the Incorporated Medical Practitioners' Association still felt 'that it is derogatory to the dignity of the profession to consult with .... homoeopathic practitioners'.[26] Scottish practitioners were no less antagonistic. The Royal College of Surgeons of Edinburgh agreed, on 16 May 1851, that 'any Fellow or Licentiate who practises [homoeopathy] or countenances others in doing so by meeting them in consultation, will justly incur the disapprobation of the

College'.[27] The Royal College of Physicians of Edinburgh took similar action, as did the Faculty of Physicians and Surgeons of Glasgow and the Royal College of Surgeons in Ireland.

The less dignified result of these kinds of resolutions was a witch-hunt, in which those suspected of dealing with homoeopaths were exposed by 'colleagues' in letters to the medical press, and were usually presumed guilty until proven innocent. One of numerous instances occurred in 1863 when The Lancet told its readership that 'we have received several letters from medical practitioners ..., strongly complaining that Dr Burrows had met in consultation a homoeopathic practitioner of Bedford on several occasions, and calling upon us to make the fact public'.[28] Dr Wharton, physician to the local infirmary, was also accused. Dr Burrows emphatically denied that he had knowingly committed the offence of which he was charged.[29] Dr Wharton, at this stage, declined to respond at all. Since Mr Coombs, the homoeopath in question, was listed in the medical directory as having graduated from the Homoeopathic College of Cleveland, Ohio, The Lancet argued that Burrows ought to have known that he was infringing the consultation ban, and that Dr Wharton's guilt was evident from his own silence. It was a shame, the journal commented, that 'one consultant [was] so oblivious, and the other so insouciant'.[30] Wharton's independent stance earnt him expulsion from the Bedford Medico-Ethical Association.[31]

The profession in Scotland adopted similar tactics. One correspondent wrote to The British Medical Journal that 'More than one Edinburgh paper, in recounting the illness and death of a nobleman last week, has referred to the frequent consultation of one of our well-known surgeons, Dr Watson, with "Dr Phillips of London"', who was strongly suspected of being a homoeopath.'[32] Again, the writer felt that 'Dr Watson ... owes it to himself to set such doubts to rest, or to afford explanation'.[33] Interestingly, the homoeopath referred to is almost certainly C.D.F. Phillips who, having later renounced homoeopathy, wrote two highly successful books on materia medica which clearly bore the imprint of his previous therapeutic inclinations. The books would not have been touched by the regular profession had Phillips not recanted. At all events, instances of 'finger-pointing', where guilt was assumed on silence, or not excused on the grounds of ignorance, continued throughout the period.

Where purely surgical issues were at stake, and no controversy over medical theory could possibly arise, the regular profession might reasonably have been expected to ignore, if not formally tolerate, instances of consultation. Such was not the case: surgeons who responded to requests for assistance by homoeopaths, even where there was no doubt that they did so in accordance with the ethical

139

imperative of helping patients in distress, were severely censured. In a contest between professional solidarity and Hippocratic ethics, regular medical organisations clearly preferred surgeons to betray their conscience. Many seem to have done so willingly.

One of the first major controversies on this issue occurred in the South Midlands area. Dr Paley and Mr Philbrick refused to meet Dr Bell in view of the consultation ban; Mr Fergusson and Mr Jackson, however, did respond to Bell's call for surgical assistance. The South Midland Branch of the BMA roundly condemned this action at its meeting in Bedford on 21 May 1858, and pointedly forwarded a copy of the resolution passed to Messrs Fergusson and Jackson, while averring that 'the very honourable conduct of Dr Paley and Mr Philbrick was beyond all praise'.[34]

A similar case occurred in 1863. Mr Corbin publicly accused Mr Foster of meeting the homoeopath Dr Ozanne. Foster freely admitted that he had done so: the meeting involved no dispute on medical issues, since 'he was required to give advice and assistance touching a mere local surgical ailment'.[35] The British Medical Journal was not impressed: 'The medical man who meets a homoeopath at the bedside of a patient, under any pretence whatever, meets a homoeopath in consultation, encourages homoeopathy, and, in the eyes of the profession, must occupy the position of one who consults with homoeopaths.'[36] Even in 1897, when Dr Jessop wrote to The British Medical Journal suggesting a review of the consultation issue,[37] the overwhelming view of correspondents, despite one or two dissenting voices,[38] was still that of 'Thrasyllus a Thrasyllo consilium petat' (like should consult with like).

Two particular cases involving the consultation issue have acquired near legendary status in the annals of British homoeopathy, and should not be passed over here. The first concerns the meeting of Drs Quain and Kidd. Kidd had certainly practised homoeopathically during his career, and was the doctor in attendance during Lord Beaconsfield's (Disraeli's) last illness. The Queen - Sir William Jenner having flatly refused to have anything to do with what he regarded as quackery - requested the attendance of Dr Quain. Quain was at first doubtful whether he should comply, but on being given a written assurance by Kidd that he was treating Lord Beaconsfield with regular medicine, on regular principles, and would be directed by Quain in the management of the case, he consented. Quain's intentions and the grounds of his action, were made clear to the RCP, which endorsed and approved his decision to meet with Kidd. In the end, the doctors failed to save Beaconsfield, but their having acted in concert excited considerable discussion. The British Medical Journal felt that since here 'circumstances were altogether altered', because, given Kidd's assurances, 'There was no question of any useless consultation, or of any want of common ground, or of any compromise between rational and irrational treatment', Quain's action was to be supported.[39] Readers' comments, however, were invited on the journal's stance. It was not slow in coming: nineteen letters were rapidly published.[40] A variety of opinions were expressed, some attacking the editorial position, some supporting it, some arguing that Kidd had shown that homoeopaths were never to be trusted (since he had promised not to practise what he professed to believe), and some suggesting that since the practice of the two schools was now so close, there was a basis for formal reconciliation, provided that the new school dropped its sectarian title.

The British Medical Journal was not prepared to go as far as this. Among the correspondents in the wake of the Quain-Kidd affair was Dr Dyce Brown, who suggested that if he was allowed to demonstrate the truth of homoeopathy in its pages, there could be no objection to consultation. The journal, however, felt 'obliged to decline renewing any discussion' on the matter.[41] Consultation was held to be useless on the a priori grounds that the two systems were opposed in theory, logic and practice. The same argument, of course, would also have ruled out consultation between Listerian and anti-Listerian surgeons - but this was an implication which the journal conveniently failed to notice.

The RCP, too, stimulated by the decision it had had to make about Quain, considered it 'desirable to express its opinion that the assumption ... by Members of the profession to designations implying the adoption of special modes of treatment is opposed to ... the freedom and dignity of the Profession ...'.[42]

The second notorious confrontation occurred in 1888. Mr Kenneth Millican was suspended from the Queen's Jubilee Hospital for having worked at the Margaret Street Infirmary, where homoeopathy was practised. Millican took his case to court, and in the first hearing was successful. An appeal was made, however, and the original judgement was reversed by a higher court. But before this happened, Millican's case had been brought before the bar of public opinion by Lord Grimthorpe's letters to The Times. These were, according to Dr Clarke:

... answered by certain members of the allopathic school, who, whilst denying the imputation of odium, approved of and attempted to justify the action of Mr MILLICAN'S intolerant colleagues. But besides attempting to justify intolerance they made an attack on homoeopathy and its professors. This attack brought to the front many champions, both medical and lay, to defend homoeopathy, whilst Mr MILLICAN maintained his original ground and pleaded for tolerance. To these the allopathists again replied, and the battle soon became general. [43]

The Times published no less than 59 letters on the issue, a mere fraction of the total number received. Eventually, the editor felt compelled to bring the argument to a close. The concluding editorial clearly demonstrated where the sympathy of the press lay: Lord Grimthorpe's original charge of odium medicum within the profession was felt to have been entirely justified by the correspondence of regular practitioners on the Millican affair. Moreover, 'When our orthodox friends descend in their wrath to the practices of the tenth rate politician, and pick up any bit of malicious gossip at second or third hand ... it is hard for the ordinary layman ... to feel very deeply convinced of the sobriety and trustworthiness of their judgement.'[44]

As the response to the Quain-Kidd controversy had shown, there were some within the profession who believed that there was a basis for reconciliation between the two schools. Feelings on this issue had been aired in the 1870s. Drs Wyld and Richardson had exchanged views in The Times. Wyld admitted that since us 'homoeopathists are gradually retiring from the use of infinitesimals, and are gradually incorporating with their practice many "orthodox remedies"' it was 'manifest that the time has arrived for a conference between the opposing schools'.[45] Dr Richardson concurred from the allopathic side. The British Medical Journal was less conciliatory, arguing that only a full and formal recantation of past folly would suffice to reopen the doors of regular medicine to homoeopaths.[46] But Dr Bradley, in a letter which candidly admitted the benefits which the regular pharmacopoeia had derived from homoeopathy, demurred. Like Richardson, Bradley wished for 'the burial of the hatchet ...'.[47] Further exchanges occurred. At length, Dr Wyld wrote to The British Medical Journal with a form of words which he felt could serve as a basis for reconciliation. Essentially, it involved a trade off: homoeopaths would relinquish their distinctive title in return for acknowledgement of the right of a doctor 'to adopt any theory or practise which he believes to be best for his patients'.[48] It was signed by many of the big names of homoeopathy, including Quin, Dudgeon, Laurie, Black, Bayes, Hale, Dyce Brown and Richard Hughes.

Again, some responding correspondents were sympathetic, others overtly hostile to any dealings with homoeopaths at all, on the grounds that they were either fools if they practised what they preached, or knaves if they did not. Nevertheless, as the Medico-Ethical Society of Manchester made clear, in a debate largely sympathetic to the cause of reconciliation, the formal relationship between the two schools had, by the 1870s, obviously reached an anomalous position:

while there is an expressed prohibition against anyone meeting a homoeopath in consulation, it is perfectly well-known that homoeopathic practitioners are being met every day by certain of the consulting physicians of Manchester. There is a strong feeling either to break down the barriers completely or make them so secure that there is no escaping them.[49]

At the 1881 meeting of the BMA in Ryde, the issue resurfaced. In the Address in Medicine, delivered by John Sayer Bristowe, he ventured to suggest that:

... where homoeopathists are honest, and well-informed, and legally qualified practitioners of medicine, they should be dealt with as if they were honest and well-informed and qualified. I shall not discuss the question whether we can, with propriety or with benefit to our patients, meet homoeopaths in consultation. I could, however, I think, adduce strong reasons in favour of the morality of acting thus ...[50]

By coincidence, as he was later to make clear,[51] Jonathon Hutchinson expressed similar sentiments in the Address in Surgery: 'it seems to me that the claims of the public should stand first, and that if a man's name is on the Medical Register, we ought to meet him, so long as the consultations result in that which we deem most for the patient's advantage'.[52]

Both speakers made the point that one of the benefits to be gained from the policies suggested would be to hasten the demise of homoeopathy, on the grounds that the tactic of concerted opposition had only served to nourish it. Nevertheless, although some doctors sympathised with Bristowe and Hutchinson, as letters to The British Medical Journal made clear, others were incensed. The Addresses had put the Council of the BMA in an embarrassing position, it was claimed, making it appear that it endorsed a policy which it in fact opposed. Bristowe and Hutchinson were quickly obliged to make it clear that no BMA officer had inspired the sentiments expressed in their speeches.[53] The British Medical Journal itself felt that both men, having talked of the fallacies of homoeopathy in their speeches, then committed a grave non-sequitur in concluding with a plea for a more relaxed attitude vis-à-vis consultation. On this, the journal felt 'neither able to appreciate the force of the arguments of Dr Bristowe and Mr Hutchinson, nor to accept their conclusions'.[54]

Local societies were also enraged. The South Midland, Bath and Bristol, South Western, and East York and North Lincolnshire branches all passed resolutions expressing their dismay at the Ryde Addresses. The South Western Branch took things further. Angered at the straws of reconciliation that were blowing in the allopathic wind, the Branch, knowing that a BMA member had been practising homoeopathically in Plymouth, demanded that the Council of the BMA enforce by-law three, and remove the doctor's name from the list of members. This demand, together with similar proposals from the Staffordshire and East York and North Lincolnshire branches, was considered by Council at its meeting on 12 April 1882. It saw no reason for reversing its opinion that expulsion of homoeopaths would only generate further support and sympathy for the movement on the ground of alleged victimisation, and resolved not to enforce the exclusion law.

C.G. Wheelhouse, President of the Council, wrote to the petitioning branches explaining the decision. Apart from the important point of not feeding martyrs to the homoeopathic movement, Wheelhouse also pointed out that since 'of thirty-one Branches, three are in favour of expulsion, one has declared against it, and twenty-seven have taken no steps', there was a strong possibility that the expulsion issue would not obtain the necessary two-thirds majority at the next meeting of the BMA.[55] The general feeling of the Association, Wheelhouse argued, was that only 'infamous conduct' was ground for expulsion: indeed, at its Bath meeting, the Association had even declined to expel a woman - a fortiori, then, it could hardly expel homoeopaths.[56]

The more radical branches, however, were still not entirely satisfied. In response the Committee of Council proposed, in its report to the general meeting at Worcester in 1882, to obtain 'a full expression of opinion on the part of the whole Association as to whether it will tolerate homoeopathy in its ranks or not'.[57] It was true to its word. Wheelhouse contacted branches by letter. Most, like those in Shropshire, Edinburgh, the South Midlands, Yorkshire, Glasgow and the Borders, supported the Council's view that known homoeopaths should not be admitted to the BMA, but members who were homoeopaths should not be expelled. This position was reaffirmed in 1895.

Ironically, then, in an area where action could have been stringently enforced - cleansing the societies of regular practitioners of all homoeopaths - prudence seems to have prevented radical measures. But this did not prevent the fight from being carried to other quarters. Parliament was one of them.

The 1858 Medical Act had originally contained a provision which would have forbidden doctors from pursuing any therapeutic system other than that legitimated by the various teaching and licensing institutions. As The British Journal of Homoeopathy noted, 'anyone who will peruse the original draft, composed by an obscure clique of conspirators, will at once perceive that one of the main objects of the legislative scheme there disclosed was to extinguish completely and forever the homoeopathic heresy'.[58] Lord Grosvenor's long established support for homoeopathic institutions, however, meant that he could hardly remain silent. He tackled the offending clause in the House of Lords. He not merely succeeded in securing its deletion, but managed to obtain the addition of an amendment to the bill - Clause 23 - which forbad licensing bodies from insisting on guarantees of therapeutic purity as a condition of graduation. A repetition of action already taken along these lines by universities such as those of Edinburgh and St Andrew's was thus no longer to be feared. Homoeopaths were in celebratory mood at the news:

... thanks to the powerful influence of our parliamentary friends, ... all the fangs of this serpent that threatened death and destruction to homoeopathy have been effectively drawn, and no ingenuity can pervert the Act into an instrument for our suppression or annoyance ... for in place of anything like this taking place, the Act expressly forbids any of the small powers it confers being employed against us on account of our adoption of a particular medical theory.[59]

This, in fact, was the second time Grosvenor had fought in parliament on behalf of homoeopathy. The first had involved a struggle to gain official recognition for the LHH's record of success in treating cholera patients. After the epidemic of 1855 in London had subsided, the President of the General Board of Health contacted all metropolitan hospitals which had been involved in receiving patients who had contracted the disease. The intention was to compile a parliamentary report detailing the recovery rate achieved by different institutions, in the hope of identifying any superior plan of treatment which could be followed in future outbreaks.

In total 1,104 patients had received regular treatment; 573 (51.9 per cent) had died. Treatment had consisted of one of the following regimens: small or large doses of calomel, calomel and opium, other mercurials, salines, sulphuric acid, chalk and opium, iron, alum and alum mixture, acetate of lead and opium, cinchona and quinine, gallic acid (from the oakgall), ammonia, brandy, ether, camphor (Cinnamomum camphora) and chloroform, cordial tonic mixture, cajeput (Melaleuca cajuputi) oil, internal stimulants, castor (Ricinus communis) oil, emetics, or olive (Olea europaea) oil.[60] When the Board of Health presented its report, however, the statistics relating to the LHH (ten deaths from 61 cases, all treated by spirit of camphor, given in the first to sixth centesimal potency), although supplied as requested, were omitted. The management committee of the hospital wrote to the President of the Board of Health requesting an explanation, especially in view of the fact that:

... the returns of this hospital prove that in an institution ill adapted from its want of space and the arrangements of its wards for the purposes of a cholera hospital that the deaths do not exceed 16.4 per cent in an epidemic in which, as the Report issued by you shows, the deaths in severe cases under the most successful treatment pursued in other metropolitan hospitals were at the rate of 36.2 per cent ...[61]

There was no excuse for the omission of the homoeopathic statistics on the grounds of unreliable diagnosis. One of the metropolitan hospital inspectors - Dr MacLoughlin, a regular practitioner - had confirmed that all the cholera cases he had observed at the LHH were genuine.[62] Lord Grosvenor, Vice-President of the LHH, raised the issue in parliament. Eventually, a separate parliamentary paper was published, in which the missing data was supplied.[63] Nevertheless, the view of the Board of Health remained that the statistics had originally been omitted because they would 'compromise the value and utility of their averages of cure' and 'give an unjustifiable sanction to an empirical practice alike opposed to the maintenance of truth and to the progress of science'.[64]

This was not the first time homoeopathy had shown its superiority in the treatment of cholera. When the disease had struck Edinburgh in 1848, the homoeopathic dispensary, where six doctors operated in rotation twenty-four hours a day, dealt with 236 cases, achieving a mortality rate of 24 per cent; the Board of Health's figures for regular treatment were 640 cases with a mortality of 68 per cent.[65] At Liverpool in 1849, Drs Drysdale and Hilbers, and Messrs Moore and Stewart, operated the same system, treating 175 people with a death rate of 26 per cent against a general rate, for all forms of treatment, according to the Medical Officer of Health, of 46 per cent.[66]

Grosvenor's campaigns stuck long in the memory of the regular profession. On standing for re-election as the representative of Westminster in 1865, The British Medical Journal advised readers that 'A man who is a quack in one thing is, in our opinion, likely to be a quack in all ...'[67] Mr Hughes - author of Tom Brown's Schooldays - who was standing for Lambeth, received the same compliment. Dr Tweedie withdrew his name from the committee appointed to further Grosvenor's election, and the journal hoped that medical practitioners in these constituencies would express their disapprobation in the appropriate manner at the polls.

Although the 1858 Act had prevented the imposition of therapeutic uniformity by licensing bodies, it did not stop claims from being lodged against homoeopaths in coroners' courts. Cases occurred both before and after the legislation was passed. If juries could be convinced that regular treatment, knowingly withheld in favour of homoeopathy, would have meant a good chance of saving the patient, verdicts of manslaughter became a possibility. An early illustration of these potential developments occurred in 1847. Thomas Hilliar, aged ten months, died under the homoeopathic treatment of Dr Norton. An inquest was held before Henry Churton, coroner for Cheshire. Post-mortem examination revealed that the cause of death had been bronchitis and pneumonia. In his address to the jury, Churton was at pains to make the point that 'prompt and powerful remedies' were required in such cases, and that 'individuals must be jeopardised by the treatment of Dr Norton', but whether the jury chose to accompany 'their verdict by any reference to homoeopathy was a question entirely for their consideration.'[68]

Fortunately for Norton the jury, probably influenced by the fact that Mr Hilliar had lost two other children from bronchitis, despite having received the kind of medical attention which Thomas had been denied, returned a verdict of death 'by the visitation of God'.[69]

A second case occurred in 1853, again involving the death of an infant. This time the coroner, Mr J.M. Churchill, was more explicit. In summing up he commented 'upon the folly of people confiding in homoeopathists', and pointed out that 'if any one died from their treatment, the practitioners would be guilty of manslaughter'.[70] Once more, however, the jury doubted whether the practitioners concerned had been solely responsible for the child's demise, and returned a verdict of 'Natural death'.[71]

William Rae, a homoeopath practising at 36, West Square, London, was not so fortunate. He had been in attendance on Mrs Betsy Poole, who died on 31 July, 1859. She had haemorrhaged seven hours after giving birth, and Rae had been unable to bring the problem under control. Following the report of Mr Bloxam, who conducted the post-mortem examination, the jury returned a verdict of manslaughter, and Rae was advised that his trial would take place at the Old Bailey. Had Rae been a qualified practitioner, the verdict might have been different. But the report makes clear that his name was not in the Medical Register, and presumably the man was therefore medically incompetent.[72]

Dudgeon reports another case: a doctor had treated a member of his family for cholera and 'It was, in truth, a glorious triumph for orthodox physic when the culprit was consigned to a cell in Newgate to await trial for his life, nominally for killing his brother, but actually for therapeutic heresies.'[73] The jury seemed to feel the same way, for the man was speedily released.

Generally, public sympathy for the medical underdog seems to have prevented juries from returning verdicts which most doctors would have liked in these cases. But where more direct action could be taken by the profession, over such issues as hospital and public appointments, and medical education, results were more tangible. Henderson and Newman had been early victims. Dr Horner was a third. Ironically, Horner had spoken at the 1851 meeting of the PMSA - but afterwards, he had decided to enquire more closely into the system which both he and his colleagues had roundly condemned. His best selling pamphlet, Reasons for Adopting the Rational System of Medicine - actually written as an explanatory letter to the Governors of the Hull General Infirmary where he worked - was the result.[74] It was to no avail. Soon after, he was removed from his post.[75]

Dr Reith suffered the same fate. In 1868, The British Medical Journal received copies of correspondence relating to his introduction of homoeopathy into the Royal Infirmary of Aberdeen, and noted that the matter had been brought before the governors. Reith soon wrote to the journal explaining his position. His research, he pointed out, had led him to the conclusion that in those diseases characterised by the dilation of the blood vessels 'medicines are to be selected for the cure, which, in their ordinary manifestation on the healthy body, cause symptoms analogous to the disease', and that 'to obtain the benefit of such powerful medicines, as aconite [Aconitum napellus] arsenic, strychnia, etc., on this principle, they must be given in fractional doses'.[76] These views, he went on, had been taught to students at the Aberdeen Infirmary, had been presented to the Aberdeen Medico-Chirurgical Society, and had been warmly received in The Edinburgh Medical Journal. Since he was now merely carrying out in practice the ideas which he had already expounded to allopathic audiences without censure, and wished to distance himself completely from the Hahnemannians, Reith could hardly see why he should suddenly be stigmatised.[77]

Reith, however had ordered the purchase of some homoeopathic medicines for the Infirmary's laboratory, and had done this without consulting his colleagues, or getting the permission of the managers. This proved to be the nub of the issue - though Reith also undermined his own defence by failing to admit from the very first that some of the dilutions he had used had not worked.[78]

The managers of the Infirmary were due to consider the re-election of the medical staff on 16 December, 1868. They were left in no doubt that if Reith was re-elected, the rest of the medical officers would resign. The governors had no alternative, and Reith lost his post.[79]

On at least once occasion, the bluff was called. One homoeopath was appointed as surgeon to the Militia of Guernsey; the other ten holders of the position threatened resignation; Colonel White, the officer in charge, remained unmoved, and the allopathic surgeons acted - or at least tried to.[80] That they were not completely successful is clear from a letter written to Colonel White in 1862, where the surgeons stated that as long as their grievances remained unredressed 'we perform under protest all the duties of the commissions we have not been permitted to resign'.[81] But the Secretary of State had made a ruling on the dispute in 1861, and as far as Colonel White was concerned, that was the end of the matter.[82]

Occasionally, homoeopaths appear to have responded to these tactics by taking an eye for an eye. The fashionable term among London practitioners for homoeopaths who practised eclectically was 'trimmers', and one Dr Bailey Eadon, as far as the Committee of the Reading Homoeopathic Dispensary was concerned, had travelled so far down this path as to lose sight of homoeopathy altogether. The committee requested, and obtained, his resignation.[83]

The dismissal of homoeopaths from hospital and other posts was matched by attempts to impede progress in terms of basic certification and higher professional honours. At one end of the scale, allopathic opposition ensured that Dr Black was refused the Fellowship of the Edinburgh College of Physicians;[84] at the other, the Universities of Edinburgh and St. Andrew's refused to grant diplomas to practitioners of homoeopathy.[85] The Court of Examiners of the Society of Apothecaries of England stated identical intentions. King's College, Aberdeen, went so far as to examine one candidate, recommend him to the senate for graduation and then, despite having established his medical competence, reversed their decision to recommend graduation on discovering the man's homoeopathic inclinations.[86]

John Marchant Davison managed to slip through the net. Admitted a member of the College of Surgeons on 5 March 1858, it was subsequently revealed, much to The Lancet's disquiet, that he was practising homoeopathically.[87] Doctors were quick to call on the College to be more vigilant. It should, they argued, require students to sign a declaration of present and future therapeutic purity before they could receive their diploma.[88]

The general torpidity of the Colleges in this respect - evidence of elite indifference to the concerns of ordinary general practitioners - aroused strong resentment. Mr Davies brought a particular instance before the BMA at Liverpool in 1859. The Edinburgh College of Physicians had created a new class of honorary Licentiateship, to which candidates could be admitted on the payment of a fee of £25 and the production of testimonials from four qualified members of the profession. One homoeopath had applied - successfully. The fact that his candidature had been supported by testimonials from two homoeopathic doctors rubbed salt into an embarrassing wound.

The College, in the face of 'some sweeping strictures' by the BMA[89], was stung into action, and 'instantly adopted measures which will give much greater ... security against such an occurrence in future'.[90]

Attempts to ostracise homoeopaths from all forms of normal professional intercourse extended, quite naturally, to the field of publication. Only very rarely were homoeopaths allowed to defend themselves or their system in regular medical journals. Indeed as Dr Drysdale, at the British Homoeopathic Congress in Birmingham (28 September, 1870) put it, 'The editors and publishers of the medical periodicals were given to understand that the slightest sign of favour, or even the commonest fairness, towards the new doctrine, was to be the signal for stopping the sale of the publication.'[91]

Pressure was even brought to bear on booksellers. One German periodical of the regular school found this action not only unnecessarily extreme but also, for the British, hypocritical. The Berliner Medicinische Central Zeitung commented:

> The agitation against homoeopathy has given rise to excesses which are more than laughable - they are utterly contemptible. At the instigation of some fanatical medical men, a large publishing house (Highley and Son) have announced that henceforward they will neither publish nor sell any homoeopathic works, and it is expected that other publishers will follow their example. This mode of attempting to stop the child's mouth is absolutely revolting, and all the more barbarous as occurring in a land where the right to give expression is sacred.[92]

Patients, too, were pressurised. When the PMSA passed its resolutions against consultation with homoeopaths, it went to some length to ensure that the public was advised of its action. The meeting agreed to insert its 1851 strictures in The Times, The Morning Post, The North British Advertiser, Saunder's News Letter and, 'in such other journals as the Council may sanction upon the recommendations of the BRANCH ASSOCIATIONS'.[93] Clearly, the intention was to deter potential patients from seeking homoeopathic assistance with the threat that regular help would not be forthcoming if they did. As Dr Cormack observed (forgetting his grammar in his passion): 'It is necessary that the public be told authoritatively ... that they must select ...'.[94]

In response to the kinds of attacks reviewed to date homoeopaths could do little other than rely on powerful friends, continue a somewhat onanistic celebration of therapeutic successes in their own journals, or stay 'in the closet'. One attempt was made to combat institutional victimisation

THE OSTRACISM OF HOMOEOPATHY 1847-1900

through the formation of the Association for the Protection of Homoeopathic Students and Practitioners in 1851 - largely as a response to the PMSA measures of that year, and to the University of Edinburgh's refusal of a degree to Alfred Pope. Its manifesto - condemning allopathic ignorance of homoeopathy and bigotry, and defending the value of consultation between doctors equal in education, science and social position - was inserted in the principal newspapers of the UK.[95] But the Association appears to have been neither particularly successful, nor long-lived. By 1867, it had apparently ceased to exist.

Accompanying attempts to frighten the public away from homoeopaths, and isolate them professionally, was a concerted effort to lampoon the system and its practitioners. This occurred at three levels: first, an attack on the character of homoeopaths themselves: second to publicise and cheer instances where homoeopathy had failed to produce results; and third, to demolish the system through theoretical critique.

The favourite double blind which the profession used to assail the intelligence and integrity of homoeopaths has already been met. One correspondent in 1877 put it like this: 'I have known homoeopathic practitioners personally and I have always taken them to be honourable gentlemen, who were subject, as I thought, to a sort of craze ...'.[96] Thus honourable homoeopaths, practising what they preached, were fools, and unworthy of professional recognition. On the other hand, the rescue of intelligence and sanity meant the sacrifice of honour: 'I for one protest ... against the recognition of any men, whether homoeopathists or anything else, on the confessed ground that they do not really practise according to the system they profess.'[97]

Some years before, in 1862, Dr Roberts had gone to the trouble of documenting the fact. Homoeopathic prescriptions, he found, 'present an astounding range of dose - from the full, indeed overfull dose of ordinary practice, to the heights serene of the sixth dilution'.[98] There is no reason to doubt Roberts's research, but insofar as homoeopaths defined themselves more as a school which adhered to a distinctive method of remedy selection, rather than of dosage, it rather missed the point.

Fools, then, or knaves: either way, homoeopaths could not be fit associates. The argument was repeated ad nauseam in the literature of the period. What made its self-righteousness even worse was the fact that, by the time the correspondent quoted above was writing - the 1870s - the same argument could be made against the regular profession. Students were being introduced to an allopathic materia medica which bore the imprint of homoeopathic research. If, on graduation, they ignored in practice what they had been taught, they were fools; if they did not, and failed to

151

acknowledge their homoeopathic debts, they were undoubtedly knaves.

The real objection was the retention by homoeopaths of a distinctive title while practising eclectically. Homoeopaths were open enough about their departure from Hahnemannian purity, and there does not seem to be any real evidence of a deliberate attempt to mislead the public. But orthodox practitioners felt that patients would regard all the successes of practice which was eclectic in posology, materia medica, diagnosis, etc., as those of pure homoeopathy, and that the system was therefore gaining medical credit which should have properly belonged to them. (Regular doctors omitted to add that by the same argument, homoeopathy's name would be tainted by the failures of mixed practice.) If homoeopathy did gain any credit from eclecticism, it was hardly fair to claim that homoeopaths had been underhanded in its acquisition. Eclecticism was not shrouded in a conspiracy of silence. Besides, when Dr Wyld made the conciliatory gesture of offering to relinquish the new school's title in return for a recognition of freedom of medical opinion, it had been refused.

One manifestation of the double blind argument was the publication of accounts which showed both the harmlessness of swallowing whole vials of homoeopathic pills, and of poisoning by homoeopathic medication. Anecdotes regarding the former were frequent. One enthusiast was:

> ... exhibiting his medicine chest, and his globules, and expatiating largely on their wonderful properties, when a gentleman, who happened to be present, in order to convince him of his folly, emptied the contents of every bottle into his hand, and swallowed them all one after another! I saw him repeatedly for days together afterwards, and I can state positively that he received no damage whatever from his supper.[99]

In the 1870s, however, allopathic journals also reported cases where patients had been poisoned by homoeopathic medication. At the meeting of the Clinical Society of London (14 November, 1873), Dr George Johnson related three instances, all involving 'Epps's Concentrated Solution of Camphor'. In the first, a young woman:

> ... having a cold and sore-throat, took in water twenty-five drops ... She went to bed, and in a short time was found foaming at the mouth, black in the face, and violently convulsed ... For several hours she was unconscious. She vomited blood-tinged fluid, smelling strongly of camphor, and had severe gastric pain. For several days she was partially paralysed, and six months afterwards she was still suffering from symptoms of

nervous derangement. The preparation which caused these serious results is a saturated solution of camphor in alcohol, the preparation being an ounce of camphor to an ounce and a quarter of spirit.[100]

In the same year, Dr Clifford Allbutt reported another case,[101] and in 1875 three more were forthcoming.[102] Though all involved camphor, the implication was that homoeopaths were generally resorting to small doses of the highly concentrated mother tinctures in order to produce dramatic effects – thus risking iatrogenic damage – while claiming the credit (if due) for the infinitesimal principle, and for homoeopathy. Homoeopathic medication was thus either innocuous or dangerous. What else, after all, could be expected from fools or knaves?

The argument was specious. To begin with, the regular profession in the first half of the century had itself defended the need for vigorous medication. Moreover, as a reading of the camphor cases reveals, the bottles were generally labelled clearly, and the doses were often taken on patient initiative, rather than on medical advice. The problem was therefore one which could be solved by increasing public awareness of the difference between potentised remedies and mother tinctures, and by ensuring that chemists labelled their products clearly. But this was not the conclusion which The British Medical Journal wished to draw. The public, instead, should be advised 'that modern homoeopaths have gone from the harmless extreme of infinitesimal dilution to the dangerous extreme of the greatest possible concentration of active and poisonous drugs.'[103]

Another area of activity which the regular profession felt compromised the character of homoeopaths was their willingness to give 'popular lectures on homoeopathy' – even to working class audiences 'at mechanics' institutions and public-houses' – and to write tracts promoting the system.[104] Both strategies smacked of advertising, and of trade, and could only be contemplated, it was felt, by doctors who had little sense of professional honour or integrity.

The second tactic adopted to attack the system and its practitioners was to give maximum publicity to those cases where homoeopathy had been tried, and found wanting. The staple diet here consisted of reports of patients worsening under homoeopathic treatment, at which point the regular cavalry would be called to save the day.[105] One of the more unusual instances, however, occurred in the veterinary field, where homoeopaths tried their system in treating cattle-plague.

Rinderpest was imported into Britain in the spring of 1865. The disease was highly contagious, usually fatal, and soon reached epidemic proportions. Although policies of slaughter, incineration and isolation were adopted, which helped to contain the problem, conventional treatment seemed powerless to cure it. The Times, having noted that 'legitimate science is beaten ...', not unreasonably suggested: 'Here, then, is just the very job for homoeopathy'.[106] At least it could do harm. The British Medical Journal was not amused. The Times' suggestion constituted, it felt, a 'shameless abuse of a learned and self-sacrificing profession'.[107]

Nevertheless an association was formed, chaired by the Duke of Marlborough, to conduct a trial of homoeopathic preventative (arsenic) and curative (belladonna) treatments.[108] The Times hoped for a successful outcome, though the paper pointed out, realistically enough, that regular practitioners would 'probably rather see all the cattle in England die outright of the plague, than be cured by homoeopathy'.[109]

The trial commenced in Norwich. The British Medical Journal recorded with much satisfaction that 'This homoeopathic experiment ... has, of course, turned out a miserable failure'.[110] The Earl of Leicester, in fact, had offered 100 guineas to anyone who could cure rinderpest. Mr Moore, having published an exhaustive pamphlet describing the homoeopathic treatment of the disease, in which he claimed a success rate of 84 per cent, took up the challenge.[111] Two regular veterinary surgeons selected 42 cattle in various stages of the disease from five Norfolk farms. Half were selected for treatment by Moore, half were assigned to a control group. All the animals died. In an understated observation, The British Medical Journal commented: 'After this experience Mr Moore declined to proceed with the competition for the prize.'[112]

At length, Marlborough's Association published its findings. The Report of the Association for the Trial of Preventative and Curative Treatment of the Cattle-Plague by the Homoeopathic Method noted that the investigation had lasted three months, that experiments had been conducted in Norfolk, Yorkshire, Cheshire and elsewhere, but that homoeopathy did not seem to be effective (the symptomatology of rinderpest being too complex for accurate prescribing). The British Medical Journal was happy to print extracts from the report, and to note its conclusion that prevention (by isolation) was the best form of cure, a position it had argued all along.[113] Homoeopathic pretensions, the journal felt, had for once been well and truly nailed.

The third level of attack consisted of theoretical rubbishing of homoeopathic principles. That homoeopathy was 'a monstrous lie, obnoxious to truth, opposed to science, and incompatible with reason' is a fair representation of the views often expressed in editorial comment.[114] But these arguments all tended to be a priori. The profession had not shown definitively that the system was innocuous. And even if it had, the fact remained that in many cases it was still superior to active drugging.

One of Henderson's colleagues at Edinburgh had been James Simpson, Professor of Midwifery. This proximity made of Simpson one of the more famous of homoeopathy's critics. His speech to the Medico-Chirurgical Society in the winter of 1851 - which afterwards appeared in pamphlet form, and then as a chapter in his larger work Homoeopathy: its Tenets and Tendencies, Theoretical, Theological and Therapeutical - was his first venture into already well-trodden ground.[115] The speech had some colourful moments. On the issue of dosage he pointed out to his audience that:

> ... if a single grain of sulphur were divided, as the homoeopathists use it and other drugs, into billionths, and if our common parent, Adam, when called into existence some 6000 years ago, had begun swallowing a billionth every second, and if he had been permitted to live up to the present time doing nothing but swallowing night and day 60 billionths every minute, he would as yet have completed only a small part of his task. It would require him to work and swallow at the same rate for 24,000 years yet to come, in order to finish one single grain of drug, which has little effect on his present descendents in doses of 25 to 50 grains.[116]

Concerning Henderson's original trial of homoeopathy, which formed the basis of his Inquiry into the Homoeopathic Practice of Medicine, Simpson gaily reported the following story. An old school friend of his had started business as a homoeopathic druggist, and had sent him a box of remedies. Simpson had given the box to his eldest son. The child, for amusement, would often open the phials of pills, mix their contents together, refill the bottles, and then place them back in the box. Henderson, on a visit to Simpson's house, and finding the latter absent, had picked up the case of remedies and, having subsequently informed Simpson of his action, reported that he had managed to obtain some good results from their use. At the time, Simpson had not told Henderson of his son's game, hoping to find a more convenient venue in the near future when he could companionably laugh his colleague out of his delusion. This, however, Simpson records, was not a wise decision in view of Henderson's rapidly developing enthusiasm for the system. He should have been told immediately.

The story was probably well-received by Simpson's audience. Henderson was quick to reply. In a letter to the President of the Medico-Chirurgical Society, which met all the issues raised by Simpson, he pointed out that although he had used a box of remedies obtained from Simpson's house,

he had not used these exclusively, but had used medicines
from at least five different sources; moreover, he had never
concealed treatment failures in the ... Inquiry and these were
reasonably attributable, he thought, to the use of medicines
from the tampered phials. [117] Regarding the sleepless Adam,
hypothetically trying to swallow one grain of sulphur,
Henderson argued that most homoeopaths recognised that
Hahnemann had indeed 'overstepped the limits of attenuation'. [118] In practice, however, they were '... descending
to the lower dilutions', [119] which made the ridicule of the
infinitesimal dose substantively irrelevant.

Soon after Simpson's 1851 speech his intended definitive
disposal of homoeopathy's credibility - Homoeopathy, its
Tenets and Tendencies - appeared. Apart from elaborating
the by now familiar criticisms, it included the novel element,
in Chapter Fourteen, that homoeopathy and witchcraft were,
if not identical, then at least analogous. Once more, in 1853,
Henderson responded to Simpson's attack, with Homoeopathy
Fairly Represented in Reply to Dr Simpson's 'Homoeopathy
Misrepresented'. [120] He was not impressed with Simpson's
efforts at all:

> ... it was generally admitted, and even by not a few of
> his own party, that in the last engagement he was very
> handsomely beaten ... Yet with the face of an old
> Hollander, here he is again with as much of the former
> tattered material as he can get to hang together, and as
> much new canvas of the same originally bad quality as
> his crippled spars will carry, trying to look as if he was
> unconscious of defeat. But the device won't do ... for
> such is the mode of attack Dr Simpson has selected, that
> almost anyone might beat him who chose to take the
> trouble. [121]

The exchanges between Simpson and Henderson were
notable as much for the way in which they indicated the
vitriol of the relationship between the homoeopathic and
regular camps as for their intellectual content. And over the
years, many other doctors joined the fray in order to defend
the regular faith. [122] Of the attacks by Drs Williams and
Bushan, Dudgeon observed that the former knew nothing
about the system he criticised, and that the latter united 'the
conflicting parts of quasi-candid examination and unreasoning
abuse'. [123] Dr Routh, in an extended statistical critique of
data supplied by homoeopathic hospitals, concluded that any
'practitioner who would attribute such cures to globulism,
must be considered as either full of simplicity, or a friend of
quackery'. [124] Homoeopathy itself could not possibly cure
the sick and so, Routh argued, putative cures had to be due
to the influence of the mind on the body, the healing power
of nature, diet, or the surreptitious use of regular

medicine. [125] Besides, he continued, since homoeopaths were poor diagnosticians, and allowed 'nothing for the different and varied circumstances under which patients are placed, as type, comfort, locality, idiosyncracy, etc.', then, 'their comparisons with allopathic practice are unfair and not to be counted upon'. [126] Dudgeon was as scathing about Routh as he had been about Williams and Bushan: the substantive conclusion that 'homoeopathic statistics must be cooked' only followed, he pointed out, if the a priori assumption that allopathy was superior was conceded in the first place - but that was exactly what was at issue. [127]

Other critical exercises from the regular school came from Drs Gairdner, Braithwaite, Barr Meadows and Sir Benjamin Brodie. Most drew forth response from the homoeopathic side - Henderson to Gairdner, Drs Bayes and Craig to Braithwaite, and Dr Sharp to Brodie. [128]

These statistical and theoretical examinations of homoeopathy covered much the same ground. As far as the latter were concerned, arguments were repeatedly put forward which strove to undermine the principles of proving, diagnosis, dosage, dynamisation and the similar remedy. Particular scorn was reserved for the records produced by homoeopathic provers. Braithwaite, for example, doubted whether anyone 'could believe that such minute ... doses could produce the huge number of symptoms recorded, and that the effects of the medicines were working some forty days or so after being taken' e.g. '"1090 symptoms as the effects of ... oyster shell; 1242 as the effects of the ink of cuttle fish; 1143 as the effects of ... quinine; 930 ... by doses of charcoal ..."'[129] The simile was also attacked as a rule of strictly limited therapeutic application. Moreover, it was argued, dynamising medicines would dynamise the supposedly inert medium, similar symptoms could indicate different diseases, and homoeopaths themselves, some felt, were also inconsistent in the application of the simile principle.

Homoeopaths such as Henderson, Bayes and Craig generally responded to these allopathic critiques by pointing out, as far as statistics were concerned, that the large number of cases involved in comparative examinations would mean that errors of diagnosis on both sides would be self-cancelling, and that deliberate falsification of returns was hardly something that professional honour would allow. And as regards the theoretical attacks, homoeopaths claimed that they missed the mark. Hahnemann, they conceded, had overstated his case. In practice, homoeopathy had changed, and criticism of Hahnamannianism did not therefore discredit the neo-homoeopathy favoured by British doctors.

These important developments are described more fully in the subsequent section. Crucially, however, regular medicine had changed too. No conception of the real difference between

THE OSTRACISM OF HOMOEOPATHY 1847-1900

the two schools - even by the late 1850s - can be gained from
an acquaintance with the allopathic literature which attacked
the new school. In response to the presence of homoeopathy,
and its popularity, regular practitioners had abandoned heroic
therapy, and covertly turned to the materia medica, and even
principles, of their rivals. This, much more than the forms of
professional and institutional reactions to homoeopathy which
have been detailed here, was responsible for its decline.

NOTES

1. Anon., 'Editorial Comment', The Lancet, vol. II
(1845) p. 354.
2. On Syme et al.'s activities among the students, see
J. D. Comrie, A History of Scottish Medicine, 2nd edition, 2
vols. (Baillière, Tindall and Cox, London, 1932), vol. II, p.
623.
3. Anon., 'Editorial', The Lancet, vol. I (1847), p.47.
4. Anon., 'Editorial', The Lancet, vol.II (1846),
p.512.
5. For these details see George Atkin (ed.), The
British and Foreign Homoeopathic Medical Directory and
Record (Aylott and Co., London, 1853).
6. See Anon., The Homoeopathic Directory of Great
Britain and Ireland (Henry Turner & Co., London, 1867).
7. Anon., 'London Homoeopathic Hospital', Annals and
Transactions of the British Homoeopathic Society and of the
London Homoeopathic Hospital, vol. V (no date) p. 272.
Curiously, the date given in this (and other) reports for the
opening of the hospital is 1853.
8. Anon., The Homoeopathic Directory ... (1867)
op.cit., p. 10.
9. See J. Gordon, A Layman's Experience of Homoeopathy (D. Wyllie and Son, Aberdeen, 1868) p. 6.
10. See, for example, George Atkin (ed.), op.cit.
11. Anon., The Homoeopathic Directory ... (1867)
op.cit., pp. 101-14.
12. See Dr Capper, 'The Progress of Homoeopathy in
England', Annals and Transactions of the British Homoeopathic Society and of the London Homoeopathic Hospital, vol.
V (no date) p. 63.
13. John Rutherford Russell, 'Address at the Second
Congress of Homoeopathic Practitioners', The British Journal
of Homoeopathy, vol. IX (1851), p. 562.
14. Anon., Homoeopathy - Report of the Speeches on
Irregular Practice (John Churchill, London, 1851) pp. 8-9.
15. R.E. Dudgeon, The Influence of Homoeopathy on
General Medicine Since the Death of Hahnemann (Henry
Turner and Co., London, 1874) p. 34.
16. Quoted by W. Bayes, Medical Terrorism in 1862
(Henry Turner and Co., London, 1862) p.12.

17. Anon., Homoeopathy - Report of the Speeches on Irregular Practice, op.cit., p. 5.
18. Anon., 'Historical Sketch of the British Medical Association', The British Medical Journal, vol. I (1882) p. 859.
19. Ibid.
20. Ibid., p. 863.
21. Ibid., p. 864.
22. Anon., 'The Profession and Homoeopathic Quacks', The Lancet, vol. I (1858), p. 538.
23. See Anon., 'Repudiation of Homoeopathy at Liverpool', The Lancet, vol. I (1859), pp. 167-8.
24. Anon., 'Reading Branch: Annual Meeting', The British Medical Journal, vol. II (1864), p. 133.
25. Anon., 'Editorial Note', The British Medical Journal, vol. I (1881), p. 653.
26. A. Brown Ritchie, 'Lancashire and Cheshire Branch of the Incorporated Medical Practitioners' Association', The British Medical Journal, vol. II (1896), p. 1350.
27. Anon., 'Consultation with Homoeopaths', The British Medical Journal, vol. I (1869), p. 106.
28. Anon., 'Alleged Consultation with a Homoeopath', The Lancet, vol. I (1863), p. 73.
29. Ibid., p. 74.
30. Anon., 'The Alleged Consultation with a Homoeopathist at Bedford', The Lancet, vol. I (1863), p. 192.
31. Anon., 'Editorial Comment', The Lancet, vol. II (1863) pp. 104-5. See esp. p. 105.
32. 'Edinensis', 'Consultations with Homoeopaths', The British Medical Journal, vol. I (1869), p. 38.
33. Ibid.
34. A full account of the case is given by Anon, 'The Profession and Homoeopathic Quacks - Meeting of the South Midland Branch of the BMA', The Lancet, vol. I (1858), pp. 563-5. The quote is from page 565.
35. Anon., 'Editorial Comment', The British Medical Journal, vol. I (1864), p. 13.
36. Ibid., p. 14.
37. T. R. Jessop, 'Consultation with Homoeopaths', The British Medical Journal, vol. II (1897), p. 1825.
38. Anon., 'Consultation with Homoeopaths', The British Medical Journal, vol I (1898) p. 344. The doctor signed himself as 'An Open Minded General Practitioner'. The remainder of the correspondence - see, for example, pages 50, 249, 402-3, 661-2 - is mostly hostile.
39. Anon., 'Consultation with Homoeopaths', The British Medical Journal, vol. I (1881), p. 650.
40. See The British Medical Journal, vol. I (1881) pp. 662, 606-7, 707, 711, 750, 784-5, 866-7, 872, 899-900, 907, 951, 987.
41. Anon., 'Homoeopathy', The British Medical Journal,

vol. I. (1881), p. 711.
42. Sir George Clark, A History of the Royal College of Physicians of London, 3 vols. (The Clarendon Press, Oxford, 1964-72), vol. III (A.M. Cooke), p. 909.
43. J.H. Clarke (ed.), Odium Medicum and Homoeopathy: 'The Times' Correspondence (The Homoeopathic Publishing Co., London, 1888), preface. Original italics.
44. Ibid., pp. 119-20.
45. Anon., 'Homoeopathy', The British Medical Journal, vol. I (1877), p. 752.
46. Anon., 'Homoeopathy', The British Medical Journal, vol. I (1877), p. 716.
47. S. M. Bradley, 'The Homoeopathic Schism', The British Medical Journal, vol. I (1877), p. 731.
48. George Wyld, 'Professional Catholicity', The British Medical Journal, vol. II (1877), p. 235.
49. Anon., 'Special Correspondence', The British Medical Journal, vol. II (1877), p. 742.
50. John Sayer Bristowe, 'Address in Medicine', The British Medical Journal, vol. II (1881), p. 261.
51. J. S. Bristowe and Jonathon Hutchinson, 'The British Medical Association and Homoeopathy', The British Medical Journal, vol. II (1881), p. 539.
52. Jonathon Hutchinson, 'Address in Surgery', The British Medical Journal, vol. II (1881), p. 310.
53. J. S. Bristowe and Jonathon Hutchinson, 'The British Medical Association and Homoeopathy', op.cit., p. 539.
54. Anon., 'Consultations with Homoeopaths', The British Medical Journal, vol II (1881), p. 410.
55. Anon., 'Staffordshire Branch: General Meeting', The British Medical Journal, vol. II (1882), p. 74.
56. Ibid.
57. Anon., 'East York and North Lincoln Branch: Half Yearly Meeting', The British Medical Journal, vol. II (1882), p. 1119.
58. Anon., 'The Medical Act', The British Journal of Homoeopathy, vol. XVI (1858), p. 530.
59. Ibid., pp. 534-5.
60. R.E. Dudgeon, 'Cholera', The British Journal of Homoeopathy, vol. XLI (1883), pp. 326-7.
61. See the reprinted correspondence under the heading 'Parliamentary Return of the Homoeopathic Treatment of Cholera', The British Journal of Homoeopathy, vol. XIII (1855), p. 679. Original emphasis.
62. R.E. Dudgeon, 'Cholera', op.cit., p. 327.
63. Ibid., p. 325.
64. 'Parliamentary Return of the Homoeopathic Treatment of Cholera', op.cit., p. 681.
65. R.E. Dudgeon, 'Cholera', op.cit., p. 324.
66. Ibid., pp. 324-5.
67. Anon., 'Editorial Comment', The British Medical

THE OSTRACISM OF HOMOEOPATHY 1847-1900

Journal, vol. I (1865), p. 568.
68. Anon., 'Inquest on the Patient of a Homoeopath',
The Lancet, vol. I. (1847), p. 422.
69. Ibid.
70. Anon., 'Homoeopathy', The Lancet, vol. I (1853),
p. 100.
71. Ibid.
72. Anon., 'Verdict of Manslaughter against a Homoeopath', The Lancet, vol. II (1859), p. 226.
73. R.E. Dudgeon, The Influence of Homoeopathy on
General Practice Since the Death of Hahnemann, op.cit., p.
10.
74. A fifth edition of 20,000 copies is listed in Anon.,
The Homoeopathic Directory of Great Britain and Ireland
(1867), op.cit., p. 119. F.R. Horner, Homoeopathy. Reasons
for Adopting the Rational System of Medicine, 5th edition
(Printed for the author?, Manchester, 1858).
75. See J.J. Drysdale, Modern Medicine and Homoeopathy (Henry Turner and Co., London, 1870), p. 9.
76. Arch. Reith, 'Alleged Homoeopathy in the Aberdeen
Infirmary', The British Medical Journal, vol. II (1868), p.
582.
77. Ibid.
78. Anon., 'Alleged Homoeopathy in Aberdeen', The
British Medical Journal, vol. II (1868), p. 617.
79. Anon., 'The Royal Infirmary of Aberdeen and
Homoeopathy', The British Medical Journal, vol. II (1868), p.
644.
80. See Edw. J. White, 'Homoeopathy and the Guernsey
Militia', The Lancet, vol. II (1860), pp. 369-71.
81. A.B., 'Homoeopathy and the Guernsey Militia', The
Lancet, vol. I (1862) p. 290.
82. Ibid.
83. Anon., 'Homoeopathic Practice', The British Medical
Journal, vol. II (1869), p. 125.
84. See the editorial remarks in W. Ameke, History of
Homoeopathy: its Origin; its Conflicts. Translated by Alfred
Drysdale, and edited by R.E. Dudgeon (E. Gould and Son,
London, 1885), p. 375.
85. Anon., 'Historical Sketch of the British Medical
Association', op.cit., p. 859.
86. Andrew Fyfe, 'University and King's College,
Aberdeen, and the Homoeopathic Fraud', The Lancet, vol. I
(1853), p. 123.
87. Anon., 'Editorial Comment', The Lancet, vol. I
(1858), pp. 393-4.
88. T.W.B., 'The College of Surgeons and Homoeopathy', The Lancet, vol. I (1858), p. 22.
89. Anon., 'Admission of a Homoeopath to the
Edinburgh College of Physicians', The Lancet, vol. II (1859),
p. 149.

90. Wm. Davies, 'Admission of a Homoeopath to the Edinburgh College of Physicians', The Lancet, vol. II (1859), p. 178.
91. J.J. Drysdale, op.cit., p. 5.
92. Quoted by J.J. Drysdale, ibid., p. 6.
93. Anon., 'Historical Sketch of the British Medical Association', op.cit., p. 859.
94. Anon., Homoeopathy - Report of the Speeches on Irregular Practice, op.cit., p. 17. Original emphasis.
95. Anon., 'Association for the Protection of Homoeo-pathic Students and Practitioners', The British Journal of Homoeopathy, vol. IX (1851), p. 694.
96. L., 'The Recognition of Homoeopathists', The British Medical Journal, vol. I (1877), p. 400.
97. Ibid.
98. Wm. Roberts, Homoeopathy as Practised in Manchester, Contrasted with its Alleged Principles (Simpkin and Marshall, London, 1862). The quotation is taken from a review of the book: Anon., 'Reviews and Notices of Books', The Lancet, vol. I (1862), pp. 358-9.
99. J. Milner, 'Homoeopathy', The Lancet, vol. I (1860), pp. 256-7. Original emphasis.
100. Anon., 'Clinical Society of London', The British Medical Journal, vol. II (1873), p. 617.
101. T. Clifford Allbutt, 'Poisoning by Homoeopathic Camphor', The British Medical Journal, vol. II (1873), pp. 679-80.
102. George Johnson, 'Another Case of Poisoning by Homoeopathic Solution of Camphor', The British Medical Journal, vol. I (1875) p. 171; A. Legat, 'Case of poisoning by Homoeopathic Solution of Camphor', The British Medical Journal, vol. I (1875), p. 243; George Johnson, 'Another Case of Poisoning by Homoeopathic Camphor', The British Medical Journal, vol. I (1875), p. 272.
103. Anon., 'Poisoning by Homoeopathic Solution of Camphor', The British Medical Journal, vol. I (1875), p. 351.
104. Anon., 'Editorial Comment', The Lancet, vol. I (1860), p. 146.
105. See, for example, John Francis McVeagh, 'Homoe-opathy', The British Medical Journal, vol. II (1873), p. 743.
106. Quoted in Anon., 'The Cattle-Plague and Homoe-opathy', The British Medical Journal, vol. II (1865), p. 589.
107. Ibid.
108. Anon., 'The Cattle-Plague', The British Medical Journal, vol. II (1865), p. 595.
109. Quoted in Anon., 'The Cattle-Plague and Homoe-opathy', The British Medical Journal, vol. II (1865), p. 589.
110. Anon., 'The Cattle-Plague', The British Medical Journal, vol. II (1865), p. 612.
111. Anon., 'Editorial Comment', The British Medical Journal, vol. I (1866), p. 154.

112. Anon., 'Homoeopathy in Norfolk', The British
Medical Journal, vol. I. (1866), p. 31.
113. Anon., 'Editorial Comment', The British Medical
Journal, vol. I (1866), p. 232.
114. Anon., 'Editorial', The Lancet, vol. I (1860), p.
98.
115. J.Y. Simpson, Homoeopathy: its Tenets and Tendencies, Theoretical, Theological and Therapeutical, 3rd edition
(Sutherland and Cox, Edinburgh, 1853).
116. Ibid., p. 12. Simpson provides other examples in
Chapter VIII and the Appendix. Simpson's billion is one
million million.
117. See W. Henderson, Reply to Dr Simpson's Pamphlet
on Homoeopathy and Second Edition of the Letter to the
President of the Medico-Chirurgical Society of Edinburgh,
with a Postscript (W.P. Kennedy, Edinburgh, 1852).
118. Ibid., p. 23.
119. Ibid.
120. W. Henderson, Homoeopathy Fairly Represented in
Reply to Dr Simpson's 'Homoeopathy Misrepresented' (Thomas
Constable and Co., Edinburgh, 1853).
121. Ibid., pp. 2-3. Original emphasis.
122. See the comments by Dudgeon in W. Ameke,
op.cit., pp. 374-5.
123. Ibid., p. 374.
124. C.H.F. Routh, On the Fallacies of Homoeopathy and
the Imperfect Statistical Inquiries on which the Results of
that Practice are Estimated (H.K. Lewis, London, 1852), p.
75.
125. Ibid.
126. Ibid.
127. See Dudgeon's comments in W. Ameke, op.cit., p.
375.
128. For the texts by Gairdner, with Henderson's
response, and by Barr Meadows, see note 59 to Chapter
Nine. For Braithwaite's A Temperate Examination of
Homoeopathy No. 3 ..., see also note 59 to Chapter Nine.
Other critical examinations in the series were W. Braithwaite,
A Temperate Examination of Homoeopathy No. 1, The Doses
and Provings, 2nd edition (Simpkin, Marshall and Co.,
London, 1859) and A Temperate Examination of Homoeopathy
No. 2, The Principles of Homoeopathy, with a Few Hints on
the Nature and Cure of Disease (Simpkin, Marshall and Co.,
London, 1860). The homoeopathic responses were W. Bayes,
"Two Sides to a Question", A Few Observations on Mr
Braithwaite's Temperate Examination of Homoeopathy (Turner
and Co., Manchester, 1860) and W.S. Craig, Homoeopathy, A
Letter in Answer to Mr Braithwaite's Temperate Examination of
Homoeopathy (Turner and Co., Manchester, 1860). Brodie's
original article and Sharp's rejoinder were subsequently put
together anonymously as Remarks on Sir Benjamin Brodie's

Letter on Homoeopathy (Henry Turner and Co., London, 1861).

129.   W. Braithwaite, A Temperate Examination ... No. 1 ..., op.cit., p. 10. The number of symptoms referred to by Braithwaite within the inset quotation marks are those quoted from homoeopathic sources by J.Y. Simpson, op.cit.

Chapter Eleven

MARRYING THE KNAVE - THE BIRTH OF
BASTARD HOMOEOPATHY

Even Simpson, in his extended and passionate critique of
homoeopathy, was forced, like Forbes before him, to concede
its implications for regular practice:

> The interesting experiment relative to the actual amount
> of the curative powers of nature, which is thus being
> carried on upon a portion of the sick part of our popu-
> lation ... will, I have no doubt, be attended with one
> beneficial result - that it will banish to some extent the
> indefinite polypharmacy and over-drugging which has
> confessedly too much prevailed in some parts of medical
> practice.[1]

Simpson was somewhat irritated by the fact that unreliable diagnosis and homoeopathic eclecticism in matters of
dosage would compromise the results of this experiment. He
did not mention the fact that the profession would probably
not have been interested in the results at all had there been
no pressure on its pocket. But once homoeopathy had entered
the medical market place as a popular force, the financial
choices facing the profession were clear; either adopt the
'young physic' of Forbes and stay in business, or adhere to
the old ways, see homoeopaths multiply, and face penury. In
the end, it was no contest.
    Indeed Forbes himself was among the first to recognise
the existence of these new developments in regular practice.
In 1857, he published Of Nature and Art in the Cure of
Disease,[2] a text which developed his earlier arguments for
greater reliance on the recuperative powers of the human
body in medical treatment. He was pleased to note that
homoeopathy had succeeded in moving the profession in this
direction:

> The favourable practical results obtained by the homoeo-
> pathists - or, to speak more accurately, the wonderful
> powers possessed by the natural restorative agencies of

the living body, demonstrated under their imaginary treatment - have led to several other practical results of value to the practitioners of ordinary medicine. Besides leading their minds to the most important of all medical studies, that of the natural history of diseases, it has tended directly to improve their practice, by augmenting their confidence in Nature's powers, and proportionately diminishing their belief in the universal necessity of Art, thus checking that unnecessary interference with the natural processes by the employment of heroic means, always so prevalent and so injurious. It has thus been the means of lessening, in a considerable degree, the monstrous polypharmacy which has always been the disgrace of our art - by at once diminishing the frequency of administration of drugs and lessening their dose.[3]

In the back of Forbes's book there are a series of reviews, appended to the text by the publisher. These are revealing. In 1846, Forbes's arguments had received a hostile press: now they were applauded. The British and Foreign Medico-Chirurgical Review wrote of the first edition of Nature and Art in 1857 that:

We cannot but believe that the courageous advocacy by Sir John Forbes of views so much opposed to the prejudices of a large class in the profession, have contributed not a little towards the reformation of the drugging system. Most sincerely do we thank him as a benefactor of his profession and of mankind. [4] The Edinburgh Medical Journal concurred. In the same year, it noted: 'This book gives explicit and coherent expression to that feeling of reaction against violent or perturbative practice, which has been going on in the profession for the last twenty-five years, and may now be considered as settled and fixed.'[5]

Neither quote mentions homoeopathy. It is significant, however, that a period of 25 years is referred to, since in 1857 this almost exactly coincided with the number of years that homoeopathic doctors had been practising in Britain.

Other critics of homoeopathy admitted similar changes. In 1859, for example, Braithwaite observed that for regular physicians 'The day has long since passed when they prescribe strong medicines.'[6] He reiterated the point in the following year: 'The public ... may rest satisfied that the modern system of medicine in the regular ranks of the profession, is to do with as little, and not as much medicine as possible; with as mild, and not with as strong medicines as possible.'[7]

Regular journals also reflected the transformation of

practice. The British Medical Journal admitted: 'How often,
now-a-days, is heard the expression - "Oh, my doctor is
almost a homoeopath; he gives so little physic".'[8] Thomas
Laycock, Professor of Clinical Medicine at Edinburgh, agreed:
'The chief characteristic of modern practice is a closer attention to the operations of "nature", and the vis medicatrix
naturae.'[9] Homoeopaths, as might be expected, used more
purple prose to describe the revolution in regular treatment.
After all, the credit, they felt, belonged mostly to them:

> Patients found that they got well with greater certainty
> and rapidity under homoeopathy and hydropathy ... so
> the old school, finding their clients leaving them in
> shoals in pure fear of their cherished methods, executed
> with wonderful quickness a turning movement ... and
> forthwith discarded their traditional methods of bleeding,
> salivation, and the like, and adopted a more or less
> expectant treatment ...[10]

That regular practitioners came increasingly to reject
heroic methods in the late 1850s is clear enough. But the
adoption of expectant approaches could only be a temporary
measure. Therapeutic nihilism was an unviable economic ethic
for those whose livelihoods depended on treating the sick.
Patients expected more for their money than just kind words,
and reassurance that careful diet and rest would allow nature
to bring them back to health. Nature might - but if it did,
then doctoring was a redundant activity. Active service was a
professional imperative, and this soon manifested itself in the
use of new supportive and restorative remedies - like cod-
liver oil, bile, pepsin, beef tea, brandy and pancreatin.
   This tendency is highlighted in the first two volumes of
A System of Medicine, edited by Sir J. Russell Reynolds,
which appeared in 1866 and 1868.[11] The Quarterly Review
noted their publication, and devoted considerable space to a
discussion of Reynolds's efforts.[12] Particular comment was
made on the extent to which the 37 contributors to the texts
(all teachers of general medicine at hospital schools) now
abjured the treatments recommended in the 1830s. Instead, in
the 108 essays comprising the collection:

> The acknowledgement seems to become daily wider spread
> that 'the man is greater than his maladies; that his
> general condition is of more importance than his
> ailments; that disease is a change in him, rather than in
> some part of him; and that no treatment can be of real
> service which sacrifies the greater to the lesser'. Hence
> we find repeated in the volumes before us so often that
> it is needless to quote instances, how in the various
> ailments discussed by various writers, 'no specific
> remedy will cure, nor must any fixed line of treatment

167

be adopted', but that in each case 'improvement in the general health is the first object to be sought'. Medicines are recommended on page after page 'to support the strength of the patient'.[13]

These ideas - a more holistic approach, and strengthening the body in its efforts to regain health - were, of course, homoeopathic, but few in the regular camp noticed or admitted it. What was admitted, however, was the need to address the pressing and embarrassing problem of why non-heroic therapy was now deemed correct, if within the space of the careers of many practising physicians, its very opposite was considered to be the optimum treatment for all inflammatory conditions.

A confession of fallibility would have been the most straightforward response. But with the reputation of the profession and of many eminent teachers and practitioners at stake, this was probably too much to bear. Instead, a number of ingenious explanations were used to show that the profession had been right all along. Thomas Laycock took the prize for inventiveness:

It must be remembered, also, that of late years a more advanced hygiene has diminished infantile mortality, and thus lives of a more effiminate and weakly class have been added to the population, while, on the other hand, a constant emigration has carried off the more masculine and stronger. In this way, the character of the more numerous middle and higher (the more protected) classes has changed somewhat of late years; so that, while they have become more imaginative, mystical, and aesthetic in arts, science, religion, and ecclesiasticism, they have for the same reason become more intolerant of copious blood-lettings, heroic doses, and all perturbative treatment.[14]

The more usual explanation for the new therapeutics was that the nature of disease had changed. As Sir Thomas Watson put it 'inflammatory diseases ... have all become less tolerant of blood-letting since the cholera swept over us in 1832'.[15] Somehow, it was argued, diseases had now become 'weaknesses', and thus strengthening, restorative and supportive treatments were called for. Violent depletion was no longer necessary - indeed, harmful. A contemporary summed up the situation as follows: whereas 'Diseases of a few years ago were characterized by plethora, erethism [over-excitement], excessive strength, and consequently required all sorts of antiphlogistic and depressing remedies', it was now the case that 'diseases are characterized by debility, anaemia, nervous exhaustion, and so forth, and consequently require tonics and stimulants'.[16]

For homoeopaths, all of this was so much humbug. As Dudgeon wrily commented:

It is not easy to understand how the 'sweeping over us' of the cholera should render pneumonia and other inflammatory diseases less tolerant of blood-letting; ... it is more likely that the 'sweeping over us' of homoeopathic knowledge, rather than of the cholera, made patients less tolerant of blood-letting, and so doctors had to give it up; and as they found that diseases did better without it, they had to alter the teachings of their text books accordingly, and they had to invent some other reason for their altered practice, and the 'sweeping over us of cholera', or the 'change of type of disease' served to save their dignity and excuse their change of front.[17]

Historians of medicine - such as Guthrie, Garrison, Major and Shryock - all record, en passant, that one effect of homoeopathy was to secure the abandonment of violent drugging and depletion.[18] What has not received its share or recognition is the debt which regular medicine owed, in the nineteenth century, to homoeopathic principles and the homoeopathic materia medica. Since allopathic writers were generally coy about the real source of the new kinds of practice which they began to recommend - for acknowledgement would jeopardise career and publication chances - this historical oversight is not surprising.

Before too long textbooks started to advocate much smaller doses, to advise remedies on homoeopathic indications and, in the search for new specifics, which followed in the wake of more passive approaches, authors turned to the homoeopathic pharmacopoeia. Such developments are reflected clearly in the work of popular writers such as Ringer and Phillips.

Sydney Ringer, Professor of Therapeutics at University College, London, wrote one of the most successful textbooks of its type: by 1880, A Handbook of Therapeutics, first published in 1869, had reached its eighth edition, and further editions followed in 1882, 1883, 1886, and 1888.[19] Reviews were enthusiastic. The second edition was greeted with the statement that 'This treatise on therapeutics at once assumed the first position on the subject in the English Language'.[20] Of the third edition, it was said that this is 'the best treatise on therapeutics we possess',[21] and of the fourth: 'The rapid sale of Dr Ringer's treatise on therapeutics speaks well for the ready appreciation by British practitioners of new views of practice ... The doctrine of the efficacy of frequently repeated small doses is an innovation.'[22]

Charles D.F. Phillips, Lecturer in Materia Medica and Therapeutics at the Westminster Hospital Medical School, also produced influential texts. Materia Medica and Therapeutics, Vegetable Kingdom appeared in 1874 and Materia Medica and Therapeutics, Inorganic Substances in 1882.[23] Again, both books went through more than one edition, the former re-appearing in 1886, and a third of the latter in 1904.

Ringer's partiality for the small dose is evident in the following examples: for diarrhoea in children, a grain of bichloride of mercury 'dissolved in half a pint of water, and of this a teaspoonful each hour';[24] for gonorrhoea, 'The following is a useful injection -: a grain of chloride of zinc ... in a pint of water ... injected every hour ...';[25] for strumous (scrofulous) ophthalmia, tartar-emetic 'may be given with advantage in doses of 1/36 to 1/48 of a grain, three or four times a day';[26] for a wheezing cough in children, the same medicine in the dose of a grain 'to half a pint of water, and of this ... a teaspoonful every quarter of an hour for the first hour, and hourly afterwards'.[27] for colic of the intestines 'small doses of opium or morphia frequently repeated';[28] and for whooping cough 'one-fiftieth of a grain of morphia every three or four hours'.[29]

Phillips held similar views. Inorganic Substances advised the following fractional grain doses of phosphorous (1/100 to 1/10); antimony (1/16 to 1/6); silver (1/6 to 1/3); arsenic (1/60 to 1/12); barium (1/16 to 1/12); cadmium (1/12 to 1/2); mercury (1/20 to 1/4); lead (1/4 to one); and tin (1/16 to 1/2).[30]

One of the later rationales given for the minute dose among homoeopaths was the fact that, as Dyce Brown supposed, medicines 'have opposite effects in small and large doses; and that the one is precisely the reverse of the other'.[31] Thus large doses gave the therapeutic indications (proving) on which drug was identified to match a case of disease, and its administration in tiny quantities, by the reverse law, would produce a curative effect. Phillips now concurred. With reference to mercury, he believed 'it is more than usually important to distinguish between the effects of small and large doses. Modern observation shows us that the former are of tonic and constructive character, whilst older records have told us only too well the fatally destructive results of the "heroic" administration of the drug'.[32]

But perhaps more important than the advocacy of the small but oft repeated dose by Ringer et al (and there were others, besides Phillips, as homoeopaths pointed out), was the extent of their debt to the materia medica of homoe-opathy. The usual lack of acknowledgement makes detailing the extent of the debt problematic. Nevertheless, it is certain that an intimate acquaintance with homoeopathic literature by such as Ringer and Phillips was responsible for the introduc-tion into British practice of much second-hand homoeopathy. (In fact, on its first appearance, Ringer's work did acknowl-

edge homoeopathic sources - but these were deleted in subsequent editions.)

Harris Coulter, focusing mainly on American medicine -
where the works of Ringer and Phillips were also popular -
lists the following remedies as passing into regular practice
from homoeopathic origins: white black and false (green or
American) hellebore (Veratrum album, Helleborus niger,
Veratrum viride); white briony (Bryonia alba); night blooming
cereus (Cactus grandiflorus); phosphorus and phosphoric
acid; poison ivy (Rhus toxicodendron); Indian cockle
(Cocculus indicus); sundew (Drosera rotundifolia); marigold
(Calendula officinalis); marijuana (Cannabis sativa); Indian
hemp (Cannabis indica); wind flower (Pulsatilla nigricans);
poison hemlock (Conium maculatum); and honey-bee poison
(Apis mellifica).[33]

Remedies already used in medicine, but whose therapeutic application was extended by homoeopaths and then
copied by regular practitioners, included: monkshood
(Aconitum napellus); deadly nightshade (Atropa belladonna);
camphor and copper sulphate (for cholera); derivatives from
the 'tree of life' (Thuja occidentalis); cantharides; copaiba
(balsam from the bark of the South American tree Copaifera
officinalis); celandine (Chelidonium majus); the 'poison nut' of
the strychnine tree; red pepper (Capsicum annum); coffee
(coffea cruda); henbane (Hyoscyamus niger); leopard's bane
(Arnica montana); ergot of rye (Secale cornutum - the ergot
coming from the fungus Claviceps purpurea, which parasitises
growing kernals of rye); preparations from the 'tree of
heaven' (Ailanthus glandulosa); and the use of small doses of
emetics (in nausea and vomiting), cathartics (in diarrhoea),
acids (in acid indigestion), and juniper berry (Juniperus
communis - used homoeopathically to avert abortion).[34]

British practitioners manifested the same proclivity as
their American counterparts for the surreptitious adoption of
homoeopathic knowledge. The British and Foreign Medicao-
Chirurgical Review was exceptional in its recognition that
'Rank homoeopathy is the cry, and Dr Ringer's fondness for
minute doses elsewhere has given apparent strength to the
accusation.'[35] Indeed, it seems to have been the only
allopathic journal prepared to admit the point. Dr Dyce Brown
wrote to The Times that 'The only journal at the time which
saw, or thought it desirable to see, the drift of this mass of
new treatment was the British and Foreign ..., which, coming
out quarterly, and long after the other favourable reviews [of
Ringer], said:- "This is neither more nor less than pure
homoeopathy".'[36]

Homoeopaths, on the other hand, were prepared to state
these developments with candour: though pleased to see
improvements in regular practice through the adoption of
homoeopathic principles they were, however, piqued at the
fact that this was generally unacknowledged, and accompanied

171

by a continued policy of professional ostracism of those who openly declared their allegiance to homoeopathic practice. Drysdale, speaking at the British Homoeopathic Congress in Birmingham (28 September, 1870), insisted that:

> ... no expensive medical work could at present be published if it contained anything favourable to homoe-opathy: accordingly the subject is entirely ignored, or, if alluded to, must be mentioned with reprobation. These books abound in plagiarisms from our school, and its influence may be seen in every page almost, yet the subject must not be named. The private and hospital practice of a physician may display in almost every prescription the fruits of knowledge gathered by our school, and yet he does not honourably acknowledge their source under the penalty of loss of his appoint-ments, expulsion from some medical societies, and general professional ostracism.[37]

And in some clinics, Drysdale continued, prescription on clinical indications alone, and the use of the Ringer-Phillips dose, had gone so far that 'we at first sight almost fancy we had got into a homoeopathic dispensary by mistake'.[38]

Other homoeopaths expressed the same sentiments. Dyce Brown, in 1875, stated that 'we find ... rising men of the "advanced" section of the old school ... employing homoeo-pathic treatment as far as they can, consistently with the retention of their professional status ..'[39]

The extent of Ringer's debt to the new school is evidenced by the fact that homoeopathic journals even felt able to advise readers that they might profitably study his Handbook. The British Journal of Homoeopathy remarked that

> An examination of this the latest systematic work on therapeutics by a professor of the dominant school shows us how rapidly the teachings of that school are converging towards the specific doctrines of the homoeopathic school: in fact, we might give many extracts from the work before us which might equally well have appeared in the work of a writer on homoeopathic therapeutics.[40]

The writer then went on to mention Ringer's use of homoeopathic indications and dosage in prescribing bichloride of mercury and arsenic, and finally concluded that 'We might multiply instances of this homoeopathic practice to any extent; indeed, were we to extract all such to be found in Dr Ringer's work, we should have to convey at least one half of it to our pages.'[41]

The reviewer's conclusion speaks for itself: no clearer testimony to the homoeopathic orientation of Ringer, and of

the new direction of regular practice, could be found.
The Monthly Homoeopathic Review felt the same way.
Citing the following remedies used homoeopathically by Ringer
- sulphides, tartar-emetic, senega (Snakeroot), bromide of
potassium, camphor, ipecacuanha, alum, iodide of potassium,
belladonna and cannabis - the writer felt that for regular
practice 'this is a great step in the right direction ... and
we heartily wish [the book] an abundant success.'[42]
Of Phillips' Materia Medica and Therapeutics, Vegetable
Kingdom the same journal commented:

Pulsatilla, hellebore, dulcamara [Bittersweet or Woody
nightshade], cocculus, chelidonium, thuja, bryonia,
spigelia [Wormgrass], juba [Squirreltail grass], rhus,
anacardium [Marking nut], cicuta [Water hemlock],
mezereum [Daphne] and others are among the medicines
in common use with homoeopathists; but with their
remedial value, those for whose edification this work is
written will now become acquainted for the first
time.[43]

Moreover, the properties of these medicines, the writer
continued 'were investigated and turned to account by
Hahnemann and his disciples', and 'Dr Phillips refrains from
stating this fact'.[44]

In the same vein, Dyce Brown asked if it was 'mere
coincidence that, till Dr Ringer's book was published,
the using of small doses of ipecacuanha in sickness, of
minute doses of corrosive sublimate [bichloride of
mercury] in diarrhoea and dysentry, of arsenic in
diarrhoea and gastritis, and cantharis in inflammation of
the kidneys, and many other bits of treatment, was
'unknown in the old school ... while these very pieces
of practice were in everyday use among homoeopaths[?][45]

Among these 'other bits of treatment' were 1/30 drop doses of
amyl nitrite to 'prevent or greatly reduce ... flushings or
heats',[46] and two drop doses of the tincture of hamametis
(Witchhazel) for bleeding piles.[47]
One writer in The British Journal of Homoeopathy illustrated these tendencies in regular medicine with a telling
fictional conversation between representatives of the two
schools:

Orthodox Practitioner - 'What medicine do you give in
inflammatory fever?'
Reputed Homoeopath - 'Usually Aconite in drop doses.'
O.P. - 'Why, that is precisely what was prescribed by
Mr Brudenell Carter in the case of Dr Anslie, as

recorded in The Practitioner for October, 1874. - What
do you give in acute gastritis?'
R.H. - 'I would probably give Arsenic in small doses.'
O.P. - 'But that is just what Dr Black recommended
some years ago in The Lancet. - How do you treat
dysentry?'
R.H. - 'Generally with small doses of Corrosive
Sublimate.'
O.P. - 'But Dr Sydney Ringer in his 'Handbook of
Therapeutics', 4th edit., p. 233, advises 100th of a
grain of Corrosive Sublimate in such cases. - What do
you give for suppuration of the cervical glands?'
R.H. - 'Very small doses of Hepar sulphuris.'
O.P. - 'That is our Sulphide of Calcium, the very
remedy Ringer advises for such cases in 1/10th of a
grain. - What is the homoeopathic remedy for whooping
cough?'
R.H. - 'Drop doses of Drosera rotundifolia as a rule.'
O.P. - 'But that is precisely the remedy lately vaunted
by Dr Murrell, who says, moreover, that small doses are
much better than large ones.'[48]

Here the conversation ceases, but its author clearly felt that
it could have gone on for pages with 'fifty other remedies for
fifty other diseases'.[49]
Lauder Brunton, physician to St. Bartholomew's and
examiner in therapeutics at the RCP, followed where Ringer
and Phillips had shown the way. Brunton explained that
clerical error was responsible for the inclusion of homoeopathic remedies in his Textbook of Pharmacology, Therapeutics and Materia Medica.[50] Dr Gutteridge was sceptical:

On reading that 'by the error of a copyist one or two
homoeopathic remedies had found their way' into Dr
Brunton's Index of Diseases', I at once reached down my
copy in order to verify this statement. I found that
aconite was very extensively advised in fever ..., that
belladonna was very frequently mentioned, and such
other well known names as arnica, bryonia, pulsatilla,
cimicifuga [Black cohosh], gelsemium [Yellow jeassa-
mine], chamomilla [Chamomile], ignatia [St. Ignatius'
bean], sanguinaria [Bloodroot], chimaphilia [Spotted
wintergreen], hydrastis [Golden seal], rhus toxicodendron, veratrum album, hamametis, veratrum viride,
phytolacca [Pokeweed] and apocynum [Indian hemp],
together with apis mellifica, grindelia [Grindelia
robusta], viola tricolor [Pansy], and thuja, were to be
found as I looked through the alphabetical arrangement.
A very good two or three it must be admitted, especially
as they are mentioned and prescribed for on directly
homoeopathic lines ... it is only fair to the public for

them to know, not to how small, but to how large an
extent one of our chief medical examiners is willing
without ... acknowledgement to borrow from his
ostracized brethren.[51]

The regular profession's general refusal to acknowledge
these claims sharpened homoeopathic discontent as the century
progressed. Soon, it became almost mandatory for every major
speech and article to rail against the injustice of continued
discrimination, while leading allopathic writers won laurels for
teaching what they professed to abjure. The columns of
allopathic journals, Dudgeon wrote 'teem with cases treated by
homoeopathic remedies'[52] Moreover: 'Black, Thorowgood and
many others recommend bits of homoeopathic practice without
mentioning the hated word. Wilks filches from us while he
abuses us'.[53] Nevertheless, while these 'converts' remained
'in the old ranks' they were 'rewarded by professorships and
the applause of orthodox journals'.[54] In America, Dudgeon
pointed out, things were very different. There, the 'Ringers,
Harleys, Wilkses, Thorowgoods and Burnesses fill chairs in
Homoeopathic Colleges'.[55]
Later on, homoeopaths added the names of
Murchison,[56] H.C. Wood Jnr,[57] and Bartholow[58] to the
list of those who ought to be brought to justice for their
pharmacological burglaries.
These claims were repeated so often that the reader of
homoeopathic material of the time soon begins to experience
either indigestion, or to suspect paranoia. The indigestion
would be justified, but the writers were not suffering from a
collective delusion. Their claims were real enough, and
occasionally regular practitioners had the grace to admit it.
When Dr Wyld was talking of reconciliation between the two
schools, S.M. Bradley wrote to The British Medical Journal
that 'it may be fairly argued that, in such works as those of
Dr Sydney Ringer and Dr Charles Phillips, we cannot fail to
see how largely beneficial an extensive knowledge of the
homoeopathic Pharmacopoeia has been to us.'[59]

Dr Alfred Pullar agreed:

In the works of our best authorities, such as Ringer and
Wood, there is ample evidence that the difference
between 'ordinary' and 'homoeopathic' treatment is by no
means so great as to preclude the possibility of useful
consultation. If we compare the chapters on many
important drugs (e.g. aconite, arsenic, antimony, belladonna, cantharides, ipecacuanha, mercury, nuxvomica)
in these text books, with those on the same medicines in
the standard modern work on homoeopathy (Hughes), we
find that there is close resemblance in the teaching. ...
we have seen that suggestions and remedies emanating

175

from the homoeopathic school are now adopted by our
leading therapeutists. The value of these new drugs,
and the successful results obtained by using old
medicines in small doses, are confirmed by our everyday
experience.[60]

The significance of these admissions should not be
underestimated, given the likely reaction from colleagues
which Messrs Bradley and Pullar risked in making them. But
it was not only lessons on drugs and dosage which the
regular profession absorbed: it also flirted with the principle
of proving.

On 17 May 1866, Dr Acland proposed to the General
Council of Medical Education that a grant of £250 a year be
made 'to try the action of remedies'.[61] The British Medical
Journal reported, however, that the Council 'only took a look
at the first round of the ladder, bud did not put their foot
on it'.[62] Nevertheless, an initiative had been made.
Homoeopaths could not help but observe that they had again
shown the way. Dr Acland, they felt, would soon realise that
'much of the work he proposed had been already well done by
many physicians during the past seventy years'.[63]

Further developments soon followed. In 1869, John
Harley FRCP, Assistant Physician to the London Fever
Hospital, published The Old Vegetable Neurotics. First
delivered as the Gulstonian lectures to the RCP in 1868,
Harley's book declared:

My object has been to ascertain, clearly and definitely,
the action of the drugs employed [hemlock, opium,
belladonna and henbane] on the healthy body in
medicinal doses, from the smallest to the largest; to
deduce simple practical conclusions from the facts
observed; and then to apply the drug to the relief of
the particular conditions to which its action appeared
suited.[64]

Subsequently, the BMA undertook trials of full doses of
mercury on animals to determine the effect on the liver and
flow of bile.[65] The British Medical Journal commented that
such research would allow medicine to get 'nearer to an exact
knowledge of the effects or changes that we should aim at
producing in order to correct any morbid action', and thus
'we shall be able to fix with confidence upon the drug (its
operation being known) that is qualified to produce the
results we desire to attain ... The haphazard of a blind
empiricism will be supplanted by a rational and scientific
treatment.'[66]

Dr H.C. Wood agreed. His Treatise on Therapeutics [67]
planned 'to make the physiological action of remedies the
principal point in discussion. A thoroughly scientific treatise

would, in each article, simply show what the drug does when
put into a healthy man, and afterwards point out to what
diseases or morbid processes such action is able to afford
relief.'[68]

Lauder Brunton, too, undertook numerous provings on
animals,[69] William Murrell investigated the medicinal properties of nitroglycerine,[70] and Alexander Burness and F.T.
Mavor published, in 1874, the results of research which bore
the revealing title of The Specific Action of Drugs on the
Healthy System: An Index to Their Therapeutic Value as
Deduced from Experiments on Man and Animals.[71]

In this field, then, thinking in the two schools had
become remarkably close. Homoeopaths agreed that experiments (or accidental poisonings) which showed the particular
organ lesions produced by drugs were a valuable guide to the
therapeutic domain of remedies, and to the extent that both
types of practitioner agreed that a small dose of the same
substance would have a reverse (tonic) effect, then the simile
principle had seemingly won joint approval. However, subtle
but important differences remained. The words which follow
the quote from Wood given above are that the 'thoroughly
scientific treatise' of which he spoke was not yet possible 'for
our knowledge is not complete enough'. This was because,
instead of using provings on 'a healthy man', experiments
were made chiefly upon animals. Toxic doses of drugs would
identify the lesions characteristic of each, and thus give some
indication of their sphere of activity in people. But homoeopaths, armed with records of symptoms experienced by human
provers, were enabled to make much finer discrimination
among remedies. Thus Wood himself argued that hyoscyamus
and stramonium could be used on the same indications as
belladonna, given the general resemblance of their physiological effects. The homoeopathic point was that symptomatic
provings individuated these drugs much more clearly and, via
the simile principle, the correct one of the three could therefore be identified for a particular patient.[72]

It is important, however, not to overstate these developments. Though as long ago as 1848, Robert Graves had
admitted that 'it is hard to expect that a remedy will cure a
disease affecting a certain tissue or tissues, unless it has
some specific effect on such tissues'[73], most of the
profession seems to have only conceded this with respect to a
limited number of diseases and affinitive medicines, such as
mercury, belladonna, strychnine, quinine and hydriodate of
potash.[74] As Dudgeon observed: 'that many diseases are
best treated by medicines which direct experience shows are
capable of acting on the same parts as are affected by the
disease' was 'a rule of practice which the majority only
acknowledge in the case of a few diseases'.[75] Thus although
the work of researchers like Harley and Wood indicated some
acceptance of the homoeopathic idea of using provings of

drugs through a simile principle, as far as most of the profession was concerned, the concession was a limited one. It was a principle which worked only with certain diseases, and it was founded on tissue lesions rather than subjectively reported symptoms. Nevertheless these developments in regular medicine did not go unnoticed by the new school. Once again, homoeopaths felt that their ideas had been justified, and angry that the point was not conceded. Drysdale commented in 1870: 'For the last sixty years the homoeopathic body have proclaimed incessantly the necessity of proving medicines on the healthy body. Lately, we have had this recommended, and grants of money proposed for its accomplishment, but no word of homoeopathy.'[76] And Dudgeon confirmed the trend:

> There is no possibility of denying the fact that the chief medical authorities of the day have for sometime past been teaching that the physiological action of drugs must be studied in order to enable us to ascertain their therapeutic powers, and that medicines must be given which have a specific action on the self same parts as the diseases for which they are remedial – this is the therapeutic principle, similia similibus curantur – in other words, homoeopathy.[77]

In a sense it was – but it was organ and tissue based, materialistic in philosophy and dose, pathological in diagnosis, and a long way from Hahnemann.

Though regular practitioners had more or less succeeded in ensuring the isolation – even, if such an awkward word may be permitted, the sectarianisation – of homoeopaths, they had not, then, refrained from epistemological intercourse with the outcasts. In short, the orthodox profession had consorted with the knave, and the union had resulted in the birth and growth of bastard homoeopathy. There can be no doubt that the practice of medicine was thereby improved. Equally, there can be little doubt that the union was promoted by financial considerations. It was a necessary investment for a healthy future once homoeopathy had exposed the redundancy of heroic therapy.

Economic necessity had thus ensured the healthy development of 'Ringerism', and had created a basis on which a formal union of the two schools could be forged. Hence the talk of reconciliation in the latter part of the century. But this came to nothing. Homoeopaths refused to admit that they had been wrong in the past, or to give up their distinctive title. To do so, they felt, would conceal forever the debt which regular medicine owed to Hahnemann. These, however, were precisely the concessions which the regular school wanted. Given the objective of securing and extending professional power by pressing claims for control over medical knowledge, and over the medical division of labour, regular practitioners could not afford to be flexible about the terms of reconciliation. Thus, despite the similarities in practice, the professional instincts of the orthodox school ensured continued separatism.

It is worth asking whether the rejection of heroic therapy would have occurred without the economic stimulus of homoeopathic competition. Almost certainly, the answer has to be 'yes', with the qualification that it would probably have taken rather longer. Advances in physiology and pathology - encouraged by the expansion of hospitals - would have tended to undercut the rationale for heroic therapy, though it is worth remarking, in turn, that these advances were also partly stimulated by competition from sectarian and quack practitioners. The profession's best defence, after all, was often thought to be the establishment of regular medicine on a sound and superior basis. And once an understanding of the role of bacteria in infectious disease had developed, treatment based on the solidist and neo-humoural pathology of people like Watson would undoubtedly have given way to the various kinds of serum therapy which later became fashionable. But homoeopaths can fairly take the credit for transforming, and indeed, improving medical practice before the scientific revolution in nineteenth century medicine had been fully absorbed by the profession. Moreover, it is salutary to recall that the biomedical model dominant in the twentieth century has not meant the end of iatrogenic damage to patients, or prevented the reintroduction of heroic methods, as in the treatment of cancer: the holistic understanding of illness still remains a powerful critique of reductionist tendencies in medicine.

As economic considerations had wrought changes in regular practice, so had they affected homoeopathy. Pure Hahnemannianism was intellectually taxing and took time to practise. It was easier on the brain and better for the pocket to think pathologically, to inform diagnosis with regular nosology, to use drop doses of mother tinctures or the lower dilutions, and to resort to palliative (regular) methods where all else failed. Moreover, to have ignored the technological, anaesthetic, prophylactic and hygienic advances made in the regular school would have been suicidal. By the end of the century, this meant that homoeopathy had become a very eclectic creature indeed.

These changes began to be signalled in the 1860s. Bayes commented that: 'I deem it my duty, as a catholic member of the medical profession, to prescribe in every case on its own merits, to the best of my judgement, whether that judgement forces me to prescribe specifically, i.e. homoeopathically, or palliatively, i.e. allopathically.'[78] Where the former was the case, medication was 'by no means confined to the use of Infinitesimals ...'[79] and 'Our assertions as to the disease producing power of medicines are based on observation and carefully conducted experiment, not with infinitesimal doses, but with strong and highly poisonous doses'.[80] Provings with attenuated remedies, then, were now apparently regarded with some scepticism. Nevertheless, at this point, there was still a public perception of difference between the two schools: some life assurance companies, at least, were prepared to offer lower premiums to homoeopathic patients, research apparently showing that they lived longer.[81]

But by 1870, Drysdale was admitting that Hahnemann's more extreme views had been 'a perpetual source of embarrassment to nearly all of us'.[82] Moreover, as far as the simile itself was concerned:

> This law applies exclusively to the vital actions of medicines when they correspond directly to the purely vital actions deranged in disease. There is, therefore, a certain field where the principle is not applicable, and there we must and do use exactly the same remedies as other medical men. Among these are all dietetic and chemical means, evacuants, stimulants, etc., which may be needed for removing exciting causes and restoring nutrition ... we are prepared to abandon attempts to treat specifically ailments which a better knowledge of their nature shows not to be within the scope of specific treatment. When the true nature of parasites was discovered, we at once abandoned the treatment of them exclusively as diseases, and began to use vermicide remedies in full dose. Likewise, we were among the very first to discern and adopt the use of carbolic acid and antiseptics.[83]

And if, Drysdale continued, agents could be found in infectious diseases to destroy 'the contagious matter within the body, we are prepared to adopt it with gladness, though it not be homoeopathic'.[84]

Gone, too, was Hahnemannian phenomenology. For Madden, homoeopathic drugs were effective because they had 'an elective affinity for certain organs'.[85] Dyce Brown concurred. The specific remedy worked 'For the obvious reason that we have got a medicine which goes direct to the seat of disease'.[86] Homoeopathy was thus a 'simple mode of stating what Dr Sharp calls organopathy'.[87] And if homoeopathy now had a pathological focus, then its practitioners, as Dudgeon pointed out, could only 'profit by the researches of the physiological school'[88], and 'employ with advantage the improved means of diagnosis afforded by the ophthalmoscope, the laryngoscope, the microscope, the stethoscope, the sphygmograph [for recording movements of the pulse], the thermometer, and chemical analysis'.[89] Moreover, he continued, 'We are at one with our old school colleagues in the

great and important division of medical treatment, hygiene, which includes diet, regimen, and all sanitary conditions.'[90]
These trends were confirmed by Richard Hughes, author of the standard work on homoeopathic practice in the late nineteenth century - A Manual of Therapeutics (1877-8) - which gave a tenchant defence of low dose pathological prescribing supplemented by auxiliary methods.[91] Among these, according to Edmund Capper, were 'poultices, eye lotions, gargles, hypnotics, soothing, antiseptically cleansing or even medicinal injections in gonnorhoea &c., parasiticides, analgesics, hydrotherapy, massage, electricity, and a host of other adjuvants ... [auxiliary methods, or substances used to assist the action of medicines].'[92]
It was vital, Bayes argued, to prevent homoeopathy from becoming a blind and dogmatic sect. Homoeopaths must 'keep themselves fully au courant with all the advances of medical science in other schools.'[93] Apparently, they had: 'I believe we may claim for ourselves that a wider eclecticism is to be found in our ranks than in any other school', he observed.[94]
In one sense, Bayes's injunction was a curious one, for the homoeopathic response to new developments in regular treatment was often that a) homoeopaths invented them first and b) that they only confirmed homoeopathic principles anyway. If nothing else, these claims probably helped to boost morale, despite the unfortunate implication that if advances in medical science only confirmed homoeopathy, then homoeopathy had no need to keep up with medical science.
A paper by Deane Butcher provides a good early example of this strategy. Two claims were made. First, that 'Dr Drysdale's tuberculinum anticipated some ten years ago ... the remedy rediscovered by Koch, and the appropriate vehicle, glycerine'[95] (Tuberculinum was one of the many homoeopathic nosodes, made from products of disease: Koch had identified the tubercule bacillus in 1882, and announced his remedy Tuberculin - which ultimately proved disappointing and even dangerous - in 1890). Second, that 'At all events, I think we may fairly take as proved, that the researches of Pasteur do support the doctrines of our school'.[96] (Deane Butcher had in mind the prophylactic/curative use of vaccines.)
The changes in homoeopathic practice signalled by Bayes, Drysdale, Madden, Sharp, Hughes and others meant that their 'school' became less and less distinguishable from regular medicine. Despite Deane Butcher's arguments, however, the major credit for the scientific breakthroughs were fairly claimed and won by the allopaths. Homoeopaths made use of these developments, just as Ringer et al had made use of homoeopathic research. The war of words between the two schools had not prevented a trade in therapeutic wares: shared exigencies of survival in the medical market place

ensured that it would flourish, and therapeutic convergence was the result.[97]

Significantly, this meant that homoeopathy lost its relative attractiveness as a therapeutic alternative to patients. Concomitantly, the incentive for doctors to declare themselves homoeopaths declined. In 1874, there were under 300 practitioners.[98] Fourteen years later, in 1888, things were much the same, with only 278 doctors listed in The Directory.[99] By 1909, numbers had shrunk to 196.[100]

Clearly, the price of convergence was decline. Homoeopaths were acutely aware that their bright hopes of earlier years had not been fulfilled. Signs of decay were everywhere. The British Journal of Homoeopathy sadly admitted in 1882 that 'We barely maintain our numbers, and seldom make a convert of any note or weight. Our journals contain little original matter; and our hospitals, when we do not lose them altogether, might as well not exist for any good they do to our knowledge of disease and its treatment.'[101] The journal itself survived for only two more years. After 42 volumes – which made it the longest surviving medical quarterly of the century – publication ceased in 1884. Now that homoeopathy had 'leavened the lump' of regular practice, and regular opposition was weakening, 'we are no longer needed', the editor believed, as 'the main object which brought us into existence' had been accomplished.[102] 'Of course', he continued, 'it will be said by our opponents that the cessation of our Journal is a proof of the decadence of homoeopathy, whereas we know that it is merely a sign that homoeopathy has entered another phase of its triumphant career for which a polemical organ is no longer needed.'[103] This was wildly optimistic: the opponents were right – there was no 'triumphant career' in prospect at all.

A task which required urgent action was the condition of the pharmacopoeia itself. When provings included the records of poisonings and overdosage 'the symptoms recorded in the materia medica were generally real effects of the drugs; now, however,' believed John Hayward, many were:

> ... more imaginery than real, and are unreliable and misleading ... to put forward long lists of isolated symptoms in mere schema form and call them materia medica, is downright disgrace to the medical men who supply them, and to the journals that publish them. Such material ought not to be admitted into our journals, much less incorporated into our materia medica.[104]

But it was. The proposal for a new journal of materia medica to improve matters did not get off the ground, with the result that the basic reference texts became increasingly confusing and labyrinthine, and seemed more and more like pharmacopoeial dinosaurs to the new generation of regular physicians.

No one wanted to listen any more. In previous years, homoeopathic education had been undertaken at the Hanover Square and Hahnemann Hospitals and when these had closed, Dr Russell had given occasional lectures at the LHH. In 1875, these had been regularised by the BHS, with Dudgeon giving the first lecture in annual courses of instruction designed for 'the honest inquirer and seeker after truth'.[105] Then, on 15 December 1876, under the stimulus of Dr Bayes, the London School of Homoeopathy was founded. The inaugral address was delivered in 1877. But 'Our School', as Dyce Brown called it, did not fair well. A struggle occurred over the legitimacy of awarding the title 'Licentiate in Homoeopathy' to successful students on the grounds that it would be contrary to the 1858 Medical Act, and would offend the RCP.[106] The BHS voted against the School's proposal. Really, it was a storm in a teacup. From the beginning there were only small audiences. In 1883, only one attender appeared. In 1884, there were none at all.[107]

Homoeopaths themselves seemed hardly more enthusiastic. Meetings of the BHS attracted scant support. As Dyce Brown dismally admitted: 'A small attendance at our only metropolitan homoeopathic society indicates a low state of the barometer of earnest enthusiasm for our cause which cannot but be injurious to our prospects.'[108]

Suggestions were made as to ways of increasing support. Calls for unity and solidarity, for further educational efforts, for more publicity, for more rigorous clinical demonstrations of homoeopathy's success and for legislative reform to ensure a place for homoeopathy on the medical curriculum, were all forthcoming at one time or another. It was to no avail. The truth was that practices were no longer to be gained, and much professional reputation was to be lost, by formal declarations of homoeopathic allegiance. And with what seemed like terminal decline, fissures began to appear among the faithful who remained.

At some point in their evolution, religious movements tend to produce sectarian reaction, with new critics claiming that the worldliness of church leaders has led to the corruption of doctrine, and that a separatist movement is necessary to restore ideological purity. If not pressed too far, this analogy is useful in understanding the split which occurred in the homoeopathic camp. According to the high dilutionist, pure Hahnemannians, the majority of homoeopaths had betrayed the Master's teachings, were practising a false medicine, were motivated by pecuniary interests, and lacked the discipline and moral fibre to acquire the demanding truths of the Organon.[109] These had to be resuscitated if homoeopathy was to save itself from an early grave: the preservation of a shining Truth by a dedicated band of followers

meant that the regular profession would eventually see the
light, and homoeopathy would then assume its rightful place
as undisputed Mistress of the Healing Art. For low dosage
eclectic homoeopaths, however, such views were hopelessly
unscientific, metaphysical, and a recipe for the permanent
closure of doors to professional credibility.
Dudgeon, in 1875, was among the first to express his
disapproval:

... we see some nominal partisans of homoeopathy developing the doctrines of Hahnemann into the most absurd
extravagancies, carrying their dilutions to the most
preposterous height, and gravely publishing so-called
provings of absolutely inert substances, such as loaf-
sugar and skim-milk, or pretending to treat their
patients with dynamized thunderbolts and diluted
moonshine. [110]

John Hayward agreed. [111] In his address to the
Liverpool Homoeopathic Medico-Chirurgical Society (7 October,
1880) he was anxious to make the point that homoeopathy,
properly applied, helped to save medical practice from the
plague of 'fashions in therapeutics' which was always rife in
the regular school. Lacking a law which matched disease and
remedy meant that, at various times, different medicines had
been fashionable among allopaths (antimony, tobacco, gold,
mercury, cinchona and phosphorous all had their day as
'universal specifics'; salicylates had been fashionable for
rheumatism, morphia for pain, bromides for nervous system,
chloral for sleeplessness etc.). Despite the insurance policy
of the simile, however, Hayward regretted that homoeopathy
was also now becoming plagued by 'fashions'. The principal
offenders were the Hahnemannians. Their crimes were
twofold. Firstly, 'Practising exclusively with the very high
and the higher dilutions'. [112] Secondly, and more
importantly, they selected medicines 'from "clinical" or cured
symptoms; that is, symptoms that are not known to have been
produced by the drug, but which have apparently been cured
by it'. [113] For Hayward, this underminded their claim to be
the true bearers of Hahnemannian doctrine, for both practices
directly contravened Hahnemann's instructions regarding
dosage (the thirtieth centesimal potency as the maximum), and
of remedy selection on the basis of provings. As Hayward put
it: 'If we are to prescribe for symptoms a medicine simply
because it has previously cured them, ... it is simple
empirical treatment, and not homoeopathy at all'. [114] Clinical
prescribing, he argued, would destroy homoeopathy if it
became standard practice. At the time, however, he took
comfort from the fact that 'In this country the votaries of
this fashion are few, and those that there are, are either men
whose education has been partial, or men whose organs of

"wonder" ... are so largely developed as to render them easily struck with the extraordinary.'[115] Hayward should not have been so sanguine. The future belonged to the Hahnemannians.

Relations between the two factions soon became strained. The Hahnemannians used terms such as 'mongrels' and 'allopaths in disguise' to describe Hughesian practitioners; in reply, the latter lampooned the alchemical nature of the opposition's remedies, cast grave doubts on the pharmacological integrity of the ultra-high dilutions, and criticised their use of unproved nosodes and their frequent selection of remedies on 'keynotes' (i.e. selecting a leading symptom - such as perspiration of the head - and always prescribing the same remedy, e.g. Calcarea, or calcium phosphate).

Doctors Skinner, Berridge, Lippe, Swan and Bayard attempted to propagate high dilutionist doctrine through a journal called The Organon. It was short-lived, probably due to dissent within the editorial camp. After the first number of volume four, it ceased publication.[116] The British Journal of Homoeopathy was pleased. Words had obviously been exchanged: 'Dr Skinner finds fault with some of the expressions in our letters as "unparliamentary and unbecoming" - we deny the soft impeachment, and think it strange that such an adept in strong language and invective should be so sensitive to a mild remonstrance in his insolent language to others.'[117]

History was repeating itself: the antagonism between the two homoeopathic camps began to assume the qualities of earlier exchanges between the regular and new schools. Though The Organon had been short-lived as a journal, the views which it espoused did not disappear. On the contrary, they gained in support. The struggle was symbolised by the exchanges between Hughes and Clarke. Hughes, editor of The Monthly Homoeopathic Review, staunchly defended low dose pathological prescribing, and only used original provings in his Cyclopaedia of Drug Pathogenesy. [118] Clarke (a one time protégé of Skinner), and editor of the rival Homoeopathic World, took up opposing views in his Dictionary of Practical Materia Medica.[119] Clarke favoured the higher dilutions in practice, used many clinical symptoms in his Dictionary, and listed them - in contrast to Hughes - anatomically when discussing a particular remedy. For Clarke, this made his text more practical to use.

The two first had sharp words on the issue of clinical symptoms at a homoeopathic congress in Paris in 1900. Afterwards, views were exchanged in The Homoeopathic World. Hughes wrote that: 'the symptomatology of your book is second-hand and vitiated; and .. its employment of clinical symptoms favours empiricism rather than homoeopathy - these are the objections which make me unable to welcome the Dictionary'.[120] Clarke's riposte was that 'your approval is the very last thing I either sought or expected. My work was undertaken because you neither would nor could do it'[121] - and he added, for good measure, that the Dictionary was 'my work and not yours. All I claim for my Schemas is that in my opinion the symptoms I have included are genuine indications of the action of the remedy.'[122]

These letters were published in 1902. Unfortunately, Hughes did not live to see his own appear in print, or Clarke's rejoinder. His death signified the closing of an era. By the end of the First World War, the views of people like Clarke were in the ascendancy.

The impetus came from abroad, via the homoeopathy of the American James Tyler Kent. From his commitment to Swedenborgian philosophy, a fervent, religious and metaphysical reinterpretation of Hahnemann appeared. The psoric doctrine was reactivated, vitalism re-emphasised, the importance of psychological and 'spiritual' symptoms in remedy selection underlined, and the use of very high potencies advocated. Margaret Tyler and John Weir studied under Kent, and became keen protagonists of his approach in Britain. Dr Gibson Miller of Glasgow was another key advocate.

That Kentianism became the homoeopathic orthodoxy is hardly explicable in terms of the possession of superior arguments vis-à-vis the technical issues of dose and clinical symptom. The reasons lay much more in the socio-medical environment in which the movement found itself by the end of the century. Practice according to the principles of Hughes was close to that of regular medicine (as he himself admitted, he tried to write 'with an allopath looking over his shoulder'). That being the case, there was little incentive to incur professional disapprobation by an overt declaration of homoeopathic faith. Fewer and fewer doctors were prepared to risk it. Those that did were of a different stamp, attracted by the spiritual and metaphysical elements in Hahnemann's work. Homoeopathy could only survive by re-emphasising its distinctiveness. Kentianism did just that, and there were just sufficient doctors attracted by its fundamentalist mysticism to keep the movement afloat.

Overall, the history of the homoeopathic movement in Britain during the nineteenth century was one of early growth and vitality, with principles vigorously defended, a maturity characterised by progressive compromise with regular practice, and an old age which heralded a hardening of metaphysical arteries. In all, there had probably been no more than 420 declared homoeopaths during the whole period.[123] But their achievements as far as the practice of medicine was concerned had been out of all proportion to their numbers. The movement repeated these successes in America - but there, its growth made its British cousin look very much the poor relation.

NOTES

1. J.Y. Simpson, Homoeopathy: its Tenets and Tendencies, Theoretical, Theological and Therapeutical, 3rd edition (Sutherland and Cox, Edinburgh, 1853), p. 188.
2. Sir John Forbes, Of Nature and Art in the Cure of Disease, 2nd edition (John Churchill, London, 1858).
3. Ibid, pp. 162-3.
4. Appended by the publisher to the second edition of Sir John Forbes, op.cit. Original emphasis. The review is dated July 1857.
5. Ibid. The review is dated November 1857.
6. W. Braithwaite, A Temperate Examination of Homoeopathy No. 1, The Doses and Provings, 2nd edition (Simpkin, Marshall and Co., London, 1859), p. 3.
7. W. Braithwaite, A Temperate Examination of Homoeopathy No. 2, The Principles of Homoeopathy, with a Few Hints on the Nature and Cure of Disease (Simpkin, Marshall and Co., London, 1860), p. 10. Original emphasis.
8. Anon., 'A Homoeopath's View of the Case', The British Medical Journal, vol. I (1866), p. 59.
9. Thomas Laycock, 'Contributions to a New Chapter in the Physiology and Pathology of the Nervous System', The British Medical Journal, vol. I (1868), p. 188. Original italics.
10. Anon., 'Allopathic Ignorance of Homoeopathy', The British Journal of Homoeopathy, vol. XXXIX (1881), p. 196.
11. Sir J. Russell Reynolds (ed.), A System of Medicine, 5 vols. (Macmillan, London, 1866-79).
12. Anon., 'Review of A System of Medicine', The Quarterly Review, vol. 126, no. 252 (1869), pp. 534-58.
13. Ibid., p. 544.
14. Thomas Laycock, op.cit., p. 188.
15. Quoted by R.E. Dudgeon, Hahnemann, The Founder of Scientific Therapeutics (E. Gould and Son, London, 1882), p. 88.
16. Anon., 'Allopathic Ignorance of Homoeopathy', op.cit., pp. 196-7.
17. R.E. Dudgeon, op.cit., pp. 23-4. Original emphasis.
18. D. Guthrie, A History of Medicine (Thomas Nelson and Sons Ltd., London, 1945), p. 220; F.H. Garrison, An Introduction to the History of Medicine, 2nd edition (W.B. Saunders Company, Philadelphia and London, 1917), p. 449; R.H. Major, A History of Medicine, 2 vols. (Blackwell Scientific Publications, Oxford, 1954) vol. II, pp. 697-8; R.H. Shryock, The Development of Modern Medicine (Victor Gollancz, London, 1948), p. 222.
19. S. Ringer, A Handbook of Therapeutics (H.K. Lewis, London, 1869).
20. Quoted by H.L. Coulter, Divided Legacy, A History

THE BIRTH OF BASTARD HOMOEOPATHY

of the Schism in Medical Thought, 3 vols. (Wehawken Book
Company, Washington, 1973-7) vol. III, p. 272.
21. Ibid.
22. Ibid.
23. Charles D.F. Phillips, Materia Medica and Therapeutics, Vegetable Kingdom (J. and A. Churchill, London,
1874); Materia Medica and Therapeutics, Inorganic Substances
(J. and A. Churchill, London, 1882).
24. S. Ringer, op.cit., p. 170.
25. Ibid., p. 177.
26. Ibid., p. 184.
27. Ibid.
28. Ibid., p. 371. Morphine - the chief alkaloid of
opium.
29. Ibid., p. 379.
30. Charles D.F. Phillips, Materia Medica and Therapeutics, Inorganic Substances, op.cit., pp. 73, 384, 414,
473, 486, 505, 672, 721, 775.
31. D. Dyce Brown, Homoeopathy in the Light of
Common Sense and Modern Science (Longmans and Co.,
London, 1875), p. 10. Original emphasis.
32. Charles D.F. Phillips, Materia Medica and Therapeutics, Inorganic Substances, op.cit., pp. 632-3. Original
emphasis.
33. H.L. Coulter, vol. III, op.cit., pp. 263-5. See also
the same author's Homoeopathic Influences in Nineteenth
Century Allopathic Therapeutics: A Historical and
Philosophical Study (American Institute of Homoeopathy,
Washington, DC, 1973).
34. H.L. Coulter, Divided Legacy, vol. III, op.cit.,
pp. 265-71.
35. Quoted in ibid., p. 273.
36. See Dyce Brown's Letter in J.H. Clarke (ed.),
Odium Medicum and Homoeopathy, 'The Times' Correspondence
(The Homoeopathic Publishing Co., London, 1888), p. 39.
Original italics.
37. J.J. Drysdale, Modern Medicine and Homoeopathy
(Henry Turner and Co., London, 1870), p. 13.
38. Ibid., p. 15.
39. D. Dyce Brown, Homoeopathy in the Light of
Common Sense, op.cit., preface.
40. Anon., 'Review of A Handbook of Therapeutics',
The British Journal of Homoeopathy, vol. XXVII (1869), p.
516.
41. Ibid., p. 517.
42. Anon., 'Review of A Handbook of Therapeutics',
The Monthly Homoeopathic Review, vol. XIII (1869), pp.
431-2.
43. Anon., 'Review of Materia Medica and Therapeutics,
Vegetable Kingdom', The Monthly Homoeopathic Review, vol.
XVIII (1874), p. 697. Italics added.

188

44. Ibid.
45. See Dyce Brown's Letter in J.H. Clarke (ed.), op.cit., p. 39.
46. See the anonymous correspondent in J.H. Clarke (ed.), op.cit., p. 76.
47. See R.E. Dudgeon, The Influence of Homoeopathy on General Medicine Since the Death of Hahnemann (Henry Turner and Co., London, 1874), p. 20.
48. Anon., 'Allopathic Ignorance of Homoeopathy', op.cit., pp.200-1. Italics as in original.
49. Ibid., p. 201.
50. T.L. Brunton, A Textbook of Pharmacology, Therapeutics and Materia Medica (Macmillan and Co., London, 1885). A second edition appeared in the same year, and a third in 1887.
51. See Gutteridge's letter in J.H. Clarke (ed.), op.cit., p. 78. Italics added.
52. R.E. Dudgeon, The Influence of Homoeopathy. op.cit., pp. 20-1.
53. Ibid., p. 25.
54. Ibid., p. 32.
55. Ibid.
56. Ibid., p. 33.
57. See William Bayes, 'Introductory Lecture', Annals and Transactions of the British Homoeopathic Society and the London Homoeopathic Hospital, vol. VIII (1876), p. 459.
58. See Alfred C. Pope, 'Presidential Address', Annals and Transactions of the British Homoeopathic Society and the London Homoeopathic Hospital, vol. X (1885), p. 62.
59. S.M. Bradley 'The Homoeopathic Schism', The British Medical Journal, vol. I (1877), p. 731.
60. Alfred Pullar, 'Consultations with Homoeopaths', The British Medical Journal, vol. I (1881), p. 907. The text to which Pullar refers is probably R. Hughes, A Manual of Therapeutics, 2nd edition, 2 parts (Leath and Ross, London, 1877-8).
61. Anon., 'Editorial Comment' The British Medical Journal, vol. II (1866), p. 45.
62. Ibid.
63. Ibid.
64. J. Harley, The Old Vegetable Neurotics: Hemlock, Opium, Belladonna and Henbane (Macmillan and Co., London, 1869), preface.
65. See D. Dyce Brown, Homoeopathy in the Light of Common Sense, op.cit.
66. Quoted by D. Dyce Brown, The Progress of Medicine (Henry Turner and Co., London, 1875), p.12.
67. Horatio C. Wood Jnr, A Treatise on Therapeutics, Comprising Materia Medica and Toxicology (J.B. Lippincott, Philadelphia, 1874).
68. Quoted by William Bayes, op.cit., p. 460.

69. See H.L. Coulter, Divided Legacy, vol. III, op.cit., p. 275.

70. See the editor's remarks in W. Ameke, History of Homoeopathy: its Origins; its Conflicts. Translated by Alfred Drysdale, and edited by R.E. Dudgeon. (E. Gould and Son, London, 1885), p. 426. Coulter's bibliography (Divided Legacy, vol. III, op.cit) cites W. Murrell's Nitroglycerine as a Remedy for Angina Pectoris (Davies, Detroit, 1882). Presumably this is the work Dudgeon was referring to at p. 426 of W. Ameke, op.cit.

71. A. Burness and F.J. Mavor, The Specific Action of Drugs on the Healthy System: An Index to Their Therapeutic Value as Deduced from Experiments on Man and Animals (Baillière, Tindall and Cox, London, 1874).

72. See William Bayes, op.cit., p. 461.

73. Quoted by D. Dyce Brown, Homoeopathy in the Light of Common Sense, op.cit., pp. 28-9.

74. See the quote from Graves, ibid.

75. R.E. Dudgeon, The Influence of Homoeopathy, op.cit., p. 24.

76. J.J. Drysdale, op.cit., p. 15.

77. R.E. Dudgeon, The Influence of Homoeopathy, op.cit., p. 19. Notice that Dudgeon uses the stronger form here - 'curantur' - which suggests that 'likes are cured by likes'. See also, however, note 21 to Chapter One.

78. W. Bayes, "Two Sides to a Question", A Few Observations on Mr Braithwaite's Temperate Examination of Homoeopathy (Turner and Co., Manchester, 1860), p. 4. Original emphasis.

79. Ibid., pp. 12-13. Original emphasis.

80. Ibid., p. 35.

81. Anon., 'Editorial Comment', The British Medical Journal, vol. I (1865), p. 543.

82. J.J. Drysdale, op.cit., p. 12.

83. Ibid., pp. 9-10.

84. Ibid., p. 10.

85. H.R. Madden, On the Relation of Therapeutics to Modern Physiology (H. Turner and Co., London, 1871), p. 45.

86. D. Dyce Brown, Homoeopathy in the Light of Common Sense, op.cit., p. 9.

87. Ibid., p. 8. Original emphasis.

88. R.E. Dudgeon, The Influence of Homoeopathy, op.cit., p. 28.

89. Ibid.

90. Ibid. Original emphasis.

91. See note 60.

92. Edmund Capper, 'Presidential Address', Journal of the British Homoeopathic Society, New Series, vol. III (1895), p. 18.

93. William Bayes, 'Introductory Lecture', Annals and

THE BIRTH OF BASTARD HOMOEOPATHY

Transactions of the British Homoeopathic Society and of the London Homoeopathic Hospital, vol. VIII (1876), p. 463. Original italics.
94. Ibid.
95. W. Deane Butcher, 'The Recent Discoveries of Koch and Pasteur as Illustrating the Law of Similars', Annals and Transactions of the British Homoeopathic Society and of the London Homoeopathic Hospital, vol. 12 (no date), p. 296. Original italics.
96. Ibid.
97. The same point is also argued by W.G. Rothstein, 'Professionalization and Employer Demands' in P. Halmos (ed.), Professionalization and Social Change, The Sociological Review Monograph, No. 20. (University of Keele, Keele, 1973), pp. 159-78.
98. R.E. Dudgeon, The Influence of Homoeopathy, op.cit., p. 32.
99. See J.H. Clarke (ed.), op.cit., p. 52. At the time, there were about 22,500 regular practitioners - see ibid., p. 102.
100. J. Roberson Day (ed.), International Homoeopathic Medical Directory (Homoeopathic Publishing Co., London, 1909), pp. 11-48.
101. Anon., 'The Transactions of the International Homoeopathic Convention of 1881', The British Journal of Homoeopathy, vol. XL (1882), p. 33.
102. Anon., 'Vale!', The British Journal of Homoeopathy, vol. XLII (1884), p. 322.
103. Ibid., p. 325. Original italics.
104. John Hayward, 'Presidential Address', Journal of the British Homoeopathic Society, New Series, vol. IV (1896), p. 72. Original italics.
105. R.E. Dudgeon, 'Lecture on the History of Homoeopathy', Annals and Transactions of the British Homoeopathic Society and the London Homoeopathic Hospital, vol. VII (1876), p. 312.
106. R.E. Dudgeon, 'The Diploma of "L.H." of the London School of Homoeopathy - A Symposium', The British Journal of Homoeopathy, vol. XL (1882), pp. 156-66. (For other contributions, see pp. 166-92).
107. D. Dyce Brown, 'Presidential Address'. Annals and Transactions of the British Homoeopathic Society and of the London Homoeopathic Hospital, vol. X (1885), p. 520.
108. Ibid., pp. 517-18.
109. See, for example, Alfred C. Pope 'Presidential Address', Annals and Transactions of the British Homoeopathic Society and of the London Homoeopathic Hospital, vol. X (1885), pp. 37-64, esp. p. 59.
110. R.E. Dudgeon, 'Lecture on the History of Homoeopathy', op.cit., p. 317.
111. John W. Hayward, 'Presidential Address', The

British Journal of Homoeopathy, vol. XXXIX (1881), pp. 26-37.
112. Ibid., p. 30. Original emphasis.
113. Ibid., p. 31.
114. Ibid., p. 34.
115. Ibid., p. 31.
116. See Anon., 'The Ethics of Mongrelism', The British Journal of Homoeopathy, vol. XXXIX (1881), pp. 270-6.
117. Ibid., p. 276.
118. R. Hughes et al. (eds), A Cyclopaedia of Drug Pathogenesy, 4 vols. (J.E. Adlard, London, 1885-91).
119. J.H. Clarke, A Dictionary of Practical Materia Medica, 2 vols. (Homoeopathic Publishing Co., London, 1900).
120. R. Hughes and J.H. Clarke, 'Correspondence - The Dictionary of Practical Materia Medica, Some Criticisms and a Reply', The Homoeopathic World, vol. XXXVII (1902), p. 164. Original italics.
121. Ibid., p. 166.
122. Ibid., p. 168. Original emphasis.
123. See Arthur C. Clifton, 'Presidential Address', Journal of the British Homoeopathic Society, New Series, vol. VII (1899), p. 3.

Chapter Twelve

FROM THE OLD WORLD TO THE NEW - HOMOEOPATHY
IN AMERICA

From its German origins, homoeopathy spread rapidly to other
countries. By 1881, as International Homoeopathic Conventions
make clear, it had won converts not only in Britain and
Ireland, but also in Austria, France, Belgium, Spain,
Portugal, Italy, Holland, Sweden, Norway, Denmark and
Switzerland. European migration had also ensured its spread
to the West Indies, South Africa, Australia, Canada, South
America, India, Mexico and the United States.[1] Nowhere
could delegates to these international meetings here more
glowing reports than those coming from America. In 1881,
there were eleven colleges producing 400 graduates per
year;[2] by 1898, America had 66 general and 74 special
homoeopathic hospitals, and the number of medical schools had
increased to twenty;[3] and by 1900, homoeopathic practitioners numbered around 10,000.[4] But from this peak the
movement, as in Britain, went into decline. Comparative
analysis shows that the reasons, in part, were the same. It
also helps to show that occupational interests and economic
exigency are key variables in understanding the reaction of
the profession to therapeutic competition. On both sides of
the Atlantic, strategies of sectarianisation helped to maintain
control over the division of medical labour, and therapeutic
reform blunted the edge of competition and sustained the
economic viability of practice.

It would be valuable to broaden this comparative analysis
through consideration of homoeopathy's career in countries
other than those of Britain and the United States. Unfortunately, this enterprise is limited by lack of secondary material
- especially in English translation - and by (traditional
reasons, these) constraints on space and time. It cannot be
undertaken here. Three excellent studies exist, however, as
far as America is concerned. Coulter's definitive work has
already been referred to in previous chapters. To this may
be added Rothstein's American Physicians in the Nineteenth
Century,[5] and Kaufman's Homoeopathy in America.[6]

Coulter's work is the most detailed of the studies, but also the most partisan; Rothstein's approach is explicitly institutional and sociological, and that of Kaufman, more straightforwardly historical. Collectively, these studies provide a comprehensive survey - to which it would be difficult to add anything really new - and the interested reader is referred to them for a more detailed discussion of the area than is proposed here. Instead, here is an overview, with this secondary material providing the basis for a comparative case study.

As in Britain, the struggle of American physicians against irregulars was waged through the organisations which the profession had developed to educate, control and represent its members. By the middle of the century, the number of licensed practitioners had expanded dramatically, and educational efforts had succeeded in standardising a routine of heroic practice. The beneficiaries of the public rebellion which followed were the various medical sects, among which the homoeopaths became the largest group. Like their British counterparts, the new school in America soon found itself ostracised by the regular profession.

Unravelling these developments must begin with an overview of the professional structures which had helped to institutionalise heroic practice, and through which the majority of practitioners strove to suppress their therapeutic rivals. Medical societies were to be an important battleground. By the 1820s, the recognition of shared economic interests had made medical societies the most significant institution in the professional lives of American practitioners. For the individual physician, membership was a mark of distinction, a source of prestige, and a passport to valued appointments, consultations and clients; for members collectively, societies performed the important function of regulating potentially destructive competition. The principal mechanism for achieving this objective was the legally conferred right of societies to license practitioners. This provided societies both with a source of income and - theoretically, at least - a way of controlling the supply of physicians through the examination of candidates by licensing boards.

Yet the effectiveness of action here was compromised in two respects. Firstly, boards had a financial incentive to pass candidates, especially in view of the fact that apprentices failed by one society could seek certification in less particular states. Inevitably, this helped to weaken examination rigour and educational standards. Secondly, the legislation which established medical societies and gave them licensing powers did little to protect physicians from the competitive inroads of those lacking formal qualifications. The strong anti-trust sentiments of most state legislatures was not sympathetic to claims for medical monopoly, and fines for unlicensed practice, even if available, were generally too small to act as

HOMOEOPATHY IN AMERICA

an effective deterrent. Even where they could be imposed, juries were reluctant to exact them. The only real privilege granted to licensed practitioners was the right to sue for the recovery of fees in the courts.

Societies were not much more successful in regulating the conduct of their own members than in securing doctors' protection from unlicensed competition. Securing adherence to codes of ethics - on consultation procedures, for example - was limited by a lack of effective sanctions, and exclusive membership policies, while raising the prestige of members, tended to undermine their practical commitment to recommended scales of charge for different forms of treatment. Non-members, after all, had no reason to abide by a society's rates, which strengthened the propensity of members to undercut each other. Ethical proscriptions on the use or sale of secret nostrums were also liable to be ignored. Manufacturers of patent remedies were not obliged to detail ingredients, and though doctors were therefore enjoined to refrain from their use, their cheapness and ready availability made them an attractive therapeutic option.

Despite these limitations, the economic benefits of membership were still sufficient to motivate physicians to found and join medical societies. This is clear from the proliferation of these institutions in the first half of the century. Not least among the rewards was that appointment to the licensing board of a society provided a valuable advert for a physician's practice and competence, and made the incumbent an especially attractive proposition as far as potential apprentices were concerned.

As in Britain, until medical schools assumed the major role in education, most physicians were educated by a system of apprenticeship. Regulated by the medical societies, the agreement between preceptor and apprentice would usually specify a period of some three years of training, with an annual fee payable for instruction received. This would vary according to the reputation of the physician concerned, but 100 dollars per year would not have been unusual. In return, the preceptor provided books and equipment, and undertook to provide the apprentice with a certificate stating that the period of training had been satisfactorily completed. Certification, however, was of little benefit to the student by itself, since a certificate would mean little to any patient or doctor who was personally ignorant of the preceptor who endorsed it. Licensing was thus popular with apprentices: a seal of approval from a society's board of censors gave a more public testimony of competence.

The two major elements of an apprentice's education were known as 'reading medicine with a doctor' and 'riding with the doctor'. In the first, as the form of words suggests, the student was supposed to study basic texts in anatomy, physiology, botany, materia medica etc., and to supplement this with general nursing, secretarial and pharmaceutical duties. 'Riding with the doctor', on the other hand, constituted the clinical element of the educational process. Here, the student would assist the preceptor during house calls and in the surgery.

Apprenticeship was popular with both doctors and students. For the former, it provided additional income and a supply of unpaid labour. For the latter, it was reasonably cheap, local and not particularly demanding. Standards of education, however, varied in direct proportion to the conscientiousness and ability of both apprentices and preceptors. Despite the supposed restraint imposed by licensing, the quality of the end product was not surprisingly variable. As medical knowledge increased in the latter half of the century, apprenticeship ceased to be a viable method of imparting an adequate education.

Ironically, it was the prospect of financial rewards from the educational process which led some physicians to develop new institutions which not only hastened the demise of the apprenticeship system, but also weakened the control of medical societies over licensing. These institutions were the medical schools. Their origin lay in the realisation by physicians that 'reading with the doctor' could be more efficiently achieved with classroom rather than practice based students. It was easy enough for a small group of physicians to obtain and equip premises - only rudimentary resources were required - and to obtain legislative approval for the award of MD degrees. Schools were thus cheap to establish and inexpensive to operate. More importantly, they were very profitable. Staff were paid from student fees, and income from teaching thus increased in direct proportion to enrolment.

Schools were not meant to eclipse the role of the preceptor entirely. Indeed, 28 months of the three years training prior to graduation were to be spent receiving clinical education while 'riding with the doctor'. The eight months at medical school concentrated instead on theoretical instruction. Here lectures, in which the medical authority of eighteenth century figures such as Cullen, Boerhaave and Benjamin Rush (1745-1813) were invoked, reigned supreme. Opportunities for practical work were severely limited.

The ease with which schools could be established, and their financial attractiveness to physicians, had a number of important effects. First, the number of schools grew rapidly - from four in 1800 to 47 in 1860.[7] Second, schools began to compete with each other for students, depressing educational standards and steadily weakening the apprenticeship system. Of the thirty schools in 1849, nineteen required evidence of certification only, with no time period specified, and seven enrolled students without apprenticeship warrants at all.[8] Third, the number of practising physicians began to climb steeply, increasing competition within the profession. Fourth, school curriculums and new textbooks ensured the institutionalisation of a routine of heroic practice among graduating students. Fifth, a new division began to emerge within the profession which mirrored the development of the consultant-general practitioner split in Britain. School physicians became wealthy, prestigious and powerful. When schools began to offer clinical training in the latter half of the century, and opened clinics, dispensaries, and advertised for patients, the resentment of ordinary practitioners sharpened still further.

Finally, since state legislatures regarded an MD degree as equivalent to a licence from a board of censors, the control of medical societies over the educational standards of the profession was progressively eroded. Soon, the apprentice trained physician was a thing of the past, and those in the profession who had qualified in this way found their status reduced. Societies lost income, prestige, and an important rationale for their existence. Not surprisingly, many local societies began to fold by the 1840s. Importantly, too, one of the unintended consequences of the new prominence of schools in medical education was to create an opportunity for empirics to campaign for the repeal of licensing laws. Once medical societies had lost control over licensing, there was little incentive to resist pressure for the suspension of restrictive legislation. By the Civil War most states had abandoned it.

It was obvious that the medical societies and schools would come into conflict. Societies wanted to protect the licensing system, and to control the number of physicians entering the profession. Schools, on the other hand, regarded their educational efforts, symbolised by an MD degree, as superior, and wanted to maximise the number of graduates. In short, the societies represented the immediate economic interests of the ordinary practitioner, while schools were the platform from which the claims of the new elite within the profession were articulated.

This interest clash helped to prompt the formation of the American Medical Association (AMA). Its immediate objective was to raise educational standards. Unfortunately, the AMA only succeeded in making a series of unrealistic proposals. The schools saw that, if followed to the letter, the AMA's recommendations would drastically reduce their intake. It was not hard to see the proposals as a thinly disguised attack on the schools in the pursuit of interests close to the heart of medical societies. Not surprisingly, the AMA's recommendations were ignored. Thereafter, the medical schools tended to regard the AMA, and its stated objective of raising standards, with some suspicion, and the two major interest groups in the profession remained more or less estranged for the rest of the century.

But if interests were in conflict, there was at least an accord as far as the actual business of practising medicine was concerned. American doctors were no less fond of vigorous treatment than their European colleagues. If anything, under the admonition of adepts such as Rush, the routine of violent depletion was pushed even further, with remedies of heroic effect permutated from an already familiar materia medica. Given the effects of poor housing, water pollution and malnutrition on general health, the endemic problems of malaria, dysentry, diarrhoea, pneumonia, influenza and TB, and the epidemic ravages of cholera, yellow fever, diphtheria, typhoid and smallpox, the profession found no reason to be idle, or to skimp on venesection or mercurialisation.

The result was a medical version of religious inquisition, with disease as the enemy, the public as its bearer, and mortification of the flesh as the price of inner cleanliness. A crucial difference remained, however. In this instance, the public could protest without risking damnation. Increasingly it did so. The first real beneficiary of this reaction was a sect whose origin lay in the indigenous tradition of botanical medicine - the Thomsonian movement. Some discussion of this sect, and its successor, the eclectics, is indispensable in appreciating the sectarian context and conflicts in which homoeopathy itself was to be enmeshed.

Samuel Thomson (1769-1843) had been a disaffected farmer with an interest in herbal remedies and a distaste, born of personal experience, for the effects of regular medicine. Around 1805, he became an itinerant practitioner. By the 1820s, he had become a successful entrepreneur and lay healer.

His system, which he had patented in 1813, is best described in his book New Guide to Health.[9] First published in 1822, the text soon became highly popular as a guide to domestic practice, and eventually ran to thirteen editions. Essentially, the principles of Thomsonism were little different to those of regular medicine - clear the system first, and then restore normal functioning with tonics. In practice, however, these principles produced a less savage system. In particular, bleeding and mercurialisation were avoided. Lobelia (Lobelia inflata) - an emetic - helped to clear the system; steam baths promoted sweating; cayenne pepper (Capsicum frutescens) warmed the body; and teas and herbal tonics, followed by wine and brandy laced with botanical remedies, helped to restore digestion and strengthen the stomach.

Thomson's basic impulse was populist and individualist. He wanted purchasers of his book to rely on themselves (and each other) for treatment, rather than the medical profession. To this end, Thomson gave advice on how his various remedies could be prepared from local herbs. Alternatively, crude ingredients could be bought from Thomson's agents, or prepared remedies obtained at the counter of local stores. Self-help and mutual aid was further promoted through the establishment of local societies. Purchasers of the New Guide automatically became members of the Friendly Botanical Society (FBS), and Thomson's agents (he had 167 by 1833)[10] helped to establish many local groups committed to the ideal of co-operation and assistance in times of sickness.

Despite the political sentiments of its founder, professionalising tendencies soon emerged within the movement. At first, full-time botanical (or root and herb doctors, as they were often known) grafted Thomson's system on to their existing methods, despite the patent protection, and pushed it to heroic levels. Soon, full-time Thomsonians began to open infirmaries and to establish medical societies and journals of their own. Conventions of the FBS began to move in the same direction, urging the establishment of hospitals and the foundation of medical schools. And though many Thomsonians urged the repeal of licensing laws - and had considerable success in achieving this objective - others were more hesitant, merely arguing for their amendment to allow those who had been certified as competent practitioners of the system to work on the same basis as regular physicians.

Eventually, Thomsonism began to fragment on this issue. Professional aspirations could only be realised through the establishment of schools empowered to grant degrees. Alva Curtis, one of Thomson's colleagues, was anxious to move in this direction. Thomson dissented, and the two parted company. Curtis established a Botanico-Medical School and Infirmary in Ohio, which received a charter to grant degrees in 1839, while Thomson attempted to rally a separatist movement. But the process of fragmentation continued. After 1838, national conventions of the FBS ceased. Thomson's wing collapsed altogether, and though a number of botanical medical schools were founded after 1845, few of these survived beyond the Civil War. Alva Curtis, however, managed to hold his particular movement together. It survived into the twentieth century as 'physio-medicalism', but the real legacy of the fragmented botanical movement initiated by Thomson was the growth, after the Civil War, of the eclectic sect.

The term 'eclectic' was coined by Wooster Beach (1794-1868). Unlike Thomson, Beach was a medical graduate. He too, however, expressed distaste for heroic practice, and turned to a variety of sources - including Thomsonism itself and botanical medicine - for fresh inspiration. The result was not so much a new therapeutic system as a hybrid of those already established.

Beach established two schools in 1827 and 1830: neither lasted long. The next venture was more successful. After the second school had closed in 1840, some of the staff moved to Cincinatti, and with local support succeeded in obtaining a charter for a new institution. Thus was founded, in 1845, the Eclectic Medical Institute (EMI). It remained open until 1939. The early history of the Institute was, to say the least, stormy. In 1850, Joseph R. Buchanan became dean. His leadership was idiosyncratic, unpredictable, and prone to ventures other than those of profitable pedagogy. Beach and others resigned, but further (and not merely verbal) disputes followed. The end result was the formation of a rival school by Buchanan in 1856. His attachment to this new institution did not last long, and the two schools merged in 1859.

These organisational upheavals were matched by an enduring therapeutic problem. The regular sect had coalesced around one medical paradigm, and by now the homoeopaths had grouped around another. Could eclecticism follow suit, and develop a coherent therapeutic approach which distinguished it from its two main rivals? The very name of the sect highlighted the dilemma involved. Little headway was made in this area prior to the Civil War. Resinoids and alkaloids of botanical drugs, developed by John M. King at the EMI, were briefly popular. But eclectics pushed these to heroic levels, reincarnated the problems of regular practice, and lost public sympathy. By the late 1850s, the sect was at a low ebb. In 1857, the National Eclectic Medical Association (NEMA) ceased to operate, and with the exception of schools in Philadelphia and Cincinnati, the movement's educational efforts collapsed, and the sect began to fragment.

From this trough, things began to improve. The impetus came from John M. Scudder (1829-94), dean of the EMI. His new system of therapeutics, developed around 1869, went some way towards solving the problem of medical distinctiveness. The heroic use of remedies was abandoned, and replaced by a system of 'specific medication'.

Eclectic practice came to be organised around four main principles: the direct action of medicines (selected for their ability to affect particular symptoms); the small dose (of, for example, botanical tinctures diluted with water); the palatability of remedies; and the choice of drugs from a wide ranging materia medica. But not all eclectics were content with these guidelines, and concrete practice varied considerably. Nevertheless, despite (or perhaps because of) its homoeopathic leanings, the reform initiated by Scudder was sufficient to bring new success. The movement experienced considerable popularity from the 1870s until the end of the century. By 1900, there were 32 state societies, the NEMA had been revived, and practising eclectics numbered around 4,000 (compared to 10,000 homoeopaths and 110,000 regulars).[11] Yet, in 1892, only ten of the 32 eclectic medical schools which had been founded were still operating - and most of these were mediocre.[12] This proved a decisive

weakness. The reform of medical education under the impetus
of Flexner and the AMA extinguished low standard institutions; the need to keep abreast of, and employ, the
innovations of the scientific revolution eroded sectarian distinctions and increased the length and cost of medical
education; and licensing requirements which demanded
concentration on the core of knowledge claimed by the regular
sect, all contributed to the decline of the eclectics. Like
homoeopathy, the strength of the movement at the turn of the
century was more apparent than real. Precipitous decline was
the future for both.

The response of the regular school to the challenges of
Thomsonism and the eclectics mirrored the tactics used
against homoeopaths. Essentially, these consisted in strategies
of exclusion and an interest in sectarian remedies to complement the momentum of therapeutic reform. Though attempts
had been made to use licensing laws against lay practitioners
of Thomson's system, these had been of little avail. Further
action was eventually made superfluous as the movement
fragmented under internal dissension. Nevertheless, the early
success of Thomsonism had focused attention on public
distaste for regular therapeutics, and increasing interest was
shown in less aggressive methods, and in the use of botanical
remedies. Similar partiality emerged for the resinoid and
alkaloid medicines developed by the eclectics. The medical
background of early eclectics, however, together with the
greater organisational strength and popularity of their movement, especially after the Civil War, elicited the more forceful
tactic of professional ostracism. Denied access to conventional
medical life, eclectics developed separate schools, journals,
societies and pharmacies. Homoeopaths were forced to do the
same.

The system was brought to America by Hans Gram, a
German physician, around 1825. He was soon followed, in the
1830s, by an ex-student of Hahnemann's, Constantine Hering,
who became the most important early pioneer and advocate of
the new approach. Some twenty years later, homoeopathy had
won a substantial following among doctors and patients.

The reasons are not hard to find. Firstly, homoeopathy
benefited from an increasingly hostile public reaction to heroic
methods. In this, its origins as a popular force resembled
those of Thomsonism - and, indeed, of other more or less
short-lived sects, such as Sylvester Graham's Popular Health
Movement of the 1830s, and 'chronothermalism' a decade later.
Secondly, and unlike the Thomsonians and later eclectics,
whose support was rooted among rural lower income groups,
homoeopathy appealed to privileged urban strata in the cities.
This was not only because homoeopaths were generally well-
educated and culturally polished physicians - no status
conscious city dweller would dream of employing 'crude
country empirics', after all - but also because the system had

the social cachet of patronage by the aristocracy and social elites of Europe.

In an overcrowded urban profession, as in Britain, the attractiveness of securing a large and financially rewarding practice by adopting - or incorporating - homoeopathic methods was considerable. Coupled with a creeping scepticism among certain physicians about the value of heroic methods, the rate of conversion among regular practitioners began to rise. Of the eighteen doctors, for example, who founded the elite New York Medical and Surgical Society in 1836, four had adopted the system by 1841.[13] Other parallels with the British case soon emerged.

Like Quin, the early homoeopaths in America - such as the New York doctors, and those who formed the Massachusetts Homoeopathic Fraternity in 1839 - sought to distance themselves from more or less unscrupulous and opportunist lay practitioners. And like Henderson at Edinburgh, they saw themselves as physicians who combined homoeopathy with the best of regular knowledge and practice, rather than as pure Hahnemannians. At the time, there were few fundamentalists; even Hering wished to distance himself from some of Hahnemann's more extreme views.

At first, regular reaction to Hahnemann's system was characterised by scepticism, slightly tempered with notes of interest. This was rapidly followed by incredulity, and then outright hostility. The 'fools or knaves' argument soon repeated itself. Nevertheless, the American profession was pinned on the horns of the same dilemma that Henderson and Forbes had identified for British practitioners. If it was argued that patient recovery, which could not be denied, was not due to the effects of the homoeopathic dose, but to the effects of nature, then the rationale for heroic medicine was removed. Jacob Bigelow, a prominent regular physician, was one of the first to draw these conclusions to the attention of the American profession.[14] Unwillingly, the lesson was absorbed. While the theoretical dismemberment of homoe-opathy, and the character assassination of its practitioners, continued to be favourite allopathic pastimes, therapeutic competition encouraged less aggressive methods. And thera-peutic reform was accompanied by the introduction of homoeo-pathic remedies into regular practice, and by interest in homoeopathic methods of identifying the sphere of drug action.

Further elaboration of these processes would tread ground which has already been covered in Chapter Eleven, and to do so again would only labour a comparison for which substantial evidence already exists. Coulter's Homoeopathic Influences in Nineteenth-Century Allopathic Therapeutics,[15] as well as Chapter Four of the third volume of Divided Legacy, contain the finer detail which the reader may wish to consult.[16]

On both sides of the Atlantic, the homoeopaths were seen as internal renegades who, if not isolated and ostracised from the profession, would shake its foundations to destruction. The Philadelphia Medical Society rapidly took action which others were soon to follow. In 1843, homoeopathic members were expelled. Attempts were also made to use the courts against members of the new school. Public sympathy, however, usually rendered these tactics unworkable.

The AMA initiated action on the consultation and educational fronts. The 1847 code of ethics argued that:

A regular medical education furnishes the only presumptive evidence of professional abilities and acquirements, and ought to be the only acknowledged right of an individual to the exercise and honours of his profession ... no one can be considered as a regular practitioner or a fit associate in consultation whose practice is based on an exclusive dogma, to the rejection of the accumulated experience of the profession, and of the aids actually furnished by anatomy, physiology, pathology, and organic chemistry.[17]

In the same year the AMA resolved to advise medical schools not to accept the certificate of any preceptors who practised an irregular system, irrespective of their possession of formal qualifications. Two years later, medical societies were advised to admit only graduates from regular schools. Both resolutions followed from the basic stance taken towards irregular practitioners in the code of ethics. In 1855, adoption of the code became a condition of membership of the AMA, and institutions which flouted it were liable to expulsion.

The response of homoeopaths to these measures was to form their own organisations. Strictly, it should not have been necessary, as a close reading of the code, and a fair examination of the actual practice of homoeopaths, would have exempted them from any penalties. After all, most did not deny the importance of the basic medical sciences, nor confine their treatment to Hahnemannian remedies. But this made them knaves in the eyes of regulars, and as sanctions began to bite, the stimulus to form rival societies, journals, hospitals etc. was enhanced. Since all these institutions were described as 'homoeopathic', the charge that their members should be debarred from the regular profession on the grounds that they were practising an exclusive dogma could be made to stick. But 'exclusivism' was not the origin of ostracism. Rather, ostracism was the cause of exclusivism.

The exclusion of homoeopaths was an obvious attempt by the regular profession to protect its right to determine legitimate medical labour. But it did not prevent the new school from flourishing. Probably a crucial difference in explaining homoeopathy's greater numerical and institutional strength in America compared to Britain was the fact that the movement was successful in establishing its own medical schools with state charters to grant degrees. Here, the wealth and influence of homoeopathy's supporters, and powerful anti-monopolist feelings, were important. These factors were also present in the United Kingdom - but here, the 1858 Medical Act probably limited their effect. Clause 23 prevented any qualifying body from imposing:

> ... upon any Candidate offering himself for Examination an Obligation to adopt or refrain from adopting the Practice of any particular Theory of Medicine or Surgery as a Test or Condition of admitting him to Examination or of granting a Certificate ...[18]

Homoeopaths had originally welcomed this measure as clear security from medical victimisation. But the other side of the coin was a restriction of educational efforts on their own behalf. After all, graduates from any British homoeopathic medical school would have had to prove proficiency in homoeopathic therapeutics and theory as a condition of receiving a certificate, and it therefore seemed that such schools would run foul of the law (not to mention the RCP). This, at least, was the view of Dudgeon.[19] Thus no medical schools equivalent to those established by American homoeopaths were inaugurated in Britain, and the movement had to depend for its support not on its own graduates, but on allopathic conversion. Consequently, its numerical strength was relatively small.

The economic effects of sectarian competition, especially from homoeopaths, and the theoretical implications of this for regular practice (reflected in the writings of figures such as Jacob Bigelow and Oliver Wendell Holmes) combined to wean orthodox physicians away from heroic therapy. This process gathered pace in the second half of the century. For a while, as in Britain, some physicians advocated expectancy. For most, however, action was an imperative of practice. New drugs were sought, and the homoeopathic materia medica, as indicated, came under scrutiny. Aconite and Veratrum viride became popular antipyretics. The use of some existing drugs in this category was extended - like quinine - and new ones developed, like the coal tar derivatives antipyrine and antefibrin, and later still acetylsalicylic acid (aspirin). Among analgesics, cocaine (Erythroxylum coca) became an alternative to morphine; chloral hydrate partly replaced opium as an hypnotic; and alcohol began to be used extensively as a tonic.

Meanwhile, the institutional apparatus of homoeopathy had been steadily developing. In 1844, the American Institute of Homoeopathy had been formed, partly to disseminate wider knowledge of the materia medica among its members, and partly to create institutional distance between lay and medically qualified practitioners. The consultation ban - strengthened by the propensity of regular physicians to expose colleagues who had wittingly or otherwise broken it - and the exlusionary policies of allopathic societies, encouraged the proliferation of rival homoeopathic organisations. Refusal of orthodox practitioners - such as those at Cook County Hospital - to contemplate working with homoeopaths, and the educational restrictions of the AMA, resulted in the formation of homoeopathic infirmaries, journals, and medical schools. With the continued financial support and sympathy of the urban wealthy, all this meant that by the end of the century American homoeopathy could boast that its doctors represented over eight per cent of all practitioners (the figures were much higher in urban states), organised into nine national societies, 33 state societies, 85 local societies, and 39 other local organisations.[20] Professional communication was taking place through 31 journals; teaching through 22 colleges; and treatment through 66 general and 74 speciality hospitals, and 57 dispensaries.[21]

The regular profession had not viewed these developments with indifference. Of the many individual struggles between the two schools, one perhaps stands out above all the others as representing the lines of battle drawn up by the antagonists.

In 1855, supporters of homoeopathy in Michigan were successful in winning the approval of the legislature for the establishment of a homoeopathic professorship at the state university. The AMA responded by threatening to withhold recognition of any of the university's graduates should the professorship be instituted. In practice, this would have meant that those graduating with a Michigan degree could not expect their right of consultation to be honoured, nor find themselves welcomed by medical societies. Understandably, the regents of the university were hesitant to proceed in the direction indicated by the state.

The legislature, however, was not prepared to let the matter rest. In 1867 and 1873, additional resolutions were passed, calling on the regents to act. The matter was referred to the state's supreme court - but to little avail. The court was unsure that it could legitimately force the university to comply.

In 1875, the state acted again. It made provision for the establishment of a new hospital for the university medical school on condition that two homoeopathic professors were appointed. In turn, the regents decided that medical diplomas would no longer be signed by medical staff, but by the university's president and secretary. This meant that regular staff would no longer find themselves in the invidious position of approving homoeopathic education, and graduating doctors who intended to practise homoeopathically. Despite the apparent ingenuity of the move, it appeared to regulars simply as a technical fix which was too economical with the truth. The fact was that regular staff would still be teaching basic medical courses to students intending to opt for instruction in therapeutics from homoeopathic professors. It could not be allowed, and the regular profession united in calls for the whole of the faculty staff to resign rather than be compromised in this way. The dean of the medical department, A. Sager, did so. But the rest of the staff were reluctant to follow suit. The profession at large was not slow to express its unqualified disapproval.

Relations between the Michigan State Medical Society (MSMS) and the legislature predictably deteriorated: in 1877, it resolved to suspend all contact with the state authority. The AMA was equally disgruntled with the MSMS. Some of its members were among the erring staff at the university and their stance, being in violation of the spirit (if not the letter) of the code of ethics, stirred the AMA into action against its Michigan constituency. It came to little. No medical organisation could realistically hope to prevail against the edicts of a democratically elected legislature, and all that the AMA's efforts to discipline the MSMS achieved was a revision of the code of ethics which, while expressing implicit disapproval of the situation at the university, was nevertheless forced to recognise its reality. Victory belonged to the supporters of homoeopathy, and regular and homoeopathic students continued to graduate from the university medical school until the end of the century.[22]

The passion which the dominant allopathic sect had vented over the Michigan affair was, by the time of its conclusion, hardly justified by the real differences between the two schools. As in Britain, homoeopaths came to have more in common with the regular school than the institutional and verbal war suggested. Homoeopathic education resembled its regular counterpart in all but the issue of therapeutics, and practitioners were quick to adopt new diagnostic techniques and technologies, and to make use of anaesthetic and antiseptic procedures. Even in the sphere of therapeutics, the imperative of providing immediate relief to patients - reducing fever and allaying pain - meant that allopathic antipyretics and analgesics were used. Reductions in allopathic dosage were matched, on the homoeopathic side, by a preference for low dilutions. Hahnemannianism became simply a method of drug selection.

Homoeopaths could not afford to ignore medical initiatives which would have taken patients elsewhere, and the growing similarity of the two schools, combined with the gathering momentum of educational reform, acted as underlying reasons for the decline of the movement in the twentieth century. Quite simply, changes in practice on both sides ceased to

make homoeopathy an attractive alternative as far as patients,
or their physicians, were concerned.

These developments were reflected in a familiar internal
schism, which further weakened the movement. Purists railed
against the corruption of Hahnemannian doctrine by 'half-
homoeopaths', especially in the medical schools. The concentration on basic medical sciences, on clinical specialities, and
the teaching of non-homoeopathic therapeutics, were all
singled out for caustic comment by those who wished to
defend the principles articulated in the Organon. In turn, the
'lows' defended their own practice by pointing to the
deficiencies and inconsistencies in Hahnemann's work. Eventually, the arguments led to an institutional split, with the
formation by the fundamentalists of the International
Hahnemannian Association (IHA) in 1880, and the appearance
of high dilutionist medical schools, such as those formed in
Chicago in 1892 and 1895.

With the dramatic decline of homoeopathy after the turn
of the century, high dilutionist views increasingly pre-
dominated. As in Britain, survival became contingent on the
re-emphasis of distinctive elements in homoeopathic
philosophy. The price was isolation, and the retreat of
homoeopathy beyond the horizon of serious medical attention.

Just as American homoeopathy had owed its position of
strength to its medical schools, so it was here that the first
signs of collapse began to occur. Scientific innovation, and
more rigorous licensing laws, began to increase the economic
pressure on self-supporting medical schools as the budgets
required to resource an adequate education rose. Weaker
institutions began to close under the impetus of AMA reform.
As Flexner concluded in his 1910 report on American medical
education: 'It has, in fact, become virtually impossible for a
medical school to comply even in a perfunctory manner with
statutory, not to say scientific, requirements and show a
profit.'[23]

In all three major sects, the number of medical schools
declined steeply after 1900. In that year, the regulars had
126 schools, 22,710 students and 4,715 graduates. The corresponding figures for the homoeopaths were: 22, 1,909, and
413; and for the eclectics: nine, 522, and 86.[24] By 1920,
the number of regular schools had been reduced to 76, the
number of students to 13,220, and the number of graduates
to 2,826. Decline had been even more precipitous for the
homoeopaths (five schools, 386 students, 97 graduates), and
for the eclectics (one school, 93 students, 30 graduates).[25]

Four major centres of homoeopathic education, in
Michigan, Boston, New York and Philadelphia, survived the
first wave of closures, but they could not, in the end, resist
the general process of decline. Michigan lost its separate
homoeopathic department at the university in the early 1920s.
The Boston school had changed its title by 1919, dropping

any reference to homoeopathy. In 1922, there were no homoeopathic graduates from the school at all. New York took similar action in 1936, and all teaching of homoeopathy ceased there in 1940. Philadelphia first reduced the number of homoeopathic courses on offer, then made them electives in the early 1950s, and dropped them altogether in the 1960s.

The atrophy of homoeopathic education was intimately connected to the therapeutic changes in the movement outlined above. The similarity of the practice of many homoeopaths to that of regular colleagues made the former less inclined to advise students to attend a homocopathic institution, and the commitment of undergraduates at these schools was increasingly focused on the core of medical knowledge required for graduation. As student interest declined, schools closed, and courses folded; in turn, the numbers of homoeopaths competent to teach the discipline fell. Once it had set in, the downward spiral could not be halted.

The practical transformation of homoeopathy had two further effects. Firstly, regulars - such as the members of the Medical Society of the State of New York in 1882 - began to argue that the consultation ban should be lifted. Secondly, co-operation among the sects on the issue of licensing led eventually to a revision of the AMA code of ethics. Both changes served to reabsorb many homoeopaths into regular life and, correspondingly, led to a widening of the theoretical gulf between those who still adhered to the system, and the rest of the profession.

Renewed interest in medical licensing had been stimulated by the steadily increasing number of new entrants to the profession in the post-Civil War period. The compulsory state licensing of all physicians, however, was complicated by the sectarian nature of the profession: single licensing boards, controlled by allopaths, were obviously seen as instruments through which the minority sects could be harassed, and were opposed by irregular practitioners. Since the AMA code of ethics forbad fraternisation - which ruled out joint boards - some states established separate licensing boards for each sect. Usually, these were none too successful: rivalry and conflict between the different boards could not be legislated away, and as in Kansas, the system proved unworkable.

It became increasingly apparent that effective legislation could only be achieved through co-operation. The prospect was distasteful to many regulars, but had to be faced. As William Osler observed: 'if we wish legislation for the protection of the public, we have got to ask for it together, not singly. I know that this is gall and wormwood to many - at the bitterness of it the gall rises; but it is a question which has to be met fairly and squarely.'[26] With the help of this new mood, states began to enact legislation which provided for sectarian co-operation in licensing. By the end

HOMOEOPATHY IN AMERICA

of the century, 33 of the 45 states with licensing laws had
effected the change.[27]
    This made for more effective control of standards, and
helped to regulate the flow of new practitioners, but it also
meant that the AMA code of ethics was now completely out of
tune with legislative reality. The sects were co-operating
every day in licensing new physicians; moreover, medical
societies had begun to follow the lead given by that of the
state of New York, and admit graduates of homoeopathic
institutions, and cede consultation rights. Inevitably, the
code of ethics had to be revised to recognise the new reality.
It happened in 1903. As long as individual homoeopaths were
prepared to discard the name, inquiries about actual practice
would cease, and normal relations would be restored.
    In part, these changes were forced by the practical need
to seek tighter control of licensing. But this is by no means
the whole story. Clearly, the reopening of normal professional
intercourse with homoeopaths was also a political strategy:
isolation and ostracism were one way of controlling therapeutic
competition, but readmittance and absorption were far better.
The few left on the perimeter - like those high potency
physicians who formed the American Foundation for Homoeopathy (AFH) in 1921 - could then be safely ignored. In over
forty years, fewer than 150 doctors took its postgraduate
course.[28]
    Rothstein argues that the ultimate cause for the decline
of sectarianism in American medicine was the development of
a scientific basis for regular practice. This meant that
techniques and procedure could receive objective validation.
The implication is that because the sects lacked this foundation, they went into decline: science for Rothstein, then, is
the deus ex machina which decided the fate of the medical
sects.
    The argument is fragile for at least two reasons. Firstly,
science was not systematically used at the time to provide a
decisive evaluation of sectarian therapeutics. Moreover, if
science had been used to arbitrate on everything which
regular physicians did at the turn of the century, they would
have been left with precious little in the way of therapeutic
resources. Secondly, it is obvious that the contemporary
version of science in medicine - i.e. practice based on a
biomedical perspective - has not extinguished interest in
systems underpinned by alternative philosophies, or extinguished the popularity of sectarian practice.
    There is no doubt that advances in the understanding of
disease process did much to enhance the prestige of the
regular profession. But this was only one of a number of
factors involved in sectarian decline. The predisposing cause
was the homogenisation of practice induced by therapeutic
competition. Among the proximate causes were: the momentum
of educational and licensing reform, which raised standards,

209

and forced weaker schools to close; the impact of the Flexner report, which highlighted the weakness of homoeopathic education, and helped to channel funds and students to regular colleges; the emphasis on a core of medical knowledge by state boards which marginalised knowledge of homoeopathic therapeutics; the revision of AMA policy on membership and consultation; the internal, political, weakness of the homoeopathic school, rooted in the individualism of its members, the high and low dosage schism, and the attractiveness of medical specialisation; and the growth of the pharmaceutical industry, which simplified general practitioner prescribing and, after an ethical accord had been reached with the AMA (on the issue of specification of drug ingredients) provided powerful financial support for the institutions of the regular profession.

The high potency wing of American homoeopathy, symbolised by the AFH, blamed much of the decline on the poor (i.e. eclectic) quality of homoeopathic education. It soon came into conflict with the AIH on this issue; while the AIH strove to stem the tide of decline by opening new colleges (attempts were made in Cleveland and Chicago towards the end of the 1920s) the AFH continued to criticise the educational effects of existing institutions.[29]

As the century wore on, further problems emerged on the educational front. In 1935, the AMA resolved that after 1 July 1938, its list of approved schools would no longer include those with sectarian titles. The result, already referred to above, was the removal of references to homoeopathy in college titles, the conversion of homoeopathic courses to an optional basis, and their final elimination.

One development, however, served to unite all wings of the profession. As in Britain, the threat of regimented state medicine grouped practitioners behind a common cause. New Deal legislation was denounced as an infringement of American (i.e. medical) liberty. Dr Lucy Herzog successfully encouraged the AIH to join forces with the AMA in order to campaign against the drift towards socialised medicine.

Encouraged by this co-operation, subsequent attempts were made to cajole the AMA into recognition of homoeopathy as a speciality in internal medicine. The IHA had voted itself and its journal out of existence in 1960, but despite this new unity in the movement, which had been forged in the hope of preserving homoeopathy through securing formal recognition of speciality status, the AMA refused to approve the request.

Despite the rebuff, homoeopaths still strove for the realisation of educational initiatives. In 1950, the AIH, under the stimulus of Dr Chal Bryant, began to raise funds in order to support a campaign for introducing homoeopathy into state medical colleges, but Bryant's death brought the effort to a close. Later, in 1967, Dr William Young proposed the

'Perpetuation and Propagation Programme', designed to fund lectureships.

By the 1960s, however, American homoeopathy was at a very low ebb. Many of its practitioners were over sixty years of age. The difficulty of developing homoeopathic expertise, its philosophical leanings, its demands on the time and energy of the physician, and regular control of the educational process, continued to make homoeopathy a discipline of interest to very few practitioners. Any revival of interest had to await a new public reaction to regular medicine. As in the nineteenth century, important factors were to be an increasing intolerance of iatrogenic damage, and recognition of the relatively limited success of medicine in combating the major diseases of the period.

NOTES

1. See Anon., Transactions of the World's Homoeopathic Convention, 26 June-1 July 1876, 2 vols. (Sherman and Co., Philadelphia, 1880) vol. II, History of Homoeopathy; and also Anon., 'The Transactions of the International Homoeopathic Convention of 1881', British Journal of Homoeopathy, vol. XL (1882), pp. 32-45.
2. See Anon., 'The Transactions of the International Homoeopathic Convention of 1881', op.cit., p. 33.
3. William G. Rothstein, American Physicians in the Nineteenth Century (Johns Hopkins University Press, Baltimore and London, 1972), p. 236.
4. Ibid., p. 226.
5. William G. Rothstein, op.cit.
6. Martin Kaufman, Homoeopathy in America - the Rise and Fall of a Medical Heresy (Johns Hopkins University Press, Baltimore and London, 1971).
7. William G. Rothstein, op.cit., p. 93.
8. Ibid., p. 97.
9. Samuel Thomson, A Narrative of the Life and Medical Discoveries of Samuel Thomson: Containing an Account of His System of Practice and the Manner of Curing Disease with Vegetable Medicine, Upon a Plan Entirely New; to which is Prefixed an Introduction to His New Guide to Health, or Botanic Family Physician, Containing the Principles Upon Which the System is Founded, with Remarks on Fevers, Steaming, Poison, etc., 8th edition (Pike, Platt, and Co., Ohio, 1832). See also William G. Rothstein, op.cit., pp. 128-40 for further discussion of Thomson's book.
10. William G. Rothstein, op.cit., p. 140.
11. Ibid., p. 226.
12. Ibid.
13. Ibid., p. 162.
14. See his 1835 Address to the Massachusetts Medical

Society: Jacob Bigelow, 'A Discourse on Self-Limited Diseases', Massachusetts Medical Society: Medical Communications, vol. V (1836), pp. 319-58. And by the same author, Nature in Disease (Ticknor and Fields, Boston, 1854).
    15. H.L. Coulter, Homoeopathic Influences in Nineteenth-Century Allopathic Therapeutics (American Institute of Homoeopathy, Washington, 1973).
    16. H.L. Coulter, Divided Legacy, a History of the Schism in Medical Thought, 3 vols. (Wehawken Book Company, Washington 1973-7) vol. III, chapter 4.
    17. Quoted by William G. Rothstein, op.cit., p. 171.
    18. Quoted by R.E. Dudgeon, 'The Diploma of "L.H." of the London School of Homoeopathy', The British Journal of Homoeopathy, vol. XL (1882), p. 157. Emphasis added.
    19. See Dudgeon's discussion, op.cit., pp. 156-66, esp. pp. 157, 159-60.
    20. William G. Rothstein, op.cit., p. 236.
    21. Ibid., p. 236, and p. 287 for the number of schools in 1900.
    22. A detailed history of the dispute may be found in Martin Kaufman, op.cit., pp. 93-109.
    23. Quoted by William G. Rothstein, op.cit., p. 293.
    24. Ibid., p. 287.
    25. Ibid.
    26. Quoted in ibid., p. 307.
    27. Ibid., p. 308.
    28. Martin Kaufman, op.cit., p. 174.
    29. See ibid., Chapter XII for a more detailed discussion of American homoeopathy after 1900.

Part IV
THE LONG WINTER: HOMOEOPATHY IN
BRITAIN AFTER 1900

Chapter Thirteen

PROBLEMS OF THEORY AND PRACTICE
IN A SCIENTIFIC ERA

In the decades after 1900, homoeopaths were acutely aware that their movement had fallen into stagnation and decline. Whenever doctors met, it was an issue which dominated discussion. As Dr McClelland put it in 1913 'the halting progress of homoeopathy' was a 'consciousness which, like a ghost, haunts all our meetings'.[1] The spectre was still there in 1926. Dr Weir, President of the BHS, remarked: 'The past session has not been outstanding. I had hoped more from it. Our roll has not increased.'[2] Six new associate members had joined the Society, but this had been balanced by the death of older members, and by the purging of those who had 'in spite of opportunities, remonstrances and pleadings, ceased to show the slightest interest in our cause or in the Society, either by attendances or by payment of fees'.[3]

The same message echoed down the years. In 1930, the then president, Dr Percy Hall-Smith, told the Society 'there is no doubt a serious crisis has to be faced. I refer to the steady decline of Homoeopaths in the provinces';[4] in 1944, Dr Wheeler was asking 'Why do we get so few recruits?';[5] seven years later, Dr Neubert claimed that few would 'disagree with the unpleasant observation that the practice of homoeopathic medicine is rapidly decreasing';[6] and in 1970, Dr Blackie's presidential address bore the by now almost inevitable title The Future of Homoeopathy because, as she said, 'of the anxiety about it in the homoeopathic world'.[7] Only by the middle of the 1970s, with the gradual rebirth of popular interest in alternative medicine, were lighter notes sounded.

The statistics bore out the pessimism. In 1901, there were 79 homoeopathic chemists, and 82 cities and towns in the UK had from one to ten practitioners each. Dr Granville Hey, who recorded these statistics in 1931, went on to ask 'Where are these now?'[8] The question was really rhetorical: what had become of the lost practitioners was not so important as the fact that they had disappeared. In 1930, the number of practising homoeopaths was under 200 (compared to a total of

39,500 regulars).[9] Inevitably, as homoeopathic practices collapsed, dispensaries closed, and hospitals came under increasing pressure as staff could not be replaced. Sometimes this resulted in the abandonment of the homoeopathic designation of the institution: the Birmingham Homoeopathic Hospital, for example, became simply the 'Midland Hospital, Birmingham', in 1930.[10] The hospital in Plymouth had already suffered the same fate in the 1920s. And with the Local Government Act of 1929, which abolished Boards of Guardians and brought Poor Law hospitals under municipal control, the Central Hospital (as the Plymouth institution had become), fearing that as voluntary hospital it would not be able to compete with those which were rate supported, agreed to amalgamate with two other hospitals in 1930.[11]

The BHS also contracted. In 1907, members numbered 202. By 1927, enrolment had fallen to 190, almost half of whom had joined in the previous century.[12] Things were no better fifteen years later. For the 1941-2 session, the Society could list only 200 members, and for 1942-3, 209.[13] Something like a third of these were associate members - LHH staff among them - and thus were unlikely to be practising homoeopathy to any great extent, or even be more than superficially interested in it.[14] In 1953-4, 221 doctors were registered with the Faculty (as the Society had become by then), and in 1954-5, 223, of which 91 were of associate status.[15] Again, any real upturn had to await the 1970s. For the 1975-6 session, the Faculty's roll totalled 306 members: by 1981-2, this had grown to 540, and by the following year to 633.[16]

With the recognition of decline came a search for causes and solutions. Among the former, commentators continued to refer to opposition from the regular profession, most concretely manifested in the refusal to cede space for homoeopathic therapeutics in medical education. Internal dissension on both medical and political issues, the retention of a sectarian title, the failure to provide convincing scientific and clinical demonstrations of homoeopathy's effectiveness and, once the National Health Service (NHS) had been established, of the difficulty of practising within the time constraints imposed by the state system, also featured prominently among the factors which homoeopaths identified as contributing to the isolation and stagnation of the movement. Occasionally, some writers hit on more fundamental issues. Dr James Watson, Honorary Physician to the Hahnemann Hospital in Liverpool, was one. He referred, in 1906, to the 'crypto-homoeopathy amongst allopaths' which 'has weakened the hold which avowed homoeopaths now have upon the minds of the laity' and, on the other hand, to the fact that homoeopaths themselves 'resort too readily, at the first sign of difficulty or of danger, to methods other than those sanctioned by our law of cure'.[17]

Quite simply, a declaration of sectarianism was no longer justified in an era when the actual practice of the two schools was close. This was the sociological background to the triumph of Kentianism. At one and the same time, it reasserted the distinctiveness of homoeopathy, and ensured its marginality. Dr Percy Hall-Smith, in 1930, was among the first to make the point:

> ... my own conviction is that our teaching is not sufficiently practical, and the approach unduly philosophical, and too far removed from the line of thought of the average doctor. ... It requires a rather special type of mind and outlook to swallow at the first blush undiluted 'Kentian principles'. The average mind trained on a more materialistic basis is liable to be repelled by such teaching at the outset ...[18]

Dr Wheeler made the same point in 1947. For Wheeler, the distinctive features of Kentianism were a refinement of the method of drug selection (i.e. an emphasis on leading symptoms to develop drug pictures of, for example, the typical 'sulphur patient', rather than detailed individual symptomatology, and the admissibility of clinical symptoms); the use of very high potencies; a scornful dismissal of the lower dilutions; and a belief in an increase of power with each successive dilution and succussion. In practice, Kentian homoeopathy was, according to Wheeler, 'slightly contemptuous of any attempt to make terms with other medical knowledge, regarding, as it were, the teaching as something so transcendental that no reasoned explanations are likely to have any validity'.[19] Kentianism, he continued, possessed 'a certain attractive semi-mystical quality', but 'it is also fairly clear that it has a limited appeal'.[20] Indeed, it left the regular school in Europe:

> ... unconverted, even indifferent. Their [the Kentians'] response is that there can be no compromise with truth. They hold themselves to possess it in a unique degree: if the medical world cannot or will not see it, so much the worse ... To the elect there is no course but to go their way ... They are willing to pipe, and if the profession will not dance their consciences are clear.[21]

Kentianism, then, was metaphysical, dogmatic, puritanical and millenial. Homoeopaths who failed to achieve results with the high dilutions lacked intellectual skill and rigour, as well as the moral fibre for the arduous task of identifying the simillimum. In short, so far as Kentians were concerned, the faithless were responsible for the corruption and decline of the movement.

217

The truth, of course, was rather the opposite. Despite Wheeler's apparent distancing of Kentianism from the moderate homoeopathic mainstream, it was a fact that high dilutionism came to be the twentieth century orthodoxy. Even in 1917, an analysis of the 1,664 prescriptions given at the LHH during the month of July revealed that 1,026 (62 per cent) were of the twelfth centesimal potency or above. At the twelfth itself, 163 had been given (ten per cent); at the thirtieth, 461 (28 per cent); at the 200th, 363 (22 per cent); and above the 200th, 39 (two per cent).[22] This high potency trend strengthened in later years.

The Kentian thrust inevitably alienated many who might otherwise have shown interest. Once again, Dr Percy Hall-Smith was keen to underline the problem. Postgraduate educational efforts had been centred on the Honyman-Gillespie and Compton Burnett lectures at the LHH, and Hall-Smith pondered, in 1931, 'what proportion of medical men and women who have attended these lectures during the last twenty years ... have been sufficiently convinced to take up the practice of homoeopathy and join this society[?]'.[23] He answered himself: 'I cannot think that the proportion is very high', and this because 'The teaching in this Hospital for many years now has been chiefly based on the principles so ably enunciated by the late Dr James Tyler Kent'.[24] Hall-Smith was in no doubt that, as far as Kentianism was concerned 'The whole conception is so foreign to the usual line of thought of the average practitioner, that, unless his case of mind is rather exceptional, there is a real danger of antagonizing him at the outset.'[25]

The Kentian orientation of many homoeopaths helped to produce a lack of interest in basic research, a complacent attitude to scientific advance in regular medicine, and an intolerant attitude to compromise. John Henry Clarke's presidential address to the BHS in 1906 caught the coming mood well:

Homoeopaths owe no allegiance to allopaths. Homoeopathy is established science. Allopathy is established nescience. The sight of Homoeopathy paying court to allopathy; of homoeopaths paying court to allopaths, is to me sickening in the extreme. It is light paying court to darkness; truth paying court to error; virtue paying court to vice. One blast of the enthusiasm of Homoeopathy should be enough to cremate such infamy in our midst.[26]

Others, however, were not so content to await the medical millenium which would follow from 'a great truth' held in splendid isolation, and strove to arrest decline through more practical endeavours. A whole range of measures were discussed. Research, designed to explain the action of

218

homoeopathic remedies in scientific terms, was advocated. The reproving of drugs with the aid of new medical technologies was called for. Suggestions were made for the establishment of research scholarships, and for the updating and simplification of homoeopathic literature for the interested student. Doctors were urged to keep meticulous clinical records, and besiege regular journals with the results. The extension of out-patient facilities at hospitals, it was argued, would help to stimulate public awareness of homoeopathy. Emphasising the financial savings to hospitals of homoeopathic treatment might elicit wider interest in the system. Amalgamation, and relinquishing the sectarian title of the school would help, so some believed, to leaven regular practice and spread homoeopathic methods, albeit covertly. Doctors were encouraged to interest members of the regular profession on a personal basis, bring them to meetings and persuade them to try homoeopathic remedies and join the Society: a 'Covenant of Extension', in which homoeopaths were invited to commit themselves to these aims, was established in 1920.

Many of these activities required funding. To this end, a 'Twentieth Century Fund' was inaugurated in 1902, with the assistance of the BHA, reformed in that year; and a 'Reconstruction Fund' was established some years later. Funds were also required to assist the educational programme. It was in this field that many homoeopaths saw the only hope of salvation. Efforts were made to diffuse homoeopathic knowledge among the public, especially through the efforts of hospitals and the BHA; suggestions were made to provide all new medical graduates, and all medical schools, with homoeopathic literature; doctors were encouraged to talk to student medical societies, emphasising the homoeopathic elements in regular treatment, such as vaccine therapy, and a more Hughesian homoeopathic perspective; generally, homoeopaths were exhorted 'to teach, to preach, to persuade, to convert'.[27]

The major focus of educational development, however, was on the institutionalisation of more formal methods. Obtaining a place for homoeopathy on the medical curriculum for undergraduates, though seen as the most desirable objective, was always recognised as unrealistic. This meant that homoeopaths had to rely on postgraduate instruction. George Burford, in 1902, called for the funding of a 'Lectureship in Materia Medica', whose incumbent would hold courses in 'successive years in the cities of London, Liverpool and Birmingham; for here are three university towns, each with its annual quota of medical graduates, and in each of these towns we have a fully equipped Homoeopathic Hospital to supply the clinical element'.[28] Nevertheless, the main objective, as Burford and others realised, was 'the securing of fair recognition by the State; in the chartered right to educate and examine in our doctrine and practice'.[29]

This objective took many years to secure. On 25 November 1943, the BHS obtained recognition from the Board of Trade as a corporate body (the Faculty of Homoeopathy), and was thereby entitled 'to grant to registered medical practitioners Diplomas, Certificates and other equivalent recognition of special knowledge in Homoeopathy'.[30] The Faculty had thus acquired the right to set the standard for postgraduate educational courses and examinations, and strengthened its position in the forthcoming reorganisation of the health service.

The first examination for the Diploma of the Faculty was held on October 4th 1944. Four candidates took two three hour papers (Principles and Practice of Homoeopathy and Materia Medica and Therapeutics), each of which was followed by a viva, together with a clinical examination consisting of one long and three short cases.[31] Three of the examinees were successful.[32] By the following day, Dr Hindmarsh and Squadron-Leader F.R. Neubert had become the first associate members to be elected to full membership by examination.[33] Prominent among the texts on which examination success had depended was the work of Hahnemann (naturally) and, significantly, Clarke and Kent.[34] Hughes was nowhere to be seen.

In the post-war period, however, when the LHH approached the London University for recognition under the British Postgraduate Medical Federation as a teaching hospital, it was turned down. Homoeopaths were alarmed by this development. The Minister of Health had indicated that the plan for the post-war health system would not discriminate against homoeopathy. Nevertheless, since the minister argued that he could not force the university to cede the recognition desired, homoeopathic teaching appeared to remain under a cloud of illegitimacy. Parliamentary pressure, however, saved most of the day. Political activity by homoeopaths and their sympathisers helped to secure the Faculty of Homoeopathy Act, which received its Royal Assent on 12 July 1950. This conferred powers on the Faculty which ensured the continuation of facilities at the LHH for research and education. The legitimacy of the Faculty's postgraduate licensing powers were thus guaranteed by Act of Parliament. Medical opposition, however, continued. Funds to support postgraduate study, provided from the public purse under Section 63 of the Health Services and Public Health Act, were controlled by the Deans of Postgraduate Medical Education, and these were still unprepared to release money for those desiring to take the Faculty's courses and examinations. Intending students could thus study for a qualification whose legitimacy was protected by parliament, but if they did so, they would have to fund it themselves, or apply for assistance from funds raised by other organisations, such as the Homoeopathic Trust. Homoeopaths have long struggled to remove this anomaly.

One of the enduring discussions among homoeopaths throughout this period focused on the issue of dosage. Ultimately, the controversy stemmed from the fact that Hahnemann had not identified a law to cover this issue equivalent to the law of the similar remedy. Although he had recommended the thirtieth centesimal potency as the upper limit, this was inconsistent with his theory of drug action, and paved the way for the high dilutionists to extend attenuation. This could reach dizzy heights indeed. As Dr Gordon Smith observed:

> But for high dilution, the man of the 200th potency is nowhere, he is still among the crudities of posology. For we have brethren who are not happy till they get to the 10,000th, and even then they are not quite at home, they deem the 100,000th a good point to start from, and hence upwards to anything you like.[35]

Given the time and equipment required for the preparation of such high potencies, a cloud of suspicion had to reign over their integrity. Gordon Smith went on to declare: 'I am satisfied in my mind that the 100,000th potency or dilution made according to, and by, the Hahnemannian method has never yet been seen on our planet', and added, for good measure, 'And if it should some day make its appearance, someone will have spent much time over its preparation which might have been employed to better purpose'.[36]

Ultimately, it had been sociological factors, rather than those of physical or medical science, which had produced the low dose regimen favoured by Hughes. Here, at least, it had been relatively easy to understand the action of remedies in terms of a material effect on body tissues and processes - and, indeed, regular medicine, through recognition of the role of vitamins, hormones and the development of vaccines, came to accept that substances in minute quantities could have profound metabolic effects. Sociological factors, however, had also ensured the subsequent drift in homoeopathy to the higher potencies advocated by Kent. With the waxing of high dilutionism, alternative explanations of drug action were clearly required. Two concerns manifested themselves. First, to provide theoretical accounts of how high potencies might work and second, to generate experimental evidence that they did.

The main stumbling block was two firmly held principles of physical chemistry. These were Avogadro's Law, and the non-specificity of sub-atomic particles. Dr Stephenson explained:

According to Avogadro the molecular weight of any material expressed in grams contains 6.12×10^{23} molecules. Theoretically, therefore, any substance diluted beyond 1×10^{-24} [twelfth centesimal potency] will contain no molecules of the original material, assuming a homogeneous mixture at each stage of dilution. Dilutions of this degree of fineness should, then, contain nothing but the liquid vehicle in which the substance was first diluted, and should act in no manner different from it. Nor can the specific action of dilutions greater than 1×10^{-24} be attributed to electrons which became separated from the diluted material and remained in solution, for the other principle already mentioned, states that the electrons from one atom differ in no manner from those of any other atom.[37]

Nevertheless, homoeopaths were convinced that clinical experience showed definite patient response to remedies in dilution far greater than the twelfth. The problem was (and still is) to square this clinical evidence with the laws of physical and chemical science. At first, in the earlier decades of the century, advances in physics were thought to point to explanations which relied on energy, rather than mechanical effect. Dr Burford provided a good example of this kind of view in his 1926 presidential address to the British Homoeopathic Congress. He spoke of:

... electrons and protons moving about in an infinite ocean of ether, and whose vibrations therein produce those ethereal undulations we call heat and light and Hertzian waves, and all the host of such. Within the octaves of these vibrations, and particularly of those in the neighborhood of the X-ray type, there is every reasonable probability we may include radiations from potencies of all sorts ... Properly, homoeopathic potencies should be envisaged in terms of modern science as the foci of etheric radiations, which, ... in the words of Sir Oliver Lodge, 'retain their vigour however diluted'.[38]

Dr W.E. Boyd's thoughts took a similar direction. He believed that where high potencies were concerned 'we are dealing with a method of releasing specific energy from specific substances which is capable of imposing its own particular properties on the diluting medium'.[39] One way of conceiving the effect of this energy was in terms of providing a stimulus to the immune responses of the body - though this was not, in fact, a view which Boyd himself seemed to favour.

Subsequently, attempts to explain the action of high potencies introduced ideas such as semiconductor activity (in lactose), and the way in which solvent molecules were re-arranged during dynamisation.[40]

Lacking expertise in physical and chemical science, it is difficult to do more than record, in summary fashion, some of the theoretical initiatives which have been taken in investigating this issue. The main point is that homoeopaths have not yet succeeded in developing a satisfactory theoretical account of the action of high potencies, despite the efforts exerted in this direction. The most recent models suggest that therapeutic activity derives from 'a structure induced in the solvent, typical for the original solute. This structure is thought to consist of water polymer chains held together by the hydrogen bonds. It has been proposed that the therapeutic mechanism is due to the interaction of the water polymer chains with peptides.'[41] But Bergholz, from whose 1985 paper this quote derives, is unconvinced that the model has any great experimental support, or theoretical justification. It could be, of course, that the effect of high potencies is not explicable in terms of the current (or any) scientific paradigm. This is a view favoured by those who are attracted to the mystical and metaphysical dynamic in homoeopathic thought. Stressing this perspective, however - and it may be defensible to do so, since the world can be rendered intelligible by 'ways of seeing' other than that proposed by Western science - is an obvious recipe for continued medical marginality.

While a workable scientific explanation for potency effect has remained elusive, homoeopaths have nevertheless been anxious to show that, whatever the mechanism of action, substances in high dilution do, as a matter of fact, affect living systems. Clinical evidence aside, three main areas of research have been initiated since 1900: investigations of the effect of homoeopathic doses on metabolic processes, clinical trails of homoeopathic drugs, and W.E. Boyd's work with the 'Emanometer'.

An early example of attempts to show the activity of potencies appeared in The British Homoeopathic Journal of 1914. The effect of different dilutions of arsenic, corrosive sublimate and nitrate of silver on the activity of yeast, measured in terms of the amount of carbon dioxide given off in a given period from sugar solution cultures, was recorded. The results are worth quoting:

(a) The activity of yeast in producing CO_2 under the influence of drugs follows (as was to be expected) the protoplasmic law of R. Arndt, viz: drugs in any concentrated form (e.g., low dilutions, 1X, 2X, 3X) exercise a retarding effect on vital activity in proportion to the concentration. In medium dilutions and higher dilutions (4X to 12C) they act as stimulants to CO_2 production.

(b) There is as yet no evidence that the stimulating effect is proportional exactly to the dilution, but in a general way as the higher potencies are reached the stimulating effect passes away. Beyond 12C, although every now and then a stimulating effect seems to be obtained, the results are not constant. There is therefore clear biological evidence of reality of potencies up to 12C ... Beyond that at present the evidence is uncertain.[42]

This research pointed the way for subsequent endeavours. Could the results be repeated and, more importantly, could the Arndt phenomenon be shown to operate beyond the Avogadro limit? Dr W.E. Boyd's work in Glasgow, which involved measuring the effect of potencies on the rate of starch hydrolysis by the enzyme diastase, seemed to confirm both phenomena. In a programme of research which lasted some fifteen years, Boyd was eventually able to conclude in 1954 that mercuric chloride in dilutions of the order of 10^{-6} 'gave a highly significant difference in the rate of hydrolysis between controls and tests, the microdoses stimulating the process. Statistically the significance is shown by the fact that a probability of <0.001 was obtained in each of the three years 1946, 1948 and 1952. The control results gave an approximately normal distribution.'[43]

Other researchers were also active in the field. In an international review of experimental literature from 1881, Dr Stephenson was able, in 1955, to identify 25 investigations into potency activity.[44] More recently, Kollerstrom has identified experimental work completed in the area for the period 1950 to 1978, and Scofield has brought the picture even further up to date with an article published in 1984.[45]

Problems of soundness of research design, execution, reporting etc., however, have plagued this large experimental effort. Kollerstrom, for example, concluded that, apart from Boyd, only two pieces of research from all those surveyed withstood rigorous critical examination, and Scofield agrees with her conclusion that most of the research does not, in fact, establish what it claims.[46] Nevertheless, just enough evidence for the activity of potencies beyond the Avogadro limit seems to exist to justify further efforts to account for the phenomenon in theoretical terms.

Further indication of potency effect - at least as far as homoeopaths were concerned - has been supplied by efforts to extend the range of drug provings. In 1904, Dr Clarke conducted a proving of radium bromide 30C. Only a small number of subjects were involved, with each recording symptoms over many days.[47] In 1940, Dr Sutherland published a fragmentary proving of 'Sulfanilamide'. Five years later, the Faculty established a drug proving committee consisting of Drs Wheeler, Fergie Woods and Kenyon. By

1962, twelve new provings had been published. Again - as with radium and sulfanilamide - an interest in new additions to the allopathic materia medica was noticeable: penicillin (Penicillium), cortisone and ACTH (Adrenocorticotrophic hormone) figured prominently on the list. Further work followed, under the initiative of Dr Raeside. For each of the twelve drugs proved between 1947 and 1962, however, the trials involved few subjects - sometimes in the absence of a control group - and were conducted over extended periods in order to obtain a symptomatology.[49] Although the remedies were given in potentised form, and provings obtained, it has to be said that critics would hardly regard the results as impressive. Regular researchers would point immediately to the number of uncontrolled variables involved, and would be reluctant, therefore, to accept the provings as hard evidence of potency activity.

A traditional objection to homoeopathy has always been that any therapeutic improvement must necessarily be due to placebo effect rather than the activity of a potentised remedy. In order to rebut this argument, homoeopaths have, over the years, organised a number of clinical trials. Some doctors, however, have always objected to this procedure on the grounds that the methodology is inappropriate: the differences among individuals, which traditional research design attempts to control by matching members of experimental and control groups, or by randomisation, so the argument goes, are just the very differences which are essential to homoeopathic prescribing. Thus while conventional research methods seek to control for 'people variance', so that the effect of a specific drug on disease can be measured against placebo, in homoeopathy it is 'people variance' which determines drug selection. Moreover, the double-blind technique to control for placebo effect eliminates the holistic thrust of homoeopathic therapy. As Dr Brieger put it:

> ... the method [of orthodox clinical trials] is not applicable. In homoeopathic practice we cannot collect a series of patients suffering, say, from asthma or migraine, or functional dyspepsia, etc., and treat alternate cases with placebo and the others with a drug. For the essence of homoeotherapy is the treatment of the individual with a remedy the symptomatology of which corresponds to that of the patient. So there is no one drug. And placebo control does not make sense.[50]

Yet others have seen conventional research methods as an essential feature of progressive homoeopathy, and as an indispensable passport to future medical legitimacy. In 1951, Dr Ledermann began a trial of high potency remedies with tubercular patients: 'Homoeopathic treatment was tested against controls and results were assessed without knowledge of whether a patient was in the homoeopathic series or the control series', but 'No absolute proof of the efficacy of homoeopathic treatment resulted'.[51] Later, in 1970, Dr Kennedy reported on the progress of a double-blind trial of arnica 200C in post-operative complications. Unfortunately, this was interrupted by administrative and organisational problems, but Kennedy was anxious for further work of this type, and spoke favourably of the mustard gas experiments of 1943, where potentised remedies (30C) had been shown useful in treatment and prophylaxis.[52] Subsequent double-blind trials of arnica by Savage and Roe, reported in 1977 and 1978, showed no significant effect.[53] Two centesimal potencies had been used: in 1977, the thirtieth, and in 1978, the 1000th.

Gibson et al., in Glasgow, however, were able to report more encouraging results. In the second part of their trial, published in 1980, 46 patients suffering from rheumatoid arthritis 'took part in a double-blind study in which homoeopathy was compared with placebo for a period of three months. The patients on homoeopathy improved significantly while those on placebo did not.'[54] More recently Reilly and Taylor, also based in Glasgow, have been working on an investigation of homoeopathic potencies (30C) of grass pollens in hay fever. Again, the trial had double-blind insurance, and the results showed 'a clinical and statistically significant effect over placebo'.[55] These sets of findings have reached a wider medical audience through publication in regular journals: those of Gibson et al., in The British Journal of Clinical Pharmacology (1980), and those of Reilly et al. in The Lancet (1986).[56]

The British Homoeopathy Research Group, first established in 1975 to pursue a rigorous scientific examination of homoeopathy, has continually encouraged work of this kind. To date, the results of double-blind trials have been as tantalising as those of research in the Boyd tradition. There does appear to be ʾsufficient evidence to suggest that potencies beyond the Avogadro limit are active, but consistent replication of successful results has been elusive. A decisive body of evidence is needed: by no means the least of the problems involved in generating it has been - and still is - access to research funds. The pharmaceutical industry, for obvious economic reasons, has not been interested and neither, in general, have universities. Homoeopathic research has conventionally had to rely on funds raised by its own organisations and charities and, of necessity, these have always been relatively limited.

The third major field of research in Britain which sought to demonstrate the activity of homoeopathic potencies was led by Dr W.E. Boyd in Glasgow. His work on diastase under the influence of potencies of mercuric chloride has already been mentioned. Boyd, however, was also keen to investigate and measure the nature of potency energy. The instrument which he developed for this purpose was known as the Emanometer – an adaptation of apparatus originally designed and used by Abrams. Boyd published a whole series of technical papers on the development of his research over a period of more than twenty years from 1922 onwards. A full bibliography is available in the obituaries to Boyd in The British Homoeopathic Journal (1955).[57]

His work appears to have been meticulous, was certainly technically complex, and is difficult for the outsider to penetrate. The gist is given by Dr Benjamin, whose remarks are quoted below. Dr Boyd:

In order to make the necessary investigations ... found that the extreme delicacy of the research could not be advanced by any of the most sensitive physical instruments so far developed in the field of modern science. The only method of detection was the use of the natural reactions of the human body.

By means of highly critical screening, both of the instrument and of the human detector, Boyd was able to demonstrate that there was a radiation from potentized medicines. He considered that this was electro-physical or electromagnetic. As his research developed he could arrange the medicines into several groups and in time he noted that it was possible to detect a similar radiation from specimens of saliva collected from his patients. When he found a patient's group he would search for a particular remedy in potency from the corresponding drug group. When he arrived at the accurate remedy it would be the homoeopathic similimum.

When such a remedy was found through Emanometer technique, and when it was exposed with the patient's saliva specimen, it produced a state of balance in the observed reactions on the human detector.

The detector stood in a close mesh copper gauze cage and, as already stated, was completely screened to prevent interference from surrounding electro-physical radiations. These reactions were superficial contractions in patches on the detector's abdominal wall. They were elicited by a delicate percussion and to do this Boyd thrust his arms through close fitting copper cloth sleeves on the side of the cage. The accurate remedy cancelled out all the reactions which he had found to be abnormally great in their intensities.

The measurement of the intensities was calculated in the length of air gap over which they could pass and that could be as much as 50 to 60cm. within the screened field of observation.[58]

Essentially, then, the Emanometer allowed potency energy to be measured by changes in the abdominal muscle tone of a human detector; diseased human products - like blood or saliva - also possessed an energy which could be registered in a similar way; when both remedy and disease product produced identical percussion patterns, the similar remedy was indicated; the exposure of both together cancelled abnormal reaction in the human detector; and the inference was that disease involved a form of electrical disturbance which could be normalised through the energy of an homoeopathic potency.

At the time, Boyd's research excited considerable interest. In 1924, his work was investigated by a commission chaired by Sir Thomas Horder, a consultant physician from one of London's medical schools. The subsequent report makes interesting reading. It noted that 'Certain substances when placed in proper relation to the Emanometer of Boyd produce beyond any reasonable doubt changes in the abdominal wall of the subject of a kind which may be detected by percussion.'[59]

Boyd's sons, however, were not so sanguine. After their father's death, they attempted to produce evidence which supported the conclusion of the Horder investigation. They did not succeed. Dr Ian Boyd concluded that 'any successful test depended on the operator rather than on the instrument', and, moreover, 'that with three human variables - the test sample, the subject and the operator - it was impossible to control the experiment satisfactorily. ... Further research on the emanometer was abandoned by us as unprofitable and that particular instrument fell into disuse.'[60] Although considerable use of the Emanometer was made during Boyd's life, it does not appear, as his son observed, to be a significant feature of homoeopathic practice today. Like the results of homoeopathic research in other fields, the Emanometer project had produced data that was suggestive and tantalising, but far from conclusive.

Though some doctors have always been concerned to use research in order to vindicate homoeopathy in terms acceptable to the regular profession, historically few initiatives have been taken to develop homoeopathy itself. This has followed from the conviction that the only real work left to do post-Hahnemann was to prove new drugs, reprove old ones, and to develop skill in applying the results according to the law of similars. One development, however, is worth mentioning - the use of potentised disease products in treatment. This, in fact, was no twentieth century development: homoeopaths had been experimenting with such substances for many years, and thus can fairly take the credit for extending the therapeutic suggestions inherent in traditional methods of smallpox inoculation before the regular profession. In 1833, Constantine Hering had developed a product called 'lyssin' from the saliva of a rabid dog, and in 1836 'anthracinum' from anthrax.[61] Another American, Swan, prepared 'tuberculinum' from the sputum of tubercular patients, and Burnett in Britain, developed a similar product, 'bacillinum'.[62] As noted, homoeopaths were pleased to record the use of these products before Koch's treatment appeared. Along with many other similarly derived remedies, homoeopaths were also using 'gonorrhinum' and 'syphilinum' - whose origin is self-evident - in the nineteenth century.[63] The extent of homoeopathic work in this area is indicated from Burnett's comment in 1890 that 'There are but few viruses known to science that I have not used as therapeutic agents'.[64] Unfortunately, however, hard evidence relating to the clinical efficacy of these remedies does not seem to be available for the period.

Remedies derived from disease products (and later, from bacteria), were known by homoeopaths as 'nosodes'. In the twentieth century, as cancer loomed increasingly large on the medical horizon, malignancy became an obvious target for such treatment. Further development of nosode therapy was undertaken in Britain first by Drs Bach and Wheeler, and then by Dr Paterson. Particular features of the Bach-Wheeler investigations were the identification of particular varieties of intestinal bacteria, the suggestion that these were responsible for many forms of chronic disease (Hahnemann's psora), and the use of bacterial nosodes (or vaccines) in treatment. Dr Wheeler reported to the Beit Research Fund in 1923 that experiments had, he felt, confirmed 'Dr Bach's original researches into chronic bacterial infections of the bowel as the prime cause of chronic disease.[65] Moreover, 'The comparison of these infections with the "psora" of Hahnemann and the suggestion that this latter is really a ... prescient conception of intestinal toxaemia',[66] were both views which, Wheeler believed, deserved serious consideration. Bach and Wheeler published the results of their research in 1925 (Chronic Disease, A Working Hypothesis), [67] and invited others to test the conclusions which they had reached during ten years of investigation. Potentised bowel vaccines first appear to have been introduced into practice in 1927.[68]

From there, the research effort was taken up by Paterson in 1928. After more than twenty years work he felt able to confirm the Bach-Wheeler hypothesis that 'the non-lactose fermenting gram negative organisms of the intestinal tract do have a role in the causation of chronic disease, and that in the bowel nosodes I find myself possessed of a new and powerful weapon for treatment'.[69]

Paterson's bacteriological research identified many varieties of intestinal bacteria. The provings associated with the nosodes were all clinical, consisting of the symptoms which patients exhibited when a particular bacterium had been isolated, or removed when a nosode had been given. These 'provings', as Paterson pointed out, complemented existing drug pictures in the homoeopathic materia medica, thus indicating associated remedies. The proper application of Paterson's work, however, demanded bacteriological examination (and incubation) of patients' stools in order to identify the appropriate nosode. Both he, and Dr Elizabeth Paterson, being well-grounded in bacteriological science, were apparently able to use the technique with success.[70] But this has tended to limit its value in general practice: indeed, by 1965, with the death of both Drs John and Elizabeth Paterson, their methods and work were discontinued at the Glasgow hospital – the centre of their research – due to the esoteric skills required to use the Paterson therapy with success.[71] And despite the lengthy record of research, and the certainty with which the results linking chronic diseases and intestinal bacteria were stated, few, apart from the homoeopathic community itself, have noted the work, or appear to have taken it seriously.

Meanwhile, therapeutic developments in regular medicine had been continuing apace. For many homoeopaths, the immediate problem was to come to practical terms with them. The response was usually one of qualified incorporation (as far as new 'curative' drugs were concerned), with the riders that they really acted homoeopathically or, somewhat later, entailed various side-effects which limited their usefulness when measured against the action of the perfect simillimum.

Where various replacement therapies were developed, such as those involving endocrine, vitamin or mineral deficiencies, homoeopaths had few qualms about their adoption. Similarly, the use of new technologies and diagnostic techniques, such as X-rays and the electrocardiograph, could be easily absorbed. Other allopathic initiatives, such as radium and X-ray treatment and allergy desensitisation, were claimed as vindications of homoeopathic principles. This, too, was the response to the wave of vaccine and serum therapy in the early years of the century, which had been promoted by Sir Almroth Wright and his colleagues in the regular school. As Dr James Johnstone observed in 1914: 'If we go back only a quarter of a century, there were not so many diseases as the fingers of the hands attributed to bacteria or invisible parasites. Today it is all the other way.'[72]

The regular rationale of stimulating immune response through the use of the organisms and toxins associated with disease, and the recognition that small doses only should be used in order to avoid aggravation, was so obviously homoeopathic, Wheeler had argued in 1912, 'that it is freely admitted by many of our orthodox brethren'.[73]

Though vaccine therapy was soon playing an important role at the LHH, homoeopaths were not slow to point out that their own nineteenth century researches had prefigured this development in regular practice, and that it was an indication that regular advances only confirmed homoeopathic theory. Bach's claim in 1919 was typical: 'it should be realised that science ... is confirming the principles of homoeopathy. To Hahnemann should fall all the honour for having anticipated science by more than a century.'[74]

Where remedies were discovered in the regular school which actually had an effect on bacteria themselves, the homoeopathic response was more problematic. In 1910, Dr Cash Reed reviewed the use of Ehrlich's 'salvarsan' (or '606') in the treatment of syphilis, and wondered whether its effects were merely symptomatic, rather than curative. In the discussion which followed his paper (delivered to the Liverpool branch of the BHS), Dr Hare claimed that the action of '606' was 'strictly in accordance with homoeopathic treatment'.[75] Dr Edmund Hughes asked for an explanation - but the discussion records no reply.[76] It would have been interesting to read it.

With the introduction of the sulphonamide drugs in the late 1930s (prontosil and M&B 693) a more promising approach to understanding the action of anti-bacterial drugs in homoeopathic terms was made. It was noted that sulphonamide drugs only possessed a weak anti-bacterial action in vitro, but that their effect was greatly enhanced in the living organism. This prompted Bodman to argue that 'it seems evident from the reports that are accumulating, that this group of drugs has little if any direct lethal action on the cocci, but alters them in such a manner that the natural defences of the body can cope with them'.[77] Thus the homoeopathic principle of advocating therapy which assisted the organism's fight against disease could be preserved even with the introduction of these new remedies. This, together with the proven effectiveness of sulphonamides and, by the 1940s, penicillin, ensured the passage of these drugs into homoeopathic practice where acute infections were encountered. Dr Sundell summarised the attitude of many when he pointed out in 1947 that:

> We must see to it that our judgement is not hampered by habit or prejudice and we must realize that our patient may justly accuse us of a breach of trust if we reject new methods of treatment which though unfamiliar, and based upon conceptions that are opposed to our adopted creed, have proved themselves in other hands to be of value.[78]

The use of sulphonamides and penicillin was, as homoeopaths freely admitted, a confession of failure to find the simillimum. But, as Dr Ross put it 'that is a difficult art and meantime one must save life. Hence sulpha drugs are some-

231

times necessary, but less often since penicillin became available.'[79]

As with previous allopathic developments, homoeopaths were prone to claim that as far as penicillin was concerned, they had (almost) been there first. In 1947, Dr McRae made the point that homoeopaths had been experimenting with penicillium and other similar moulds as long ago as 1935, and had sufficient funds and research facilities been available 'we should have known a great deal more about its adaptability to our practice long ago'.[80]

For homoeopaths, then, the new antibiotics were seen as valuable stand-bys in the emergency of acute infections. But approval was definitely qualified. From the early days, homoeopaths underlined the record of iatrogenic damage, the proneness of patients to repeated infections after antibiotic treatment, and the problem of increasing bacterial resistance. Belief in the safe, gentle and complete cure obtained from the correct homoeopathic remedy remained untarnished.

Confidence in the ultimate superiority of homoeopathic therapy, and the belief that eventually the regular profession would be led to admit it as a result of research and the problems associated with allopathic practice, manifested itself in two related concerns within homoeopathy: first, a desire to highlight homoeopathic elements in regular literature and research and, second, to point up the iatrogenic dangers associated with orthodox medicine.

Homoeopathic belief in the gradual confirmation of their principles by developments in regular practice has already been noted with respect to vaccine and serum therapy. With the introduction of antibiotics, this could be less confidently asserted. Nevertheless, homoeopathic journals throughout the period were keen to scan allopathic literature for more reassuring evidence. 'Emetine' was an early example: used in the treatment of amoebic dysentry, The British Medical Journal had also noted, in 1917, that it could cause diarrhoea. The editor of The British Homoeopathic Journal soon drew this to the attention of readers.[81] Thereafter 'Critical Digests from Medical Literature' became a notable feature of the journal.[82]

From the 1920s onwards, attention was increasingly drawn to the other major factor presaging the hoped for homoeopathic dawn - iatrogenic damage. Partly this was held to be the result of an aggressive pharmaceutical industry and partly, also, of the desire of patients and doctors for easy solutions: patients were morally culpable for not caring more for their own health, and doctors were similarly castigated for opting for the simplification of therapeutics by reflex drug prescription rather than treating the individual patient. Dr Dishington in 1929 despaired that:

Five hundred tons of aspirin are consumed in one year in our country, and to judge from the expensive advertising of other drugs, this sapping of the vitality of our race is a more than ordinary profitable business. Deaths are common from over-dose or from an error in prescribing, yet we are complacent. Today we are living in a dark hour, and this drug consuming is the black spot on the fair page of twentieth-century progress.[83]

The introduction of each new major group of drugs into regular practice came to be evaluated in similar terms.[84] In the early 1960s, after the thalidomide disaster, and in the wake of prolonged experience with antibiotics and tranquillisers, the editor of The British Homoeopathic Journal was driven to observe that 'In Semmelweiss's time hospitals were breeding houses of septicaemia. They are again. Today embryos are being deformed and adults are having all their finer human imaginative faculties atrophied by drugs, sedatives, tranquillisers and the rest.'[85] Following up the point, Dr McAusland demanded: 'What is the matter with us that we need all this doping?'[86] Not very helpfully, he suggested that what was lacking was more self-discipline. But, as his subsequent remarks showed, there was clearly more to the general problem than this. 'We must', he argued:

... prevent medicine from running riot and becoming insane - by over-dosing and by poisoning our fellows: the needless druggery that goes on is wickedly enormous. ... we allow ... dangerous drugs to be consumed in vast quantities. Our foodstuffs are chemically botched up, our water is flouridated. ... There must be much chronic chemical absorption [from food and the environment].[87]

The 'greener' elements in McAusland's remarks introduced a theme - the ecological critique of industrial capitalism - which subsequently assumed greater prominence in homoeopathic writing as the holism of its medical philosophy, particularly when interpreted through the work of Rudolf Steiner, was extended to a macrocosmic level. Further discussion of this issue would be inappropriate here, however. It is taken up again in Chapter Fifteen.

A final topic which merits attention concerns the attitude of the regular profession towards its old rival during this period - especially in view of the rapid therapeutic developments which had taken place since 1900. Only fairly recently have indications of more sympathetic views begun to emerge (see Chapter Sixteen). But there were some sporadic signs of greater tolerance and even interest in earlier years of the century. As the data on BHS membership shows, however, this was not matched by any significant increase in the number of regular converts to the homoeopathic cause.

Things had looked more optimistic in 1932. During that year, The British Medical Journal had indicated that its hostility toward homoeopathy in the previous century was now no longer justified: 'In more recent years a wider view has been taken, and it has been realized that in medicine there is no orthodox doctrine, but that when once a man has obtained a registrable qualification in the usual way he is entitled to hold his own opinions on therapeutics.'[88] This attitude was matched by concrete action. Sir John Weir was invited to present a paper on The History of British Homoeopathy in the Last Century at the centenary meeting of the BMA. In the same year - 1932 - Weir also lectured to the Royal Society of Medicine on An Explanation of the Principles of Homoeopathy. These courtesies were reciprocated: Alexander Cawadias was invited to speak to the BHS on Neo-Hippocratic Tendencies in Modern Medicine.

Briefly, these moves resulted in greater interest in homoeopathy. Attendance at homoeopathic courses rose in 1933 to the point where it was 'greater than could be dealt with efficiently along the lines on which classes have been conducted in the past'.[89] The main reasons for the 'definite desire on the part of the "old school" towards a better understanding of, and with, our own body', were attributed by homoeopaths to the growing realisation of the 'unsatisfactory state of modern therapeutics' among regular colleagues, and to 'the recognition of Homoeopathy in the highest quarters of the land'.[90] Presumably, this latter referred to Royal patronage. At the time, Weir was Physician in Ordinary to HRH the Prince of Wales, and to the King and Queen.

But then came penicillin and its derivatives. Interest waned once more in homoeopathy, and older less tolerant attitudes resurfaced. In one sense, homoeopaths were their own worst enemy. Frank Neubert pointed out the problems from the orthodox point of view in 1946. Homoeopathic case reports, he argued, were too often unsubstantiated by clinical and laboratory evidence; homoeopaths themselves were too prone to pseudo-scientific philosophising in order to explain the simile and the infinitesimal dose; and the school's literature, he felt, was of a quality which generally did more harm than good to homoeopathy's reputation.[91] Some homoeopaths, such as William Gutman, agreed.[92]

The brief thaw of the 1930s was not, then, maintained. By the early 1950s, medical opposition was still sufficiently pervasive to motivate the London University - as already noted - to refuse recognition of the LHH as a teaching hospital, to lead the BMA to prohibit the formation of a homoeopathic section in its ranks, and to encourage the RCP to retain its policy of refusing membership to homoeopaths.[93] Even the LHH, until considerable pressure had been exerted in 1955 by the Management Committee, the Medical Advisory Committee, and the Council of the Faculty of Homoeopathy, had had to advertise, under the constraint of the Regional Hospital Board, for 'Consultants in General Medicine', rather than for 'Consultant Homoeopathic Physicians'.[94] Moreover, a field trial of potentised poliomyelitis vaccine, organised by one homoeopath in 1958, elicited so many objections from local GPs that the Medical Officer of Health concerned was forced to broadcast a warning. Its substance was that the tablets were useless.[95] Despite some evidence of changing attitudes, most doctors would probably still endorse this view in the 1980s. After 150 years the medical legitimacy of homoeopathy remains, as far as the bulk of the profession is concerned, in question.

NOTES

1. See George Burford, 'The International Homoeopathic Council: its Being and Doing', The British Homoeopathic Journal, vol. III (1913), p. 241.
2. John Weir, 'The Present-Day Attitude of the Medical Profession Towards Homoeopathy', The British Homoeopathic Journal, vol. XVI (1926), p. 262.
3. Ibid., p. 263.
4. Percy Hall-Smith, 'Facing the Facts', The British Homoeopathic Journal, vol. XXI (1931), p. 10.
5. Anon., 'Discussion on the Aims and Objects of the Faculty of Homoeopathy', The British Homoeopathic Journal, vol. XXXIV (1944), p. 22.
6. Frank Neubert 'A Constructive Policy for Homoeopathy', The British Homoeopathic Journal, vol. XLI (1951), p. 160.
7. Margery G. Blackie, 'The Future of Homoeopathy', The British Homoeopathic Journal, vol. LX (1971), p. 1.
8. C. Granville Hey, 'The Present Position and Future of Homoeopathy in Great Britain', The British Homoeopathic Journal, vol. XXI (1931), p. 371.
9. See Anon., 'British Homoeopathic Congress', The British Homoeopathic Journal, vol. XXI (1931), p. 395.
10. Edwin A. Neatby, 'Homoeopaths in Birmingham', The British Homoeopathic Journal, vol. XX (1930), p. 183.
11. Philip McK. C. Wilmot, 'Some Details of the History of Homoeopathy in Plymouth', The British Homoeopathic Journal, vol. XX (1930), p. 347.
12. See the list of members names prefixed to: Journal of the British Homoeopathic Society, New Series, vol. XV (1907); The British Homoeopathic Journal, vol. XVII (1927).
13. See the membership figures given in the secretary's report to the Annual Assembly of the BHS: The British

Homoeopathic Journal, vol. XXXIV (1944) at p. 65.
14. See Anon., 'Editorial', The British Homoeopathic Journal, vol. XXXII (1942), p. 57.
15. See the membership figures given in the secretary's report to the Faculty: The British Homoeopathic Journal, vol. XLV (1955), p. 38.
16. See the membership figures given in the secretary's report to the Faculty: The British Homoeopathic Journal, vol. 71 (1982), p. 220 and vol. 72 (1983), p. 244.
17. James Watson, 'The Resources of Homoeopathy', Journal of the British Homoeopathic Society, New Series, vol. XIV (1906), pp. 69-70.
18. Percy Hall-Smith, 'Facing the Facts', op.cit., p. 12.
19. C.E. Wheeler, 'Presidential Address to the International Homoeopathic League', The British Homoeopathic Journal, vol. XXXVII (1947), p. 118.
20. Ibid.
21. Ibid.
22. Anon., 'A Census of Drugs', The British Homoeopathic Journal, vol. VII (1917), p. 307.
23. Percy Hall-Smith, 'An Introduction to a Discussion on Homoeopathic Medical Education and the Provision of Medical Personnel', The British Homoeopathic Journal, vol. XXII (1932), p. 8.
24. Ibid., p. 9.
25. Ibid.
26. John Henry Clarke, 'The Enthusiasm of Homoeopathy', Journal of the British Homoeopathic Society, New Series, vol. XV (1907), p. 18.
27. Stuart McAusland, 'Future Possibilities', The British Homoeopathic Journal, vol. LIV (1965), p. 1.
28. George Burford, 'Homoeopathy: Its Polity and Policy', Journal of the British Homoeopathic Society, New Series, vol. X (1902), p. 23.
29. Ibid., p. 19.
30. Quoted from the memorandum of the Faculty of Homoeopathy by Sir John Weir, 'Presidential Address', The British Homoeopathic Journal, vol. XXXIV (1944), p. 8.
31. See the examination syllabus given in the president's report to the Extraordinary General Meeting of the Faculty of Homoeopathy, The British Homoeopathic Journal, vol. XXXIV (1944), p. 194.
32. See the examination results given in the president's report to the first Annual General Meeting of the Faculty of Homoeopathy, The British Homoeopathic Journal, vol. XXXIV (1944), p. 195.
33. Ibid.
34. Agnes Moncrieff, 'Diploma Examination Syllabus', The British Homoeopathic Journal, vol. XXXVI (1946), pp. 85-6.

35. R. Gordon Smith, 'The Homoeopathic Dose Question', Journal of the British Homoeopathic Society, New Series, vol. XIV (1906), p. 113.

36. Ibid., pp. 113-14.

37. James Stephenson, 'Substances in Dilutions Greater than 10^{-24}, The British Homoeopathic Journal, vol. LXII (1973), p. 3.

38. George Burford, 'The Mathematics of Homoeopathy', The British Homoeopathic Journal, vol. XVII (1927), pp. 20-1.

39. W.E. Boyd, 'Potency Variation', The British Homoeopathic Journal, vol. XXVII (1937), p. 91.

40. See D.S. Rawson, 'A Scientific Approach to Homoeopathy', The British Homoeopathic Journal, vol. LXI (1972), pp. 116-22 and A. Kumar and R. Jussall, 'A Hypothesis on the Nature of Homoeopathic Potencies', The British Homoeopathic Journal, vol. LXVIII (1979), pp. 197-204.

41. W. Bergholz, 'Homoeopathic Dilutions - High Potencies, A Physician's Dilemma', British Homoeopathy Research Group, Communications, No. 13 (February 1985), p. 27.

42. Anon., 'Biological Experiments', The British Homoeopathic Journal, vol. IV (1914), p. 283.

43. W.E. Boyd, 'Biochemical and Biological Evidence of the Activity of High Potencies', The British Homoeopathic Journal, vol. XLIV (1954), p. 7.

44. See James Stephenson, op.cit.

45. Jean Kollerstrom, 'Basic Research into the "Low-Dose Effect",' The British Homoeopathic Journal, vol. 71 (1982), pp. 41-7; A.M. Scofield, 'Experimental Research in Homoeopathy - A Critical Review', The British Homoeopathic Journal, vol. 73 (1984), pp. 161-80. Both Kollerstrom and Scofield mention other literature surveys of potency activity besides that of Stephenson.

46. See Jean Kollerstrom, op.cit., p. 42 and A.M. Scofield, op.cit., p. 161.

47. John H. Clarke, 'Radium as an Internal Remedy in Cancer and Diseases of the Skin, with Provings and Cases', Journal of the British Homoeopathic Society, New Series, vol. XVI (1908), pp. 210-43.

48. Allan D. Sutherland, 'Sulfanilamide - A Fragmentary Proving', The British Homoeopathic Journal, vol. XXX (1940), pp. 286-92. 'Sulphonamide' had made medical headlines in the regular school from about 1935 onwards.

49. See J.R. Raeside, 'A Review of Recent Provings', The British Homoeopathic Journal, vol. LI (1962), pp. 188-96.

50. Johana E.G. Brieger, 'Methodological Obstacles in Homoeopathic Research', The British Homoeopathic Journal, vol. L (1961), pp. 240-1. Original Emphasis.

51. E.K. Ledermann, 'Homoeopathy Tested Against Controls in Cases of Surgical Tuberculosis', The British

Homoeopathic Journal, vol. XLIV (1954), p. 88.
52. Charles O. Kennedy, 'A Controlled Trial', The British Homoeopathic Journal, vol. LX (1971), pp. 120-7.
53. R.H. Savage and P.F. Roe, 'A Double Blind Trial to Assess the Benefit of Arnica montana in Acute Stroke Illness', The British Homoeopathic Journal, vol. LXVI (1977), pp. 207-13, and by the same authors 'A Further Double Blind Trial to Assess the Benefit of Arnica montana in Acute Stroke Illness', The British Homoeopathic Journal, vol. LXVII (1978), pp. 210-22.
54. Robin G. Gibson et al., 'The Place for Non-Pharmaceutical Therapy in Chronic Rheumatoid Arthritis: A Critical Study of Homoeopathy', The British Homoeopathic Journal, vol. 69 (1980), p. 121.
55. D. Reilly and Morag Taylor, 'A Double Blind Placebo Controlled Study Model for Assessing Homoeopathy Using Homoeopathic Mixed Grass Pollens 30C in Hay Fever', Midlands Homoeopathy Research Group, Communications, No. 11 (February 1984), p. 68.
56. R.G. Gibson et al., 'Homoeopathic Therapy in Rheumatoid Arthritis: Evaluation by Double-Blind Clinical Therapeutic Trial', The British Journal of Clinical Pharmacology, vol. 9, No. 5 (May 1980), pp. 453-9, and David Reilly et al., 'Is Homoeopathy a Placebo Response? Controlled Trial of Homoeopathic Potency, with Pollen in Hay Fever as Model', The Lancet, vol. II (1986), pp. 881-5.
57. T.O.R. et al., 'Dr William Ernest Boyd', The British Homoeopathic Journal, vol. XLV (1955), pp. 27-8.
58. Alva Benjamin, 'The Presentation of Our Case', The British Homoeopathic Journal, vol. LV (1966), pp. 218-9.
59. Quoted by Alva Benjamin, ibid., p. 217.
60. Ian Boyd, 'Empirical Medicine versus Rational Medicine', The British Homoeopathic Journal, vol. LX (1971), pp. 21-2.
61. See Sir John Weir, 'British Homoeopathy During the Last Hundred Years', The British Homoeopathic Journal, vol. XXIII (1933), p. 6. Weir uses the term 'mad' to describe the dog: presumably he meant 'rabid'.
62. Ibid.
63. Ibid.
64. Quoted by Sir John Weir, ibid. Since the first virus was not discovered until 1892, Burnett's use of the term is somewhat misleading.
65. C.E. Wheeler, 'A Report on Chronic Intestinal Toxaemias and their Relation to Homoeopathic Prescribing', The British Homoeopathic Journal, vol. XIII (1923), p. 278.
66. Ibid.
67. E. Bach and C.E. Wheeler, Chronic Disease, A Working Hypothesis (H.K. Lewis & Co., London, 1925).
68. See John Paterson, 'The Role of the Bowel Flora in Chronic Disease', The British Homoeopathic Journal, vol.

XXXIX (1949), p. 4.
69. Ibid.
70. See William Lang, 'Perennial Problems', The British Homoeopathic Journal, vol. LIV (1965), p. 85.
71. Ibid.
72. James Johnstone, 'The Evolution of Homoeopathy', The British Homoeopathic Journal, vol. IV (1914), p. 346.
73. Charles E. Wheeler, 'The Scientific Basis of Vaccine Therapy as a Homoeopathic Procedure', The British Homoeopathic Journal, vol. II (1912), p. 358.
74. Edward Bach, 'The Relation of Vaccine Therapy to Homoeopathy', The British Homoeopathic Journal, vol. X (1920), p. 76.
75. Wm. Cash Reed, 'An Introduction to a Discussion on the Treatment of Syphilis', The British Homoeopathic Journal, vol. I (1911), p. 162.
76. Ibid., p. 163.
77. Francis Hervey Bodman, 'The Present-Day Confirmation of the Homoeopathic Approach', The British Homoeopathic Journal, vol. XXIX (1939), p. 6.
78. C.E. Sundell, 'Homoeopathy and Modern Therapy', The British Homoeopathic Journal, vol. XXXVII (1947), p. 259.
79. T.D. Ross, 'Homoeopathy and Modern Therapy', The British Homoeopathic Journal, vol. XXXVII (1947), p. 263.
80. W. Ritchie McRae, 'Presidential Address to the British Homoeopathic Congress', The British Homoeopathic Journal, vol. XXXVII (1947), p. 241.
81. Anon., 'Drug Pathogenesy and Cure', The British Homoeopathic Journal, vol. VII (1917), pp. 305-6.
82. See, for example, Anon., 'Critical Digests from Medical Literature', The British Homoeopathic Journal, vol. XXI (1931), pp. 289-91 and Anon., 'Orientations', The British Homoeopathic Journal, vol. XXII (1932), pp. 90-2.
83. Thomas M. Dishington, 'Presidential Address', The British Homoeopathic Journal, vol. XIX (1929), p. 337.
84. See, for example, Alva Benjamin, 'The World's Present-Day Need for Homoeopathy', The British Homoeopathic Journal, vol. XLV (1956), pp. 182-92.
85. Anon., 'Editorial', The British Homoeopathic Journal, vol. LI (1962), p. 226.
86. Stuart McAusland, 'Presidential Address', The British Homoeopathic Journal, vol. LII (1963), p. 220.
87. Ibid., p. 221.
88. Quoted by Sir John Weir, 'Homoeopathy: An Explanation of its Principles', The British Homoeopathic Journal, vol. XXII (1932), p. 359.
89. D.M. Borland, 'The Present and the Future', The British Homoeopathic Journal, vol. XXIV (1934), p. 6.
90. Anon., 'Editorial', The British Homoeopathic

Journal, vol. XXIII (1933), p. 111.
    91. See William Gutman's reply. 'The Homoeopath Looks at the Orthodox Practitioner', The British Homoeopathic Journal, vol. XXXVII (1947), p. 49, where he summarises Neubert's objections – and agrees with them.
    92. Ibid.
    93. See Alva Benjamin, 'Presidential Address', The British Homoeopathic Journal, vol. XLII (1953), p. 169.
    94. See W. Ritchie McRae, 'The President's Review of the 12th Session', The British Homoeopathic Journal, vol. XLV (1955), p. 5.
    95. See D.M. Foubister, 'Correspondence', The British Homoeopathic Journal, vol. XLVIII (1958), pp. 310-11.

Chapter Fourteen

SOCIAL ISSUES AND POLITICAL CONCERNS

In the nineteenth century, the main opponents of homoeopathy had been the organisations of regular medicine, and its most valuable friends in securing the right to practise had been found in parliament. After 1900 homoeopaths, on occasion, had to struggle with both the profession and government. Legislative initiatives which threatened homoeopathic practice do not seem to have stemmed from any real parliamentary vindictiveness: rather, they seem to have followed from the fact that homoeopathy had been largely forgotten, and when new government measures were being constructed, the implications for homoeopathic practice were simply ignored. The introduction of the NHS was one threat - but the first was Lloyd George's National Insurance Bill of 1911.

Three issues concerned homoeopaths: the threat of exclusion from providing medical services under the new scheme on the grounds that they practised a special system of medicine, the possible elimination of the right to dispense medicines, and the fear of being forced to accept claimants who did not want to be treated homoeopathically. In 1911, the BHS and BHA circulated a letter to the Chancellor of the Exchequer and various members of parliament in which the first two of these worries were forcefully expressed.[1]

Traditionally, homoeopaths had dispensed their own medicines. As the legislation stood, however, no medical practitioner would be allowed to do this, except under exceptional circumstances. Thus where no homoeopathic chemist was locally available to patients, doctors would not be able to prescribe their preferred remedies - unless this particular circumstance could be made to fall under the exceptional clause. This matter, together with the problem of whether or not homoeopaths would be forced to accept patients who wanted regular treatment, was raised by the joint efforts of the BHA and BHS during the passage of the National Insurance Act through parliament. Homoeopaths, however, no longer had to fear complete exclusion from the Act's provisions - any registered practitioner could be included on the lists of doctors prepared by the Insurance Committees. Homoeopaths hoped that careful negotiation with these bodies, who assisted in the administration of the legislation under the Insurance Commissioners, would produce 'some workable solution' of the two remaining difficulties.[2]

In this, they were successful. Negotiations with the Insurance Committees in Doncaster, Northampton, Nottingham, Surrey and the West Riding soon resulted in permission for 'homoeopathic doctors to dispense their own medicines and to receive the capitation grant for doing so, there being no homocopathic chemist on the panel or within two miles.'[3] Moreover, 'At least one Insurance Committee - that of Birmingham - has allowed a homoeopathic practitioner to limit his list of insured persons, thus securing that he shall have none but such as desire homoeopathic treatment.'[4] In the end, the outlook was more promising than had been feared: homoeopaths were confident that other committees could be persuaded to follow the policies which some had already adopted.[5]

While government legislation could potentially restrict homoeopathic practice, it at least did not threaten the physical safety of doctors themselves. The outbreak of war in 1914 introduced this new and alarming possibility. Doctors and nurses from the LHH went to the front to offer their services. Together with the provincial hospitals, the LHH was put on a war footing. Free beds were offered to the armed services, and the BHA organised fund raising to help hospitals equip themselves to meet the new demands imposed by civilian and military casualties. By 1915, grants had been made to eight hospitals taking in British or Belgian wounded.

In the same year, the International Homoeopathic Council inaugurated a movement to establish a hospital in France for the sick and wounded. A meeting of interested subscribers met at the LHH on 12 February under the presidency of Lord Donoughmore: it was informed that preliminary agreement had been reached for the purchase of a suitable hospital building at Neuilly, near Paris. It was proposed that the Board of Management of the new hospital - an Anglo-French-American venture - would have that already running the LHH as a basis. The hospital, after some initial difficulties, opened later that year, with a number of British homoeopaths among its medical staff. Dr Burford was soon able to report that 'The hospital was continually full of French sick and wounded soldiers, about 50 per cent being the latter. The results were uniformly good, and had made a great impression on the French military authorities. There was a strong feeling of desirability for a similar institution nearer the fighting line.'[6] The BHS strongly encouraged its members to volunteer for periods of service at Neuilly in order to maintain a strong British presence: after all, it was the Society's membership which had played a major role in funding the institution and 'It would be a thousand pities if they as British homoeopaths let it slip out of their hands now.'[7]

As reports from doctors who had served at the front and/or treated wounded soldiers in British hospitals make clear, surgery was an obvious essential for many casualties. Homoeopathic remedies were thus largely confined to post-operative treatment. Septic gunshot wounds, for example, were treated with fomentations of calendula; painful amputation stumps with lotions of hypericum (St John's wort); sinuses (burrowing ulcers) with silica 200C; ununited fractures with symphytum (comfrey) 6C and 30C; trench fever with belladonna 30C and gelsemium 30C; and gas poisoning with phosphorus 30C or sulphur 30C.[8]

Though homoeopaths had long regarded themselves as a radical school of medicine, there was definite evidence of cultural lag in other attitudes. They shared a number of traditional prejudices with the regular school during this period. It is impossible to resist mention of Dr Vincent Green's remarks on adolescence, and on women. 'A word', he told the BHS in 1913, 'must be said on the subject of onanism.'[9] Actually, he proceeded to say a great many. The following is an example of his sentiments:

> Apart from the effect upon the individual, which varies enormously, the seriousness of the vice lies in the effect upon the next generation, incomplete maturity of mind and body so often showing itself. It is one of the easiest and most spontaneous of vices, and in very young children is said to be more frequent among girls than boys.[10]

This was curious indeed. Was this last observation mere hearsay, or had Dr Green personally investigated the matter? Besides, it was generally supposed that it was males who had a natural sexual appetite - an appetite which, if unbridled, would lead to debility. The civilised man was sensibly continent. Still, the fragile sexual identity of men has always tended to produce two opposing images of women: the angel, the real woman, who has no sexual feelings, and is no sexual threat, and the whore, the sexually accomplished woman, who is. Men have valued the one, and despised the other, and the need to defend the myth of masculine sexual superiority probably lies at the bottom of both attitudes.

But to return to Green. Onanism, he believed, was encouraged by dummies, thumb-sucking, precocious mental development, hereditary tuberculosis, skin diseases, constipation, irritating urine, laziness and over-eating.[11] Given the responsibility of parents to future generations, the pubescent child should be discouraged from the habit by 'Early rising, cold baths, washing without wiping', and by 'filling up every moment with interests and tasks that are active and absorbing'.[12]

Successfully dissuaded from masturbation, the next problem facing young women was menstruation. This phenomenon, Green argued, 'makes a profound impression on the girl's mind and constitutes a strain upon her mental faculties'.[13] Hence girls should 'do hardly any steady work for a year before and a year after puberty. Their work should be adjusted to the law of their nature.'[14] Moreover:

> reliable data are available which conclusively show that the more scholastic the education of women the fewer children they have, the more severe parturitions, and the less their ability to suckle, which simply amounts to this: Nature has decided that the highly-educated woman is unfit and accordingly, is eliminating her. [15]

There was more to come: 'the feminist who would educate every girl with the view of making her a self-sufficient wage-earner, able to compete with her brother, is breeding temperamental neuters'.[16]

By this time five per cent of the Society's membership consisted of women. There were nine in all. Unfortunately, their reaction to Green's remarks, is not recorded. Like many colleagues in the regular school, however, Green was clearly - if not self-consciously - using medical theory to legitimate established social relationships. Men controlled the world of wage and salary earning, and benefited from the unpaid domestic services of women. There was no reason why things should change as far as men were concerned, especially when the domestication of women was so obviously good for their health.

Gender aside, government moves to promote public health were in everyone's interest. These had begun in the early nineteenth century, stimulated by the cholera epidemic of 1831. Subsequently, the Public Health Service developed in two directions - the establishment of the Poor Law Medical Service, and the passing of various Public Health Acts. These empowered local authorities to appoint a Medical Officer of Health, whose job would be to administer government health legislation. Mainly these laws involved protecting the community from the spread of infection from the sick. Increasingly, doctors became involved in the service. And with the development of postgraduate courses, public health started to become a medical speciality. As one doctor who had recently completed a Diploma in Public Health told the BHS in 1914: 'My opinion is that this study is of the highest possible service to most of us who follow a general line of practice, and that it will become a necessity prior to appointments in more branches of preventive medicine and Government work, &c., than obtains today.'[17]

Soon after the end of hostilities in 1918, a Ministry of Health was created, and a Minister of Public Health appointed. The BHS wished these new efforts in preventive medicine well. It was less than keen on the fact that the Chief Medical Officer's memorandum to the Minister of Health – which outlined the basis of the department's work for the future – omitted to mention Hahnemann in its discussion of important figures in the history of the prevention of disease.[18]

Given Hahnemann's own interest in this work, the Society could do little but applaud moves to improve public health. But its concrete involvement in preventive medicine appears to have been small. As long, it felt, as 'we see multitudes of patients before us ... who desire and need cure', the Society's founding rationale, it felt, would still be required.[19] Prevention was important – but it ought to be left to others, since 'the British Homoeopathic Society stands for the cultivation and development and elaboration of curative medicine as long as it is needed'.[20]

Needed it certainly was. A series of epidemics erupted after the war. In 1918, influenza struck. The mortality rate was severe: in Oxford, for example, it reached 74 per 1000 at its height.[21] Homoeopaths appeared as powerless as anyone else to reduce it. A large increase in venereal cases, caused by the return of infected soldiers, was also feared among the public. Dr Boyd pleaded for 'a serious effort to investigate the result of homoeopathic treatment of both gonorrhoea and syphilis'.[22] It was presumed that homoeopaths would certainly lose all venereal patients to the regular camp unless this was done, as orthodox remedies, such as NAB (Novarsenobillon), were producing 'some startling results'.[23] Nothing, however, seems to have followed from Boyd's exhortation other than an injunction from Dr Goldsborough for doctors to educate the public in the principles of self-restraint.[24]

Homoeopathic response to increasing twentieth century mortality from cancer may be cited as a final example here. In the 1930s the Cancer Commission was established, charged with developing better understanding of the disease and improving forms of treatment. The successes of the nineteenth century, however, could not now be repeated. Then, the superiority of homoeopathic treatment over regular therapy had been clearly demonstrated with respect to epidemics such as cholera. Now orthodox practice had changed, and the profile of disease was gradually being transformed. No doubt homoeopaths scored individual successes with influenza, venereal disease, cancer and the like – but their overall record no longer seemed so obviously better than anything achieved by conventional methods. Valid and reliable statistics could correct this judgement but, if extant for the period, further research than has been possible here would be required to obtain them.

In the nineteenth century, though mesmerists and hydrotherapists had also offered alternative forms of treatment, homoeopathy had certainly been regular medicine's main competitor. After 1900, other therapeutic rivals appeared. Faced with the reality of their own contraction and decline, homoeopaths found themselves unable to extend a warm welcome to these new systems. A Plea for a Thorough and Unbiased Investigation of Christian Science, written by 'an Inquirer' around 1913, received a contemptuous reception: 'The real argument of the book is, that, holding its fundamental assumptions, matter is to be regarded as nothing and disease non-existent.'[25] This was a rather ironic judgement from a school of medicine which itself used non-material doses of medicine.

Edward Bach - whose work on chronic disease with Dr Wheeler has already been noted - also developed, in later years, a phenomenological approach. Heal Thyself, a small book which explained his new position, appeared in the early 1930s. Homoeopathic reviewers were not impressed. Bach, it was argued, had drifted into 'metaphysical speculation and dogmatism'.[26] Again, in view of the latter influences of Steiner on many homoeopaths, this was ironic.

Osteopathy received a scarcely less friendly greeting. One editorial remarked: 'To be a homoeopath is necessarily to be a physician or practitioner of medicine. To be an osteopath is not'; and went on to argue that osteopaths should 'be obliged to go through the mill of a complete curriculum of medical education before being legally qualified to practise ... for the simple reason that diagnosis of the whole case is imperative before any treatment whatever is undertaken'.[27] The point may be well taken, but it was precisely the control over the educational process exerted by the regular profession which represented the principle mechanism for ensuring therapeutic uniformity, and for containing the medical appeal and claims of rival therapeutic systems. The defence of the existing educational process was also, for homoeopaths, a recipe for ensuring their own marginal status within medicine.

In the 1980s, however, a new climate appears to be emerging. Regular practitioners themselves seem to be showing more interest in what are now referred to as 'complementary therapies', and homoeopaths, on the whole, are in favour of eclecticism.[28] A 1982 survey of British homoeopaths found strong support for the use of a range of treatments - including osteopathy, accupuncture, yoga and herbalism - and many doctors had recommended these therapies to their patients.[29]

The 1980s have also seen the continuation of royal sympathy and support for homoeopathy, a tradition the origin of which lies in the nineteenth century with Queen Adelaide

(1792-1849), her niece Princess Mary Adelaide (1833-97), and Queen Mary (1867-1953).[30] In 1918, Dr Weir was appointed physician to King George V and Queen Mary.[31] Later, he was invited to hold the same position for their sons Edward (later Duke of Windsor) in 1923, and George VI, in 1936.[32] In 1951, Queen Elizabeth II continued the tradition of the Weir appointment.[33] He was succeeded in the post by Dr Margery Blackie in 1968, and by Dr Charles Elliot in 1980.[34] Currently, the Queen Mother is patron of the BHA and Queen Elizabeth of the Royal London Homoeopathic Hospital (RLHH) - the prefix having been obtained in 1948 at the instigation of King George VI who himself had become patron in that year.[35]

Homoeopaths have always been proud of their royal affiliations. Those within the regular profession who regard homoeopathic practice as absurd are no doubt thankful that they have not been publicly required to draw the logical conclusion about the mental faculties of the royal family.

One piece of history which the homoeopathic community would probably rather leave in the cupboard concerns the Twelfth International Homoeopathic Congress. It was held in Berlin, 6-15 August, 1937 under the presidency of Dr Rabe and the patronage of Reichsminister Rudolf Hess, Deputy Führer. A number of British delegates, including Dr Paterson, were present. The congress sent 'respectful greetings to Adolf Hitler' by telegram, and wished to 'thank him for the benevolence the Reich government shows to Homoeopathy'.[36] The addresses by Hess himself, by Dr Wagner, head of the German Physicians' Organisation and by Mr Schmierer, head of the German Druggists' Organisation, all contained predictable political messages.[37] The theme of the new German physician, serving the interests of state and people, was prominent. Dr Wagner averred that 'National-Socialist physicians ... do not recognise any form of medical dogmatism. We are ready to adopt what is right and good for our people ...'.[38] No one needs reminding of what this came to mean in practice. Understandably, then, the patronage of Hess is not often referred to in homoeopathic testimonials. The royal family is a rather safer and more respectable advertisement.

With the declaration of the war soon after the congress of 1937, the LHH became part of the Emergency Medical Service involved in the treatment of civilian and air raid casualties. The building itself was severely damaged by bombing. The west wing of the nurses' home and the pathology department were completely lost. Throughout the repeated air raids, and during the actual bombing of the hospital itself, the staff acquitted themselves with great distinction, and won recognition for their efforts in the award of four George medals and one MBE.[39]

Coping with the exigencies of war was a major preoccupation during these years. Thoughts were spared, however, for the period of social, economic and political reconstruction which would follow the cessation of hostilities. Here, increasing anxiety was felt for homoeopathy in the proposed state medical service.

Worries were expressed as early as 1941. Thomas Robertson, noting that homoeopaths were people 'who have been specially filtered out by temperament', and that they were physicians who were 'fundamentally individualistic', feared the survival of medical liberties and freedoms in a system where 'state control of everything and everybody was the rule'.[40] The Scottish branch of the BHS, having listened to these presidential sentiments, subsequently adopted the following resolution: members

> view with anxiety, the trend towards state control, of the General Medical and Hospital Services, and they call upon the British Homoeopathic Society to take steps to define the position of its members and to ensure the continuation of the right of medical men to independent judgement, in matters of treatment.[41]

The first step which the Society took was to write to the Ministry of Health in an attempt to obtain clarification of the position of homoeopathic hospitals in the post-war scheme. In addition, a move was made to quantify the demand for homoeopathic treatment, in order to build up evidence which could be used to substantiate a claim for special consideration. Members were circulated with a questionnaire requesting information on the number of patients they had treated in the three years to 1939.[42] It was at this time, too, that the 'incorporation' movement was initiated. As Dr Miller Neatby put it: 'If we are "incorporated", we get a legal status which should enable us to put some extra ferro-concrete on the homoeopathic "pill-box"'.[43] Clearly, homoeopaths felt that the state system was going to place the movement under seige.

By January 1944, the BHS was still uncertain of the precise implications of the government's plans. At the time, the relevant White Paper had still not appeared. Ernest Brown, however, had - as Minister of Health - made some reassuring noises: any scheme, he had remarked, would necessarily preserve the patient's right of choice of physician, the importance of the personal relationship between doctor and patient, and the doctor's freedom to decide on treatment.[44] But homoeopaths remained nervous. Any state intervention, it was feared, would produce regimentation - and put the unique character of homoeopathic diagnosis and consultation in jeopardy. Specific proposals which were being aired were the cause of further anxiety: matching the supply of physicians by area with demand could prevent homoeopaths from establishing practices in areas which had already been deemed to be adequately serviced by regular practitioners; placing hospitals in particular regions under a central board could force homoeopathic hospitals to adopt a role which would be anathema, and could deprive them of the right to appoint staff; and doctors could be forced to abandon homoeopathic practice if the number of patients which they needed to accept for financial survival under the state scheme was too large.[45]

During 1944, the Society began to initiate moves to obtain recognition within the BMA as a special group. This would have strengthened homoeopathy's claims for special consideration in the profession's negotiations with the government. But despite continuous efforts over the coming years, these hopes were frustrated.

By April 1944, the White Paper had appeared, and some of the 'worst' was known. The Faculty launched on the first of a series of lengthy discussions on the proposed legislation. Dr Paterson initiated the proceedings. There could be little disagreement, he felt, with the general objectives of the scheme. These were set out in paragraph one of the White Paper: in future, people would be ensured of 'all the advice and treatment and care which they may need in matters of personal health; that what they get shall be the best medical and other facilities available', and 'that their getting these shall not depend on whether they can pay for them'.[46] All admirable enough, Paterson felt: the problems for homoeopathy, however, came with the concrete proposals for implementing the scheme. In particular, concern was expressed about the proposed limitation of area from which a general practitioner in the scheme could take patients (people often travelled long distances to secure homoeopathic treatment), about access to homoeopathic consultants (if the general practitioner was to act as a gatekeeper, could patients obtain access to a homoeopathic consultant where regular doctors refused approval?), and about recognition of teaching facilities at homoeopathic hospitals, as the White Paper proposed to focus all consultant and teaching services on the hospital system. This latter was crucial. If homoeopathy was to survive, the legitimacy of homoeopathic teaching and qualifications had to be protected within the new scheme, which meant in turn that the special character of homoeopathic hospitals had to be retained, as well as their right to maintain control over the appointment of staff.[47]

Paterson's view was that homoeopaths would have to fight for the best deal possible within the scheme. To stay outside would mean - since the service was to offer the best service available - that homoeopathy would rapidly appear to be second rate, even quackery.[48] Other contributions to the discussion raised a host of more or less technical issues, and expressed more or less alarm at the future. Subsequently, Dr Julian wrote to his member of parliament, requesting his assistance in clarifying the future of homoe-opathy with the Minister of Health, Henry Willinck. Willinck's reply was, for the most part, sympathetic and reassuring. The BHA, and other homoeopathic representatives, met Mr Willinck's secretary, with much the same result. A meeting was suggested with the Minister himself, with the promise that 'if there was anything in the White Paper against Homoeopathy, it would be considered'.[49]

On 21 November 1944, a deputation consisting of Drs Weir, Bodman and Templeton met the Minister. A memor-andum, consisting of a total of 59 points expressing the principal causes of concern, and main recommendations for the protection of homoeopathy, was presented.[50] The memor-andum proposed that the consent of the Central Medical Board should not be required before a doctor could set up in practice and that homoeopathic physicians and hospitals should be represented on the Central Health Services Council, the Central Medical Board, and the local Health Services' Councils; it pointed out that general practitioners in the scheme would suffer financially because of the relatively small number of patients which they could treat homoeopathically; it argued that the staff of homoeopathic hospitals should be appointed by those institutions rather than have restrictions imposed by the local Health Services Council; that the Faculty's qualification be deemed sufficient for these posts; that homoeopathic physicians did have the right of con-sultancy status; and that homoeopathic hospitals should be recognised as teaching centres.

Though the Minister demurred on the suggestion that the Faculty's diploma was perhaps of a sufficiently high standard for staffing hospitals, the deputation nevertheless felt that they had had 'a very friendly and cooperative hearing, and that the Minister and his advisers appreciated the special difficulties of homoeopathic practitioners, and were anxious to fit them inside the scheme'.[51] At the time, it had seemed to the Minister and his advisers that many of the problems which had been raised were related to the view that Homoeopathy was a speciality, and that 'if Homoeopathy were included amongst the specialities that would solve most if not all our difficulties'.[52] Unfortunately, however, the scheme for specialities had not, at the time, been finalised.

Soon, a new difficulty presented itself. The LHH, striving to cope with the additional financial burden of repairing war damage, was in debt. By 1945, it was living on an overdraft, and Sir Clarence Sadd, the honorary treasurer, launched an appeal to save the institution. As he made clear, it would be disastrous if the hospital was lost when homoe-opathy was already struggling to defend itself within the new health service.

With the end of the government, and the election of a

Labour administration in 1945, it appeared increasingly likely that homoeopathic hospitals would not be allowed to continue as voluntary hospitals within the state scheme - unless a solid case for special treatment could be made. As one editorial made clear, the collection and tabulation of clinical evidence would be an important element here, and members of the Faculty were invited to forward clinical reports.[53] Individualistic convictions of therapeutic superiority had traditionally led to apathy in compiling such data, and the request only highlighted the point.

By 1946, it was clear that the National Health Services' Bill would be passed. As the Act finally stood, it confirmed many of the worries of the previous five years.[54] There was no specific provision for homoeopathic representation on the Health Service's Council, the central body which would advise the Minister on the operation of the service. Voluntary hospitals could not refuse to be incorporated into the scheme. Regional Hospital Boards, with the assistance of universities, would appoint Hospital Management Committees and hospital staff. General practitioners wishing to enter the scheme once in operation would have to apply to the Medical Practices' Committee, which would approve the application only if the number of doctors in an area was deemed inadequate. But Dr Paterson found room for optimism: since homoeopaths could join the scheme, they would need access to homoeopathic hospitals. In turn, these would need to be staffed, which would mean a need for candidates with homoeopathic qualifications, and thus a need for a recognised and legitimate teaching role. Since the Minister was in overall control of the service, he or she would be led logically from the fact of homoeopathic general practice to the defence of homoeopathic hospitals, teaching and qualifications - and the Faculty would no longer be at 'the mercy of the universities or the British Medical Association'.[55] Paterson's evaluation proved to be prescient - in the end, something very like his prediction came to fruition.

On 12 March 1946, a second deputation from the Faculty went to the Ministry of Health. Again, reassuring noises were made: Sir Arthur Rucker 'was not impressed by the difficulties' which the legislation posed for homoeopathy.[56] The Minister, he observed, could direct Regional Boards to appoint Faculty qualified homoeopaths to relevant hospitals. The deputation was also advised that general practitioners could not deny patients an introduction to a homoeopathic consultant if they wished it; that patients would not be prevented from such consultation, or hospital admission, even if it involved travelling to other regions; and that doctors were free to seek financial compensation for the limited amount of homoeopathic health service work which they could realistically do by taking private patients. Subsequently, on 23 May, Mr Bevan, the Minister, gave an 'absolute guarantee' that Regional Boards would be obliged to respect the special character of homoeopathic institutions.[57]

Meanwhile, the BHA had also been active, hoping to impress the Minister with the concerns of the homoeopathic laity. Deputations visited the Ministry of Health in June 1946, and March 1947. Concern was expressed about a range of issues, among them homoeopathic representation on the various bodies established by the Act, and the thorny problem of education.

Here, things had arrived at an inconsistent position. Homoeopathic hospitals were recognised under the scheme, and the Faculty's qualifications were regarded as essential for staff appointments. Hence a strong claim could be made for recognition of the LHH as a teaching hospital. But on this matter the Minister felt compelled to bow to the universities. They would decide which hospitals could be so regarded. And, as already noted, Sir Francis Fraser, head of the British Postgraduate Medical Federation, declined to sanction the Faculty's application for recognition of the LHH by the London University. The old prejudice remained, and was able to bite under ministerial respect for autonomy in matters academic.[58] At the time, the BHA undertook to pressure members of parliament to redress the anomaly.[59] Little headway was, or has been made. Homoeopathy continued to be available through the NHS but, despite further efforts in 1975 and 1979, it remained the one area where training for such provision was not publicly financed.

A few days before the Act came into operation, the Faculty held a final discussion.[60] The president noted that 'the Minister had recognised the Homoeopathic Hospital, has given it the status of a group, with its own Board of Management',[61] and that this was indeed valuable security. The educational issue was still live, however, and the right of doctors to dispense their own medicines - in doubt again, despite the experience of the Lloyd George legislation - was a further worry. Doctors were particularly anxious that they would have to rely on regular pharmacists for homoeopathic remedies.

In the end, consistent political pressure saved the day. When the Faculty met in the following year (1949), the President, Dr Paterson, was able to answer his own question about the position of homoeopathy in the state medical service with the assurance 'that Homoeopathy is accepted under the National Health Services' Act'.[62] The Faculty, he observed, had been granted no privileges 'but it has been given all the facilities which are available to other departments' - excepting in the area of postgraduate education.[63] And in the following year, the independent existence of homoeopathic medicine, teaching and research was finally sealed by the Royal Assent to the Faculty of Homoeopathy Act.

For the general practitioner, however, the NHS was

always to be an inhospitable environment for homoeopathy. The need to maintain a large list of patients in order to secure a reasonable income reduced the amount of time available per patient for all doctors. Consultation times hovered around the five minute mark.[64] Regular practitioners found it difficult to cope. For those attempting homoeopathic work, it was even worse. Even before the NHS, the busy homoeopathic general practitioner found little enough time to develop and use high potency skill with patients - now it was almost impossible. The result was an increasing reliance by homoeopaths on regular medication in health service work - especially the antibiotics.[65]

Though some hope for alleviating this structural problem was seen in the development of computer technology from the 1960s onwards, which could speed up selection of the simile, many homoeopaths continued in mixed practice (i.e. private and public sector work) as a way of preserving homoeopathic skills.[66] A survey of homoeopaths in 1982 found that respondents took almost four times as long over a homoeopathic consultation (a mean time of 41 minutes) as over one where orthodox remedies were to be recommended, that 70 per cent of all respondents (N=189) engaged in private work, and that there was a highly significant difference between the number of homoeopathic remedies prescribed in private versus NHS work.[67]

The political recognition of homoeopathy within the NHS did not, by any means, bring an end to problems. A renewed period of struggle was heralded by the loss of sixteen doctors in an air crash at Staines in June 1972, and by efforts to save A. Nelson & Company, the main UK supplier of homoeopathic remedies, which had run into difficulties, and was up for sale. Two years later, in 1974, the NHS was reorganised. The RLHH lost its group status (and so its independent management committee, as it had been the only hospital in the group), and its endowed funds, which were taken over by the newly created Area Health Authority. This was regarded as a 'political disaster'.[68] Other homoeopathic hospitals were similarly threatened by these new measures. One of them, the Hahnemann Hospital in Liverpool, did not survive. It closed in May 1976.[69]

A subsequent proposal to open a Department of Homoeopathic Medicine in the new Royal Liverpool Hospital was met with great hostility. The doctors concerned expressed their belief that patients, staff and especially undergraduates should not be exposed to unorthodox systems.[70] Mr Tom Ellis took up the matter as a member of parliament, and obtained the acknowledgement that 'homoeopathy was a legitimate form of medical practice' from the Under Secretary of State for Health.[71] This was all very well, but the government remained committed to the view that it could not intercede on matters requiring purely medical decisions.

On these grounds, Ministers refused to bring pressure
to bear on the Council for Postgraduate Medical Education to
release funds under Section 63 of the 1968 Act to support
general practitioner training in homoeopathy. The most that
the Minister, Mr Roland Moyle, could offer in April 1979 was
advice that the Council might reappraise the situation if there
were evidence of sufficient demand.[72] Letters duly arrived
by the bundle. The Council remained unmoved.

During 1978-9, it began to emerge that the future of the
RLHH itself was in danger. The BHA immediately launched a
campaign to publicise the threat, linking it with evidence of
strong demand for homoeopathic treatment, and growing
interest in the system from regular doctors. In March 1979
the support of 230 members of parliament was enlisted for the
'Early Day Motion 449 on Homoeopathy'.[73] This produced a
demand for a debate on homoeopathy in the House of
Commons.[74] Roland Moyle was also invited to attend a
public meeting, chaired by Mr Ellis, in the Grand Committee
Room of the House. Six hundred people attended. A resolution was passed calling on the government to cease its
apathy in the matter of homoeopathy, and to guarantee the
future of the RLHH. Mr Moyle gave the sought for assurance
that the hospital would stay open.[75]

Parliamentary pressure was maintained in July 1979 when
Mr Ellis presented a nation-wide petition, organised by the
BHA, to 'lie upon the table' in the House of Commons. It
contained 116,781 signatures.[76] The text, which urged
parliament to apply pressure on the Secretary of State for
Health to safeguard homoeopathic institutions and to recon-
sider neutrality on the Section 63 issue, was read to the
House.[77] As a result, Mr Ellis obtained an interview with
the new Minister of State for Health, Dr Gerard Vaughan,
persuading him to see the president of the Faculty, and other
homoeopathic representatives. The meeting took place on
8 August, 1979.[78] The Minister afterwards invited the
submission of problems in writing, together with proposed
solutions, and promised further contact.[79]

In the same month, however, the Camden and Islington
Area Health Authority, having been informed by a cost
conscious government to cut its expenditure by two million
pounds, ordered the closure of five of the ten wards of the
RLHH. Frantic attempts to contact the Minister were
frustrated. He was on holiday. The wards were due to be
shut down on 24 September. On the morning of that day the
Minister, having just returned, ensured that the Area Health
Authority received a partial holding order. Only two of the
wards were closed. Once again, the institution had survived.
With a Conservative administration still in office (1987) -
despite its commitment to containing public expenditure - the
immediate future of the hospital now seems reasonably secure.
Royal patronage, after all, is a trump card for homoeopaths

254

in dealing with a 'traditional' Tory government.

But one major - and possibly catastrophic threat - is still on the horizon. According to the Medicines Act of 1968, which came into force in 1971, all proprietary and natural medicines sold to the public must, as their licences fall due for renewal, undergo tests of safety and efficacy. The review of product licences for homoeopathic drugs is due in the 1990s by the Department of Health's Committee on the Review of Medicines.[80] Financing and organising the trials will be a huge problem. If mounted, many homoeopaths will be forced, de jure, to abandon their rejection of randomised double-blind tests. Certainly, any results would testify to the safety of homoeopathic products. Efficacy is another matter. The threat of legislative annihilation is thus accelerating the research effort. In turn, this has thrown into new prominence a basic dialectic within homoeopathy - the dialectic of science and metaphysics.

NOTES

1. The letter is given in Anon., 'The National Insurance Bill', The British Homoeopathic Journal, vol. I (1911), pp. 388-9.
2. See Anon., 'The National Insurance Act and Homoeopathic Practitioners', The British Homoeopathic Journal, vol. III (1913), p. 136.
3. See the letter by W. Lee Mathews et al., 'The British Homoeopathic Association (Incorporated), National Health Insurance Act', The British Homoeopathic Journal, vol. III (1913), p. 382.
4. Ibid., p. 383.
5. Ibid.
6. See the summary of Dr Burford's speech given in the report of the meeting of the British Homoeopathic Society, The British Homoeopathic Journal, vol. V (1915), p. 520.
7. See the summary of Mr Caird's remarks on the hospital given in the report of the meeting of the British Homoeopathic Society, The British Homoeopathic Journal, vol. V (1915), p. 558.
8. See F.J. Wheeler, 'Notes from the Southport Cottage Hospital', The British Homoeopathic Journal, vol. VIII (1918), pp. 58-60.
9. Vincent Green, 'Adolescence', The British Homoeopathic Journal, vol. III (1913), p. 495.
10. Ibid.
11. Ibid.
12. Ibid.
13. Ibid., p. 496.
14. Ibid., p. 497.
15. Ibid., p. 498.

16. Ibid.
17. Conrad Theodore Green, '"D.P.H." Work is of Great use to the General Practitioner', The British Homoeopathic Journal, vol. IV (1914), p. 157.
18. Anon., 'Our Society and General Medicine', The British Homoeopathic Journal, vol. X (1920), pp. 58-9.
19. Anon., 'The Forward Movement of Our Society', The British Homoeopathic Journal, vol. X (1920), p. 148.
20. Anon., 'Our Society and General Medicine', op.cit., p. 59.
21. John McLachlan et al., 'A Discussion on "The Treatment of Influenza and its Complications as seen in the Present Epidemic"', The British Homoeopathic Journal, vol. IX (1919), p. 5.
22. Wm. E. Body, 'Correspondence', The British Homoeopathic Journal, vol. IX (1919), p. 30.
23. Ibid.
24. Giles F. Goldsborough, 'Health: its Promotion by Public Ministry', The British Homoeopathic Journal, vol. IX (1919), p. 57.
25. Anon., 'Review of A Plea for a Thorough and Unbiased Investigation of Christian Science. By an Inquirer. London: J.M. Dent and Sons Ltd.' The British Homoeopathic Journal, vol. III (1913), p. 369.
26. Anon., 'Review of Heal Thyself: An Explanation of the Real Cause and Cure of Disease. By Edward Bach ... The C.W. Daniel Company'. The British Homoeopathic Journal, vol. XXI (1931), p. 183.
27. Anon., 'Osteopathy and Homoeopathy', The British Homoeopathic Journal, vol. XVI (1926), pp. 195, 198. Original italics.
28. On regular interest see, for example, David Taylor Reilly 'Young Doctors' Views on Alternative Medicine', The British Medical Journal, vol. 287 (1983), pp. 337-9.
29. See Phillip A. Nicholls, Homoeopathy and the British Medical Profession: the Sociology of a Medical Pheonix (Unpublished Ph.D Thesis, University of Nottingham, 1984) Table 29, p. 372.
30. See the diagram Anon., 'The Royal Connection', Homoeopathy, vol. 37 (1987), p. 21.
31. See Anon., The Homoeopathic Handbook (Wigmore Publications Ltd., London, 1984), p. 40.
32. See Anon., 'The Royal Connection', op.cit.
33. Ibid.
34. Ibid.
35. Ibid.
36. Anon., 'The Twelfth International Homoeopathic Congress', The British Homoeopathic Journal, vol. XXVII (1937), p. 308.
37. Rudolf Hess, 'Address', The British Homoeopathic Journal, vol. XXVII (1937), pp. 314-16; Dr Wagner, 'Address

by the Head of the German Physicians' Organization', The British Homoeopathic Journal, vol. XXVII (1937), pp. 316-18; Mr Schmierer, 'Address by the Head of the German Druggists' Organization', The British Homoeopathic Journal, vol. XXVII (1937), pp. 318-19.

38. Dr Wagner, op.cit., p. 316.

39. A.C. Young, 'A Short History of the Hospital', The British Homoeopathic Journal, vol. LXI (1972), p. 32.

40. Thomas Robertson, 'Homoeopathy and Post-War Reconstruction', The British Homoeopathic Journal, vol. XXXII (1942), pp. 115, 112.

41. Ibid., p. 117.

42. See the report of the discussion at the meeting of the BHS, 'Post-War Planning', The British Homoeopathic Journal, vol. XXII (1942), p. 87.

43. T. Miller Neatby, 'The Homoeopathic Problem of the Hour - A Rejoinder', The British Homoeopathic Journal, vol. XXXII (1942), p. 126.

44. Sir John Weir, 'Presidential Address', The British Homoeopathic Journal, vol. XXXIV (1944), p. 9.

45. See ibid., pp. 9-10.

46. Quoted by Dr John Paterson. See the report of the 'Discussion on White Paper' at the meeting of the Faculty of Homoeopathy, The British Homoeopathic Journal, vol. XXXIV (1944), p. 122.

47. Ibid., pp. 124-6.

48. Ibid., p. 126.

49. See the report of the discussion on 'The Government White Paper' at the meeting of the Faculty of Homoeopathy, The British Homoeopathic Journal, vol. XXXIV (1944), p. 145.

50. Sir John Weir et al., 'Deputation from the Faculty of Homoeopathy to the Right Hon. The Minister of Health, 21st November 1944', The British Homoeopathic Journal, vol. XXXIV (1944), pp. 202-11.

51. Ibid., p. 210.

52. Ibid.

53. Anon., 'Editorial', The British Homoeopathic Journal, vol. XXXV (1945), pp. 113-14.

54. See the report of the 'Discussion on National Health Services' Bill' at the meeting of the Faculty of Homoeopathy, The British Homoeopathic Journal, vol. XXXVI (1946), pp. 118-29.

55. Ibid., p. 121.

56. See the report on the 'Deputation from the Faculty of Homoeopathy: Impressions of Interview at Ministry of Health March 12th, 1946', given to the meeting of the Faculty of Homoeopathy, The British Homoeopathic Journal, vol. XXXVI (1946), p. 130.

57. Quoted by Sir John Weir, 'Valedictory Remarks on Relinquishing the Office of President of the Faculty of Homoe-

opathy', The British Homoeopathic Journal, vol. XXXVI (1946), p. 149.

58. See the report of the 'Deputation to the Minister of Health of the British Homoeopathic Association', given to meeting of the Faculty of Homoeopathy, The British Homoeopathic Journal, vol. XXXVII (1947), pp. 150-1.

59. Ibid., p. 150.

60. See the report of the 'General Discussion of the National Health Service Act as it Affects Homoeopathic Practice', held at the meeting of the Faculty of Homoeopathy, The British Homoeopathic Journal, vol. XXXVIII (1948), pp. 191-9.

61. Ibid., p. 191.

62. John Paterson, 'Valedictory Address', The British Homoeopathic Journal, vol. XXXIX (1949), p. 223.

63. Ibid.

64. William Lang, 'Perennial Problems', The British Homoeopathic Journal, vol. LIV (1965), p. 87.

65. See, for example, Hugh L. MacKintosh, 'Homoeopathy in General Practice', The British Homoeopathic Journal, vol. XLII (1952), pp. 153-4.

66. For computer initiatives see, for example, Rudolf Pirtkien, 'Homoeopathy and the Computer', The British Homoeopathic Journal, vol. LVII (1968), pp. 140-3.

67. See Phillip A. Nicholls, op.cit., Table 35, p. 291; Table 22b, p. 345; Tables 33 and 34, p. 388.

68. M.C. Barraclough, 'Quis Seperabit?', The British Homoeopathic Journal, vol. 69 (1980), p. 58.

69. Ibid., p. 59.

70. Ibid., pp. 59-60.

71. Quoted in ibid., p. 60.

72. Ibid., p. 61.

73. Anon., 'News from the Faculty and the Trust', The British Homoeopathic Journal, vol. 69 (1980), p. 118.

74. See Phillip A. Nicholls, op.cit., p. 399.

75. Ibid., p. 400.

76. Anon., 'News from the Faculty and the Trust', op.cit., p. 118.

77. Ibid.

78. Ibid., p. 119.

79. Ibid.

80. See Anita E. Davies, 'The Media and Homoeopathy', British Homoeopathy Research Group, Communications, No. 14 (August 1985), p. 1.

Chapter Fifteen

MAKING IT MYSTICAL - THE METAPHYSICAL FACE
OF HOMOEOPATHY

From the very beginning, homoeopathy has been Janus faced.
In one direction it has looked towards scientific inquiry and
empirical proof, in the other, towards religion, metaphysics
and mysticism. The origin of this dialectic lies in the double
orientation of Hahnemann's original work: while claiming
serious consideration as a rational system of therapeutics
based on the observed effects of drugs in health and disease,
it also advanced a metaphysical theory of illness and of the
action of medicines.

Put this way, however, the question is posed rather
than answered, for the problem remains of accounting for the
scientific-metaphysical axis within Hahnemann's writing itself.
A number of factors seem to have been involved here.

Firstly, Hahnemann himself had powerful religious convictions.[1] These had helped to focus the basic therapeutic
problem - how to heal the sick - in metaphysical terms. For
Hahnemann, it was a 'shameful blasphemous thought! .. that
the wisdom of the Infinite Spirit animating the universe would
not be able to create means to relieve the sufferings of
diseases which He, after all, allowed to arise'.[2] Remedies,
then, there must be for people's ailments. The problem was to
find them, and to apply them correctly. God had given people
the intelligence to solve the riddle. So far, doctors had
failed. Hahnemann, however, believed that through rational
experimentation he had discovered the answer. Similia
similibus could thus be seen not merely as an empirical
principle, but as a Divinely ordained law of cure. And the
power of the 'Infinite Spirit animating the universe' could be
unlocked by potentising medicines in a way which would allow
them to affect the vital force which animated people in health
and disease. Homoeopathy, then, laid strong claims for
clerical sympathy. As has been seen, they did not go
unanswered.

Secondly, it needs to be remembered that Hahnemann
lived at a time when German idealist philosophy was in its
ascendancy. Among the major philosophical figures which

Hahnemann could count among his contemporaries were Schelling (1775-1854), Fichte (1762-1814), Goethe (1749-1832), Hegel (1770-1831), and Kant (1724-1804). German thinkers strove, as Shryock put it, to 'create constructive philosophies that would at once bring all of art and all of science within the compass of an idealistic Weltanschauung'.[3] These efforts affected many areas of academic endeavour in German universities, and medicine was not excepted.

The Naturphilosophie of writers such as Schelling and Goethe was particularly important. Their influence helped to produce a situation where physiological research was conducted with philosophical intent. Johannes Müller (1801-58), for example, felt that 'physiology and philosophy must be made one', and that the objective of physiology was to 'study living phenomena as a whole, in terms of a grand concept of life which unified and gave meaning to the data of experience.'[4] Though Muller subsequently recorded many outstanding achievements in medical research, he never lost his Naturphilosophie conviction that biological phenomena were irreducible to matters of physics and chemistry. Life in all its forms had a purposeful nature: it was possessed of some innate vitalistic principle.[5]

To what extent this intellectual climate directly affected Hahnemann is hard to say. But the idealist concept of a universe which was purposeful, meaningful, teleological and, above all, vitalistic, resonates as strongly with Hahnemann's work as it contrasts with more mechanical and materialistic cosmologies. Moreover, the problem of explaining potency energy within this latter paradigm has periodically created more or less dissatisfaction among homoeopaths with a 'soulless' view of the universe, and has sometimes resulted in outright hostility to the imperial claims of scientific method as epistemological arbiter (and also to the destructive effects of unchained reason on the integrity of the environment).

A third source of metaphysical currents within homoeopathy may be traced via German freemasonry and Rosicrucianism, to the alchemy of Paracelsus.[6] Hahnemann himself was a mason, and it seems clear that masonic societies in Germany had a strong historical affiliation with alchemy. According to Lenning and Mossdorf the lodges were 'only a modern reshaping of the societies which dropped the deprecated names of the alchemists in order to appear in a new dress'.[7] Certainly, strong similarities exist between Hahnemann's work and that of Paracelsus. Hahnemann, though, does not acknowledge the connection, and it could be that a masonic pledge of secrecy accounts for the fact.[8]

The connection between alchemy and freemasonry was strengthened by Rosicrucianism. The Rosicrucians broke into freemasonry in the second half of the eighteenth century and, as Withers remarks, it appears 'that Hahnemann's own initiation coincided ... exactly with the period of upsurging

THE METAPHYSICAL FACE OF HOMOEOPATHY

Rosicrucian influence'.[9] Again, there was a Paracelsian presence in Rosicrucian doctrines, and it seems unlikely that Hahnemann could have avoided noticing it.

But what was the Paracelsian-homoeopathic connection? For Paracelsus, all the possible diseases which could afflict people (collectively, the iliadus, to use his term) were the product of three fundamental materials or principles - salt, sulphur and mercury. Withers takes up the story from there:

> ... the iliadus was thought to be a reservoir of potential forms in which all the different elements in man were assimilated. Provided these elements were integrated correctly, health was ensured. Under these circumstances, none of the individual elements would be visible. In ill-health, however, one of them breaks loose from the iliadus and can be seen. The resultant disease is then presented in the image of the unbound element. This element itself corresponds to an external element in nature. Thus the disease may appear in the form of a specific mineral or substance. It is from this same substance that a remedy can be prepared to cure the disease homoeopathically.[10]

Moreover, Paracelsus believed 'that man contained within him (the microcosm) all the forms of external nature (the macrocosm)'.[11] This 'enabled the physician to gain knowledge of both remedy and patient through what he called "experience" ... The key to this mode of experience lay in the outward characteristics of the remedy, which were thought to reveal something of its inward properties.'[12] These properties were grasped more intuitively than rationally, or deductively. Hahnemann himself was dismissive of this 'doctrine of signatures', but, ironically, many latter-day homoeopaths - especially in the second half of the twentieth century - have returned to it under the influence of the microcosm-macrocosm idea, and the work of writers such as Jung and Steiner.[13] The result has been the appearance of heavily symbolic, almost mythological, drug pictures where remedies - such as sepia (cuttle-fish ink) - are described less in terms of provings, than 'understood', or imaginatively felt, in terms of the form and function of the organism or mineral from which they have been derived. In this way, homoeopathic medicines have come to be seen not merely as pharmacological chemicals, but also as agents derived from a vitalistic and meaningful universe, whose use can be discovered by imaginative reflection, based on teleological convictions about the cosmological significance of structure. Gynaecological analogy, for example, indicates the therapeutic domain of mollusc remedies. Sepia turns into a female medicine. As Dr Twentyman put it: 'It was not accidental that Venus came ashore in a scallop shell.'[14]

More of this later. At present, it is more important to follow
up the connection between homoeopathy and the occult in the
nineteenth century.

Though Hahnemann himself was dismissive of Paracelsian
influence, others were less shy of the connection. The
Hermetic Order of the Golden Dawn - a magical society - was
founded in 1888 by Dr Wynn Westcott. A number of British
homoeopaths were members. The order was Rosicrucian - and
so linked to alchemy, to medicine and to Paracelsus.

The Rosicrucian Manifestos had been published in
Germany in the early seventeenth century. They supposedly
described the career of Christian Rosenkreutz, a German
monk who had acquired alchemical and medical knowledge
during Eastern travels. On his return, Rosenkreutz had
formed a secret brotherhood. His writing, together with
contributions from other members of the movement - and also
from Paracelsus - was buried with him in a secret vault when
he died. The discovery of the tomb led to the publication of
the Manifestos and, indirectly, to the formation of the Golden
Dawn Order the following century.

Rosenkreutz had been a physician, and Rosicrucians
were supposed to earn a living by practising medicine. It was
not surprising, therefore, that doctors interested in
Paracelsus and the occult joined Wescott's society. Many were
also interested in homoeopathy. Of these, Dr Edward Berridge
was the most prominent. His short-lived journal, The
Organon, and its reception by the Hughesian camp, have
already been noted in Chapter Eleven.

It was through the Golden Dawn Order - or rather
through its breakup - that homoeopathy was led to its first
connection with Steiner. Unfortunately, Dr Westcott had
forged the particular Rosicrucian documents on which the
society had been founded. When this became clear, it dis-
integrated. But Dr Felkin, convinced that a true coterie of
savants must exist somewhere, began a series of travels
throughout Germany in order to try to discover them. This
eventually led him to Steiner. The founder of anthroposophy,
however, was none too receptive, and refused to make Felkin
his British representative. Nevertheless, this first contact
eventually bore fruit though not, apparently, through the
efforts of Felkin. Steiner's work bore a similar metaphysical
and mystical stamp to that of Paracelsus, and many homoeopaths in Britain later came to see anthroposophy as a new
way of interpreting homoeopathy which would rescue it from
stagnation, and save it from the dismissive claims of materialistic science.[15]

However, even before Steiner's work had begun to
fertilise (or corrupt, depending on the point of view adopted)
British homoeopathy, another metaphysician had penetrated,
and helped to recast Hahnemannian doctrine - Swedenborg.

Emmanuel Swedenborg (1688-1772) - whose country of origin needs no elaboration - was a person of many talents. He was, variously, a politician, an engineer, a scientist, and a philosopher. He was also a mystic and a clairvoyant, who believed himself to be in contact with a spirit reality denied to ordinary people. Like Steiner afterwards, Swedenborg's philosophy has to be understood in terms of claimed paranormal abilities to contact an extra-sensory reality.

No attempt will be made here to give a complete summary of Swedenborg's work. It would be misplaced and, perhaps more pertinently, less than circumspect for the writer to do so. Some indication, however, of his major concerns, and of those elements of his ideas which seem to be of importance as far as homoeopathic thought was concerned, are called for.

Two main foci of interest for Swedenborg were the nature of the physical universe, and the nature of people. He explored both issues in a way which materialist philosophers would find anathema. His approach was teleological, and turned on discovering the purpose in creation. Swedenborg's account of the origin of the universe is rooted in a complex mathematical analysis of the creation of matter from motion and points of force under Divine guidance. The next philosophical task - developing an understanding of that most complex of creations, people themselves - was predicated on the solution of the first. By pressing into service the 'doctrine of use', Swedenborg hoped to ascend from anatomical study to a knowledge of the immaterial principle which governed the physical body. The end-product of all this was a conception of the soul as spiritual in form, given life by the Creator, operating via the mind, and permeating the whole of the organism. The soul was able to effect the body through the mediation of an immaterial spiritual fluid or force, derived from the original motion from which universal matter was derived. This 'fluid' was physically omni-present, receptive to life, and gave life to tissues.

Just as each stage in the derivation of matter itself was understood as a formative descent of higher degrees of reality to lower, so the soul was held to create and inform the building of the body. The two processes were parallel, and everything in the material universe - minerals, air, fluids - was represented in the physical composition of the organism. The blood itself Swedenborg called the 'corporeal soul', as the body received nourishment from it. Above all these processes was the guiding influence of Divine wisdom.

Gardiner summarises as follows:

> It will be seen that this philosophy involves a descent of the infinite by a series of degrees of modification ... until matter is produced ... Influx from the higher degrees into the lowest can then mould these latter into living forms, the last and highest of which is the human

form. When this is complete the soul can dwell in it fully and influx then proceeds directly through the soul and mind into the living body. The ultimate end of every created thing is Use. Nothing is formed that is not of use, and the form given to each .. is most perfectly adapted to the use it has to perform. These uses are not performed in watertight compartments, but interact with each other throughout the created universe. There is a mineral atmosphere, a vegetable atmosphere, an animal atmosphere, and a human atmosphere, each acting and reacting on the others by a universal influx from the Infinite for its end of use, and this is the cause and origin of the equilibrium, stability and order of the cosmos. In his later theological works, Swedenborg describes how the heavens are maintained in the same equilibrium, and his influx of the Divine Power (which is Divine Love) through the heavens descends through corresponding degrees there, and how there is a correspondence between all things in heaven with those of the material universe, and that it is this influx that is the ultimate cause of the creation of the infinite variety of forms ... [16]

The response of the sceptic to this cosmogony and cosmology is obvious enough. Specifically, there seem to be no compelling reasons why Swedenborgianism has any higher claims to serious consideration than any similar system. If it is accepted, it has to be accepted as a matter of faith. Here, however, its philosophical coherence is less a matter of concern than highlighting the ideas which homoeopaths found attractive. In Swedenborg's scheme, the universe appears as a dynamic entity, permeated by a Divine force which gives meaning and structure to the material world, and finds expression in the transubstantiation of Idea into purposeful forms. It is a cosmology of vitalism, teleology, and of correspondence, where the individual microcosm mirrors the macrocosm and stands at the pinnacle of the heirarchy of forms impressed from Divine Idea. In short, it is a sort of Platonic and Aristotelian reinterpretation of Genesis - which is exactly what the psychic sensitivity of Swedenborg had revealed it ought to be.[17]

A church, founded to celebrate and promulgate Swedenborg's teaching, was established in Britain after his death. This 'New Church' rapidly fragmented into a number of sects: on export to America, the doctrine underwent the same process. By the late eighteenth century, however, Swedenborgianism had taken root in several American cities. When homoeopathy also emerged, the two systems found a natural complement in each other. Swedenborgians welcomed Hahnemannian vitalism, and homoeopaths found in Swedenborgianism a metaphysical system which made cosmological and religious sense of Hahnemann. Potentisation was an obvious candidate for reinterpretation as a reversal of the Swedenborgian energy to matter thesis, while the doctrine of use and of correspondence buttressed the appeal and divine status of the medical simile.

Indeed, many of the leading American homoeopaths in the nineteenth century were Swedenborgians - most notably, Hans Gram and Constantine Hering. Boericke and Tafel - the leading homoeopathic drug manufacturers and publishers - was also owned by Swedenborgians.[18]

But in Britain, despite the more mystical leanings of Dr Berridge and others, the dominant homoeopathic orientation at this time was pragmatic, scientific and empirical. This was nowhere better exemplified than in the work of Hughes and Dudgeon, which distanced itself from those very qualities and aspects of Hahnemann's work which Swedenborgianism found attractive. Only when the sociological climate was more propitious - a climate born of therapeutic convergence, homoeopathic decline, and the need for a more distinctive doctrine as a banner for sectarian survival - did Swedenborgianism find a more receptive audience. The American James Tyler Kent (1849-1916) was the intermediary in this process and, as noted, Drs Margaret Tyler, Weir and Gibson Miller were the main protagonists of Swedenborgain homoeopathy in Britain. It was not long before Hughesian orthodoxy was routed.

The distinctive and dogmatic quality of Kent's approach has already been illustrated. Its high potency prescribing was instilled with a fervour born of missionary certainty, and a new moralistic twist to a revivified theory of chronic disease was linked to Hahnemann's miasm theory. Swedenborg's view that the human body was the physical expression of a soul which guided the pressing of immanent form into matter allowed his homoeopathic followers to see disease as the blight of a corrupted spirit. Disease was a moral as well as a physical problem, and treatment of the mind and soul an integral aspect of the therapeutic endeavour (hence the emphasis on mental symptoms in Kentian homoeopathy).

The three miasms of which Hahnemann had spoken were 'syphilis', 'sycosis' - both venereal infections - and 'psora', really any kind of itchy skin eruption whose remittence or suppression later manifested itself by accounting for some seven-eighths of all forms of chronic disease. And, as Campbell explains, whereas 'For Hahnemann the miasms had been acquired "infections" ... for the Swedenborgians they were moral taints passed from generation to generation, and psora in particular took on some of the characteristics of Original Sin.'[19]

Though Kent makes few explicit references to Swedenborgianism in his writing, he was nevertheless prone to the pedagogic averral that the principles of the Organon were in

perfect accord with this philosophy. Kent's principal works -
Lectures on Homoeopathic Philosophy, Lectures on Homoeopathic Materia Medica, and the Repertory of the Homoeopathic
Materia Medica - do not show him to have been a particularly
attractive character.[20] The dividing line between the confident, caring physician, and the dogmatic authoritarian,
moralistic preacher, was often breached, and the metaphysical
inspiration of his thought frequently obtrusive.[21] For Kent,
homoeopathy was religiously ordained, religiously inspired,
and disease appeared as the physical retribution of a moral
order transgressed by the thoughts and actions of the
corrupt. In short, Kent would have made Karl Popper -
whose epistemological defence of the 'open society' and of
critical rationalism has had a profound effect on the
philosophy of science in this century - blanch.[22] It is
doubtful whether even Kent could have found a remedy to
restore his colour.

Yet Kent's work was eventually victorious in Britain.
Faculty members were expected to study it in order to qualify
and, as Dr Mitchell observed in 1976, 'We [Kentians] are now
the official voice of British homoeopathy, and, ... we
sincerely believe ourselves to be the chosen people who are
correctly interpreting Hahnemann's teaching.'[23]. The
'chosen people' had been fortified in a long period of
stagnation by the prop of Kentian certainty, and the more
immediate quality of his drug pictures, but there is no doubt
that the therapeutic arrogance which was its inevitable
accompaniment helped to perpetuate isolation, and to stultify
research.

This heady metaphysical brew was given a further twist
by those homoeopaths who turned to the work of Rudolf
Steiner (1861-1925) and his school. Like Swedenborg, Steiner
was clairvoyant (or claimed to be), and used these powers to
penetrate beyond the normal sensory world to discover and
describe a 'higher' reality. The result was the system known
as 'anthroposophy', in which the alchemical orientation of
Paracelsus, the theory of formative influences, and the
doctrines of correspondence and use, were revitalised. The
BHS seems to have been first addressed on the work of
Steiner by Dr James Turner in 1939.[24] From 1960, the
anthroposophical position became increasingly prominent in the
Faculty's journal.

Steiner wrote and lectured widely. Those who are
interested in a comprehensive picture of his particular metaphysical trip - and the author must confess a reluctance to
be among them - are recommended to contact the Anthroposophical Association.[25] All that can be done here is to
note a few influential ideas.

Steiner had originally been a follower of theosophy - a
movement founded in the second half of the nineteenth
century which accepted the idea of 'prana', or life energy.

He split with theosophy in 1909, and founded the Anthroposophical Society: Steiner meant the term to stand for
'awareness of one's humanity' or spirituality.[26] Though not
medically qualified, he nevertheless went on to write on the
therapeutic implications of his system. A number of books
appeared - among them The Anthroposophical Approach to
Medicine.[27]
    It is perhaps as well to begin with Steiner's concept of
the person. This consisted of a physical body, an etheric
body (a system of formative forces), an astral body (emotions
and drives) and an ego (self-consciousness).[28] Possession
of the latter distinguished people from animals.
    Conventionally, life is held to have emerged (somehow)
from the chemical and physical material and properties of the
universe. Steiner reverses this formula. According to Engel
'The whole evolution of the earth, with all its complicated
developments, is regarded as a process of materialization of
spiritual forces. This process may take place either directly,
or, more typically, through the agency of living organisms.'[29] Thus, as far as people are concerned, it would be
the etheric body which governed the deposition of tissue and,
through a process of materialisation, the structure, form and
function of organs. Immediately, then, it becomes possible to
see homoeopathic potentisation as a reversal of this 'spirit
into matter' formula (we have been here before): thus the
etheric forces of plant remedies can be released to exert a
spiritual effect.[30]
    Though Steiner conceded that conventional pathological
investigations were useful, he argued that disease and remedy
needed to be studied together. The key here was to recognise
the relationship between physiological and pathological processes, and their counterparts in the natural and spiritual
worlds. An example helps to clarify matters. A patient
suffering from anaemia may have the symptoms suggestive of
the homoeopathic remedy ferrum met. Engel takes up the
story:

> But a reflection on what iron does in nature, the import-
> ance of iron to human endeavours, in industry, for
> example, or in warfare; the kind of spiritual forces out
> of which iron has materialized; all these considerations
> can tell us more than the microscope and the haemo-
> globinometer. They can tell us that iron draws the
> human ego down to earth in a particular way, and helps
> the spiritual nature of man to work through the power of
> his will, and to make his mark on the earth.[31]

The therapeutic application of remedies can thus be
understood by an anthroposophical appreciation of their
origin, form and function in nature. And since 'the same
spiritual forces that have become material in the evolution of

man have also materialized elsewhere in nature', and since a
kinship exists 'between certain processes in the human
organism and certain substances in nature', the medical simile
is deduced as the law of cure.[32]

We have been here before too ... Steiner's work licensed
the mystical, imaginative, dynamic description of remedies,
and the law of correspondence, in the same way as that of
Paracelsus and Swedenborg. It is really nothing more than a
sophisticated version of the magical simile, and the doctrine
of signatures, all over again.

Steiner supported homoeopathy, and hoped that his work
would help to develop the system. He suggested new remedies
(such as iscador - mistletoe - for cancer), new ways of
potentising remedies - in particular, through using the
medium of living organisms, such as plants - and the use of
remedies in combination or in unpotentised form (the body
would do the rest).

The anthroposophical influence appears to have been
powerful enough, according to Dr Mount, to promote a degree
of conflict at the RLHH in the 1970s.[33] Dr Rose felt, in
1981, that it was highly off-putting to regular doctors who
attended the Faculty's courses to find themselves confronted
with anthroposophical work: it would, he predicted, lead to
an atrophy of new recruits, and drive homoeopathy into the
hands of the unqualified.[34]

There is no doubt that, under the editorship of Dr
Twentyman, The British Homoeopathic Journal became increasingly sympathetic to anthroposophically inspired views and
articles. Some quotes from the editor are worth recording to
give the flavour of the period:

Nature ... calls to our souls for a solution to its riddle
in terms of meaning and significance. All outer natural
processes find themselves again within our organisms and
whereas they appear separated, exteriorized and
analyzed outside in Nature, they are to be found
interiorized and synthesized within us. We are the
wholes whose parts are spread out around us in Nature.
When we seek for significance it is the relationship of
parts to the whole which will reveal it to us.[35]

Another 1974 piece argued in a similar vein:

It should be possible to study a metal, for instance,
more fully when we have learnt to know its manifestations in Man, in his soul and spirit and physiology.
From the metal as known in the human sphere it should
be possible to interpret its nature down to its appearance within the mineral kingdom as well. What I am
proposing is to reverse the habits in which we have
been overeducated. The more perfect expression or

revelation of the metal will be manifest in the human realm. The lower can be understood from the higher, but the higher cannot be explained from the lower. ... Then we must try and re-establish the knowledge of soul forces as real agents, and observe how they express themselves firstly in our own organisms but also physiognomically in animals. Ferocity has built the Tiger, cunning the Fox, timidity the Rabbit ... In this way we can relearn how qualities, emotions, thoughts act into and within the whole organic realm and observe them in their objective operation as well as in our subjectivity. When we have discovered the correspondence between an innerly experienced emotion or qualitative reality and its activity in Nature our knowledge takes a real step forward and the world begins again to sing with meaning. We must, in short, school ourselves to recognize the same melody in its various manifestations or metamorphoses, in Nature, in Man and even again in the Cosmos.[36]

A third, and rather earlier example, may perhaps be permitted. The year is 1961:

The real essence of biology is form and function. One cannot explain the physiognomic form of a tiger by natural selection, nor the multitudinous mysterious patterns of behaviour that natural history has unveiled. Function creates organism and organ. Function precedes, and we confirm this every time we use restoration of function to speed a healing process. We know today, from radio-activity that so-called matter is only the frozen forces of the cosmos, and we should recognize also that organs and organisms are condensed functions, processes, or uses. Gradually we can begin to see that Man is the only complete organism and that other natural forms are fragments or partial organisms or organs, and a certain absurdity becomes apparent in expecting to solve the problems of human biology by microscopic cellular research. Man himself is a macroscopic cell, in which we can observe with our unaided senses the cellular processes, and in him alone a real wholeness manifests.[37]

Reading through the journal during this period is a surreal experience for the outsider. It is like entering a different world. People become a kind of metaphysical Russian doll, in which the mineral, plant and animal kingdoms are all represented; remedies are understood in terms of armchair speculation related to the principles of correspondence and use; and the world is a place of magical, astrological and symbolic influence. As one editorial put it:

... homoeopathic drug pictures are graspable as symbols and the homoeopathic remedies are real living symbolic powers which heal and unite the divided functions. In saying this, one runs the danger today that one is implying that a homoeopathic remedy is only eye-wash, and acts only, as placebo also acts, as a medium for the symbol-dominated doctor-patient relation. If, however, Nature herself works imaginatively and her forms are living, real symbolic powers, then the remedy becomes when intuitively chosen a perfect medium of the healing forces. [38]

The work of Dr Hélan Jaworski, Dr Karl König, and Wilhelm Pelikan, which figured prominently in the journal during this period, indicate all these anthroposophical tendencies. [39]

König, in what was meant to be a quite serious discussion of diabetes, wrote:

... the regular process of menstruation is the living memory of that cosmic event which Rudolf Steiner describes as the expulsion of the moon from the earth. Something which happened once to the whole of the earth repeats itself monthly, so that the female organism undergoes a constant softening process which keeps it as 'heavenly' as possible. For that reason menstruation occurs in a 28-day rhythm, this being the period of a moon cycle.

It now becomes obvious [sic] why in women latent diabetes does not manifest in the acute form before the menopause; through the cessation of the monthly period the hardening forces of hereditary dispositions become so powerful that they lead to the outbreak of the disease. [40]

König also illustrated the anthroposophical approach to embryology. The 'spiritual germ', he said, comes 'from the all-embracing vastness of the universe', and:

... getting smaller and smaller as it passes through the spheres of the planets, gathering itself through Saturn, Sun, Mercury and Venus, arrayed in astral body and spiritual germ, the Ego, or I, enters into the sphere of the Moon. And there, at the moment of physical fertilization, the spiritual germ drops away from astral body and ego. This creates a vacuum and causes another group of beings, the original Teachers of mankind who dwell on the Moon, to weave an ether-body for this human being, putting it together from light and warmth, sound and life. [41]

This metaphysical and astrological language also informed the understanding of drugs. Dr Turner, for example, presented the therapeutic indications of copper and tin as follows:

> Copper related to the sulphur in the bowels of the earth, and related in us to sulphur which inflames the metabolic system, and tin related to silica in nature, and related in us to silica and the form-giving force, copper and tin, Venus and Jupiter, are the two sculptors who mediate between the flaming metabolic system and will on the one side, and the freezing form-giving and thinking nervous system on the other.[42]

These bewildering views were compounded by other propositions: the heart, for example, was held to be an organ of balance; blood had the power of spontaneous movement; the liver was the organ of depression; and cancers were displaced sensory organs.[43]

Dr Twentyman's argument that the study of soul forces should involve their expression in animals was buttressed by a series of articles on animal symbolism – of the bee, the toad, the tortoise, the dog, slugs, snails and the crab.[44] Other articles discoursed on radiesthesia as a diagnostic technique and its relation to potency energy and selection, on colour as a healing agent, and on disease and reincarnation.[45] To this, many readers were no doubt receptive. One survey, published in 1962, had already established that eighty per cent of British and American homoeopaths who had graduated from regular medical schools belonged to religious minorities and/or believed in reincarnation.[46]

One further current in homoeopathic thought during this period should be mentioned – Jungian analysis. The holistic perspective had always suggested reciprocal relations between mental and physiological disease. Moreover, Jung's theory of archetypes could be pressed into service on behalf of the doctrine of correspondence.[47] Since Jungian analysis held that mental disorders could be traced to the repression or malintegration of archetypal ideas within the patient's psyche, homoeopathic symptom taking could be seen as a process which assisted the patient to come to conscious terms with the problem. In short, symptoms could be seen as a symbolic representation of the repressed archetype itself, and the remedy – its correspondent in the natural world – as a mirror in which patients could see themselves. Acceptance of the remedy was thus a process of self-recognition which would restore archetypal harmony, and relieve mental and/or physiological distress.[48]

A sense of confusion at the results of Steiner's influence on homoeopathic thought is justified. Straightforwardly, it is confusing to anyone unaccustomed to his approach. This certainly includes the author, who is unable to take it seriously (and who, moreover, feels that this does it no great disservice): nevertheless, apologies are due for any mis-representation which has occurred as a result of frustration experienced in reading the material.

One positive result of Steiner's work, however, was a sharpening of homoeopathic consciousness about the patho-logical effects of science and technology in the modern world. Sometimes this was also conjoined with a recognition of the feminist point that a full explanation of this phenomenon must take on board the fact that science is a predominantly masculine activity.

The reasons for this 'greening' of homoeopathic thought are not difficult to find. People were, anthroposophically, the expression of a living and vital cosmos, in which the whole creative process was represented. Microcosm and macrocosm were intimately connected. And the 'self-awareness' of which Steiner spoke in coining the title of his school involved recognition of this fact, and recognition by people of their spiritual and emotional, as well as rational, complexity. Science and technology, on the other hand, represented disembodied reason. Dismissive of the spiritual dimension of people, of holistic perspectives, and of the idea of a vitalistic cosmos, it instead manipulated, dominated and threatened to destroy a living planet. Unchained rationality was one dimensional understanding, and the consumption ethic of industrialism one dimensional being. Together, these were responsible for pathological consciousness in a pathological world.

From about 1960 onwards, editorials repeatedly dis-coursed on the peculiar insanity which characterised twentieth century existence. One early example, from 1961, catalogued the themes which others were to elaborate:

... the over-treatment practised in ... [Hahnemann's] day is exceeded by the pandemic of synthetic poisoning around us. The situation is worsened by the ever-increasing destruction of living nature engineered by modern methods of agriculture which is littering the countryside with the corpses of birds and animals and insects. A fundamental undermining of the health of Man and Nature is going on under the direction of an economic system which makes financial profit its sole guiding principle. Greed and fear of one's neighbour are the inner meaning of this situation, and a terrifying psychosomatic world experiment on the social organism is presented to our gaze.

The guidance of medicine has fallen to the forces of scientific materialism, with its one-sided emphasis on the measurable and techniques of measurement. But we are not only measurable – we are also the measurers. This measuring, calculating mentality of modern science, the attitude of the bourgeois writ large, despises everything coming tenderly into existence. It wants the dead, finished corpse of the living to pull to pieces and measure, and so it furnishes us with terrifying nightmare phantasmagorias of a dead, meaningless cosmos, and a blind, chance-directed nature. It admits only its abstract measurements as real and dismisses imagination, inspiration, intuition, the forces of the heart, as useless for probing the mysteries of existence. That such one-sidedness, such overweening pride of the mere male intellect has produced a world torn and divided, has produced in the unconscious a dangerous and volcanic situation already manifest in two world wars, is undeniable and evident.[49]

This is certainly powerful and effective writing. Homoeo-paths had arrived at an assessment of science as rationalised irrationality which bore a striking resemblance to the con-clusions of the Frankfurt school of critical Marxism.[50] The route adopted to reach this conclusion, however, was very different. For homoeopaths, the critique of science was underpinned by the anthroposophical-Platonic principle of a bridge between the worlds of people and nature forged from the activity of living Idea, and expressed through the symbolism of homoeopathic drug pictures; for Marxists, the critique was developed from the concepts of knowledge as commodity, alienated labour, ideological control, and the Weberian account of science as a rationality of means which discounted ends or values. But whatever the route adopted – whether homoeopathic, Marxist or feminist – the point that twentieth century science is largely life denying and life threatening, rather than life enhancing, rings true. The future, in a very real sense, depends on the resolution of this pathology.

For anthroposophically inspired homoeopaths, however, the problem with scientific rationality is not merely a question of reconnecting it with a sane discussion of values. The 'problem' is that it is irrelevant to homoeopathy. Scientific research is redundant because, as one editorial put it, it is a waste of time 'trying to secure recognition by those whose talents and training make such recognition impossible'.[51] The Janus face of homoeopathy thus continues to look in two directions, and a rift remains between those who would interpret the system through a metaphysical cosmology, and those who seek to win its legitimacy through the application of conventional research methods. Dr Charles Elliot pointed to the schism in 1986, when he referred to the continued appearance of articles on anthroposophy in the Faculty's journal. Scientifically inclined homoeopaths, he felt would find these alarming, and he went on to make his own position very clear: 'Should the Faculty of Homoeopathy be serious in its quest for absolute proof it must follow that it declares its interest by ... the removal of such material from its official publication'.[52] But for many, allowing homoeopathy to fall 'to the forces of scientific materialism, with its one-sided emphasis on the measurable and techniques of measurement', would be to deprive it of its magic, its mystery and its attraction.[53] One thing, however, is becoming increasingly clear: whatever the particular orientation of homoeopaths themselves, the 1970s and 80s have ushered in an era when the confidence of patients in conventional medicine appears to have been damaged. The result has been an increasing popularity of complementary techniques, a popularity in which homoeopathy has shared.

NOTES

1. See Anthony Campbell, The Two Faces of Homoeopathy (Jill Norman, London, 1984) Chapter 3.
2. Quoted in ibid., p. 43.
3. R.H. Shryock, The Development of Modern Medicine (Victor Gollancz, London, 1948), p. 161. Original italics.
4. Ibid., p. 165.
5. Ibid., pp. 166-7.
6. See Anthony Campbell, op.cit., Chapter 9, esp. p. 114.
7. Quoted by R.J. Withers, 'Towards a Psychology of Homoeopathy and the High Potencies', The British Homoeopathic Journal, vol. LXVIII (1979), p. 142.
8. Ibid.
9. Ibid.
10. Ibid. Original italics.
11. Ibid.
12. Ibid., pp. 142-3.
13. Ibid., p. 143.
14. L.R. Twentyman, 'Sepia in the Male, or the Male in Sepia', The British Homoeopathic Journal, vol. LXIII (1974), p. 271.
15. See Anthony Campbell, op.cit., Chapter 9, esp. pp. 114-17, from where much of the discussion of Westcott, Rosicrucianism and Felkin derives.
16. Harold Gardiner, 'Swedenborg's Philosophy and Modern Science'. The British Homoeopathic Journal, vol. XLIX (1960), p. 201.
17. See Anthony Campbell, op.cit., Chapter 7, esp. p. 91.
18. Ibid., p. 93.
19. Ibid., p. 94.

20. James Tyler Kent, Lectures on Homoeopathic Philosophy (Sett Day and Co., Calcutta, 1961); Lectures on Homoeopathic Materia Medica (Boericke and Tafel, Philadelphia, 1905); Repertory of the Homoeopathic Materia Medica (B. Jain, New Delhi, reprinted 1974).

21. See Anthony Campbell, op.cit., Chapter 7, esp. pp. 95–104.

22. See, for example, the arguments in Karl R. Popper, Objective Knowledge: an Evolutionary Approach (Clarendon Press, Oxford, 1972).

23. G.R. Mitchell, 'Hughes, Hahnemann and the Half-Homoeopaths', The British Homoeopathic Journal, vol. LXV (1976), p. 129.

24. James F.G. Turner, 'Rudolf Steiner – A Fresh Outlook on the Etiology of Disease', The British Homoeopathic Journal, vol. XXXIX (1939), pp. 157–68.

25. Anthroposophical Association, Rudolf Steiner House, 35 Park Road, London NW1.

26. See Brain Inglis and Ruth West, The Alternative Health Guide (Michael Joseph, London, 1983), p. 74.

27. Rudolf Steiner, The Anthroposophical Approach to Medicine (Anthroposophical Publishing Co., London, 1928).

28. Brian Inglis and Ruth West, op.cit., p. 75.

29. Peter B. Engel, 'Rudolf Steiner's Medical Thinking and its Relationship to Homoeopathy', The British Homoeopathic Journal, vol. L (1961), p. 186.

30. Ibid., p. 187.

31. Ibid.

32. Ibid., p. 188.

33. Lambert Mount, 'Reflections on Homoeopathy', The British Homoeopathic Journal, vol. LXVI (1977), p. 65.

34. B.S. Rose, 'The Future', The British Homoeopathic Journal, vol. 70 (1981), p. 172.

35. L.R. Twentyman, 'Sepia in the Male', op.cit., p. 268.

36. L.R. Twentyman, 'The Place of Homoeopathy in Modern Medicine in the Light of History', The British Homoeopathic Journal, vol. LXIII (1974), p. 91.

37. L.R. Twentyman, 'Presidential Address', The British Homoeopathic Journal, vol. L (1961), p. 211. Italics added.

38. Anon., 'Editoria', The British Homoeopathic Journal, vol. L (1961), p. 72.

39. See, for example, Hélen Jaworski, 'The Biological Plan', The British Homoeopathic Journal, vol. XLVIII (1959), pp. 33–8; 'The Sponges – Their Significance', The British Homoeopathic Journal, vol. XLIX (1960), pp. 279–89; 'Fishes, Crustaceans, Bryozoa – Their Significance', The British Homoeopathic Journal, vol. LII (1963), pp. 58–69; Karl König, 'Embryology and World Evolution', The British Homoeopathic Journal, vol. LVII (1968), pp. 27–35, 111–21 and vol. LVIII

(1969), pp. 103-11; Wilhelm Pelikan, 'Archetypal Relations Between Plant and Man', The British Homoeopathic Journal, vol. LIX (1970), pp. 163-8; 'The Lichens', pp. 103-7; and 'Disease Process and Medicinal Plant', pp. 169-73.

40. Karl König, 'Diabetes Mellitus', The British Homoeopathic Journal, vol. LIV (1965), p. 162.

41. Karl König, 'Embryology and World Evolution', The British Homoeopathic Journal, vol. LVIII (1969) op.cit., p. 104.

42. Anthony Turner, 'Venues and Jupiter', The British Homoeopathic Journal, vol. LXV (1976), p. 181.

43. Geoffrey Douch, 'The Heart as an Organ of Balance', The British Homoeopathic Journal, vol. LXVII (1978), pp. 100-3; Leon Manteuffel-Szoege, 'On the Movement of the Blood', The British Homoeopathic Journal, vol. LVIII (1969), pp. 196-211; Geoffrey Douch, 'Depression and the Liver', The British Homoeopathic Journal, vol. LXV (1976), pp. 230-3; L.R. Twentyman, 'Neuro-Sensory Aspects of Malignant Disease', The British Homoeopathic Journal, vol. LXVII (1978), pp. 149-64.

44. Patricia Dale-Green, 'Apis Mellifica', The British Homoeopathic Journal, vol. XLVIII (1959), pp. 236-48; 'Bufo Bufo', The British Homoeopathic Journal, vol. XLIX (1960), pp. 54-68; 'The Tortoise', The British Homoeopathic Journal, vol. LI (1962), pp. 272-9; 'The Healing Lick and the Rabid Bite', The British Homoeopathic Journal, vol. LIII (1964), pp. 51-9; E.L. Grant Watson, 'Animals in Splendour and Decline', The British Homoeopathic Journal, vol. LV (1966), pp. 112-21.

45. A.T. Westlake, 'New Factors in the Twentieth-Century Disease Pattern', The British Homoeopathic Journal, vol. LIV (1965), pp. 180-9; A.M. and O.E. Scarlett, 'Colour as a Healing Agent', The British Homoeopathic Journal, vol. XXXII (1942), pp. 174-5; Arthur Guirdham, 'A Theory of Disease', The British Homoeopathic Journal, vol. LVIII (1969), pp. 173-81.

46. Marcia Moore and James Stephenson, 'A Motirational and Sociological Analysis of Homoeopathic Physicians in the USA and UK', The British Homoeopathic Journal, vol. LI (1962), pp. 297-303, esp. p. 299.

47. See R.J. Withers, op.cit., p. 145.

48. Ibid., pp. 146-9.

49. Anon., 'Editorial', The British Homoeopathic Journal, vol. L (1961), p. 71. Italics added.

50. For a useful discussion of the school's work see e.g. David Held, Introduction to Critical Theory, Horkheimer to Habermas (Hutchinson, London, 1980).

51. Anon., 'Editorial', The British Homoeopathic Journal, vol. LII (1963), p. 80.

52. Charles Elliot, 'Homoeopathy: Science or Philosophy?', British Homoeopathy Research Group, Communi-

cations, No. 16 (October 1986), p. 46.
  53. Anon., 'Editorial', The British Homoeopathic Journal, vol. L (1961), p. 71.

Chapter Sixteen

A NEW SPRING? MEDICINE, HOLISM AND
THE COMPLEMENTARY THERAPIES

In 1975, Ivan Illich published a powerful sociological critique of modern medicine.[1] Medical Nemesis left a lasting impression in medical and academic circles. Working the concept of 'iatrogenesis' through at three different levels - clinical, social and cultural - Illich announced that 'The medical establishment has become a major threat to health. The disabling impact of professional control over medicine has reached the proportions of an epidemic.'[2] Though other academics disagreed with Illich's analysis of the causes of the threat - Marxists, for example, relating the problem ultimately to the imperative of capital accumulation, and feminists emphasising the issue of masculine control, and its implications for medical views of women and the treatment which they received - few were prepared to challenge the conclusion that something was radically wrong with the profession and practice of medicine in the advanced societies of the late twentieth century.[3]

The 1970s also witnessed a renaissance for alternative medicine. In 1964, Brian Inglis had published a small book called Fringe Medicine.[4] At the time, the subject was something of an esoteric interest - a point reflected in the use of the term 'fringe' in the title. Twenty years later, the same therapies are often called 'complementary', which perhaps reflects the change of public and professional attitudes which has occurred during the period. Precise measurement of the change in public attitudes to, and demand for, complementary therapy (CT) since the 1960s is, however, difficult. The main stumbling block is an absence of data against which to compare contemporary surveys. Nevertheless, such evidence as is available suggests that popular demand for these forms of treatment is strong, and that among certain members of the public, confidence in conventional medicine has fallen.

The marketing research company - Taylor Nelson Medical - which has been monitoring changes in public perceptions of doctors and medicine for some time, found that the proportion of people who 'said that they trusted the doctor to know what they needed' had fallen, according to their sampling, from

52 per cent of the population in 1978 to 39 per cent in 1980.[5] Twenty-two per cent also stated that they had 'less faith in doctors than they used to'.[6] Another survey, organised by the Threshold Foundation in 1980, estimated that the number of consultations with complementary therapists was growing at around ten to fifteen per cent per year.[7] In February 1986, the Consumers' Association asked 'nearly 28,000 members whether they had used any form of alternative or complementary medicine during the previous 12 months. About one in seven said they had.'[8]

From this list of users - nearly 4,000 - the Association drew a random sample, and forwarded a more detailed questionnaire in order to elicit further information. In total, 1,942 people responded. In descending order, the types of practitioner most frequently consulted were osteopaths (42 per cent), homoeopaths (26 per cent), acupuncturists (23 per cent), chiropractors (22 per cent) and herbalists (eleven per cent).[9] Eighty-two per cent of respondents claimed to have been cured, or derived some benefit, from the practitioners consulted.[10] Psychological, pain or joint problems were the most common disorders for which people had sought help.[11] Eighty-one per cent of those who had sought conventional treatment for their condition reported that 'they were dissatisfied because they had not been cured, only got temporary relief or couldn't be treated'.[12]

As far as homoeopathy itself is concerned, these data support the more impressionistic view of homoeopaths themselves that demand for their services has grown: in 1982, 95 per cent of respondents who answered a survey question on this issue felt that patient demand had, in their experience, expanded.[13] This is reflected in competition for service. As the chairperson of the BHA reported in October 1986 'three months is not an unusual period of time to wait before you can become a new patient of many of the doctors on our lists'.[14]

A final piece of evidence which tends to support the impression of a new popularity for CT is the extent of media interest. Homoeopathy and other techniques have received radio and television coverage. The most recent example of the latter was the BBC television series The Healing Arts, which ran during the summer of 1986. Newspaper coverage has also been frequent. All the serious dailies, for example, gave space to the BMA's report on alternative therapy (May 1986), and to the rejoinder and critique of this report by the British Holistic Medical Association (BMHA), which appeared the following July.[15]

It is, then, difficult to avoid the conclusion that, as The British Homoeopathic Journal put it in 1978, 'There has arisen during the last few years a very remarkable and widespread interest in Alternative Therapies ...'.[16] The next problem is the obvious one of accounting for this social change. Three issues seem to recur in the various commentaries which have explored the problem: the impersonality of much conventional treatment, its inability to cure, improve or relieve a range of modern ailments, and the dangers of iatrogenic complications.[17]

The Consumers' Association, in an earlier (1981) survey, found that 'two-thirds of those who had received alternative medicine during the last five years said that they had been having treatment with conventional medicine, but that it was not helping or they did not like it - because of side-effects, for example.'[18] As already noted, these findings were supported by the same group's 1986 survey. In a study of 500 consecutive new medical out-patients at the RLHH, published in 1981, the main reasons for seeking homoeopathic treatment again focused on issues of dissatisfaction with conventional medicine, and a wish to avoid regular drugs.[19] A later survey of UK homoeopathic practitioners confirmed these findings: the two main reasons which new patients gave for turning to homoeopathic medicine were 'no help or improvement from allopathic regimen' and 'dangers and side-effects of allopathic drugs'.[20]

If some patients are registering some dissatisfaction with regular treatment by turning to non-orthodox practitioners, then the fault should not be attributed solely to the wrong-headed belligerence of individual members of the regular profession. This is far too simplistic. What needs to be examined is the relationship between medical theory and the socio-economic context which shapes its expression. Historically, social and economic factors have played an important part in the rejection of holistic and vitalistic medical theories, and favoured instead the adoption of disease orientated, active, oppositional therapy by those who strove to earn a livelihood from the practice of medicine. The development of medicine as an important area of capital accumulation in the twentieth century - through the development and sale of technologies and drugs - has provided an important economic underpinning to this approach. Moreover, the institutional structure of health care, represented by an underfunded NHS, leaves little room for patient centred approaches, and the contemporary profile of disease, in which chronic non-responding conditions, exacerbated by an ageing population, loom large, has made the medical mission one of disease management rather than cure. Collectively, these factors have helped to institutionalise and reproduce a medical setting which is technological, impersonal, rushed and drug orientated. A mounting toll of iatrogenic damage has been the result. Thalidomide made a powerful impression on public consciousness. More recent iatrogenic scandals have involved the butazone drugs (Butazone, Butazolidin, Butacote, Tanderil, Tandacote) as well as products such as Zomax,

Zelmid, Osmosin, Opren, Flosint and Eraldin. Melville and Johnson claim that 'Drug-induced disease leads to many deaths. In both the United States and Britain it has been calculated that more people are killed each year by prescribed drugs than by accidents on the roads. The figures for the maimed and injured may be proportionately higher.'[21]

More recently, public concern about the quality, effectiveness and safety of aspects of regular treatment - concretely manifested in a willingness to seek alternative therapy - has been matched by signs of changing attitudes among general practitioners. In 1983, <u>The British Medical Journal</u> published the results of a survey by David Taylor Reilly of general practitioner trainees' views on alternative medicine.[22] Of 86 respondents, eighteen doctors were using one or more alternative therapies, and seventy indicated a wish to train in at least one of them. Moreover, 'A total of 31 trainees had referred patients for such treatments; 12 of these doctors made referrals to non-medically qualified practitioners.'[23]

A survey of general practitioners in the Potteries area in 1985 produced similar results. A total of 162 doctors were contacted. The response rate - 38 per cent - was low, but of those who agreed to participate:

> ...substantial numbers of doctors gave positive therapeutic evaluations of alternative therapies, and were prepared to refer patients to practitioners of these treatments. Support was also found for the incorporation of CTs into medical education; for the registration of lay therapists as 'Professions Supplementary to Medicine'; and for opportunities to receive training in alternative treatments. Doctors felt that patient demand for, interest in and knowledge about CTs had increased during the last 15 years, and that similar changes were apparent within the medical profession itself.[24]

In the same year, a survey of 145 general practitioners in Avon produced comparable results. Over half the doctors thought osteopathy, chiropractice, accupuncture and hypnosis were useful, with over a third endorsing homoeopathy. One third of participants stated that they had received some form of training in one or more CTs.[25]

Nationally, it seems that around 2,000 doctors - about seven per cent of the whole profession - have received training from the associations representing hypnosis, accupuncture, manipulation and homoeopathy.[26] Reilly concluded from his own survey, and from these national figures, 'that alternative methods of treatment are currently being used to complement orthodox medicine and an expansion in their use appears imminent'.[27]

This conclusion is perhaps a little optimistic. Though undeniable signs of change are visible among general practitioners, powerful opposition to CT from the elite of the profession remains. The climate of growing interest in these forms of treatment, and the presidential impetus of Prince Charles during 1982-3, were strong enough to motivate the BMA to establish a working party to report on 'possible methods of assessing the value of alternative therapies', but its conclusions were largely dismissive of the value of the therapies themselves.[28] Indeed, the report rather assumed what it supposedly set out to question. It begins with an account of the rise of scientific medicine, and concludes with the point that 'The fundamental division separating orthodox from alternative approaches to medicine is the scientific principle which underlies the former, and the testing of theories by systematic observation which that principle implies.'[29] The implication that regular medicine is scientific, and that anything else in the therapeutic field is not, was especially ironic in view of the fact that many orthodox procedures and practices have been adopted without the randomised double-blind assurance of efficacy which the report argued should be applied to CTs.[30]

The BHMA - a group founded in 1983 by doctors interested in encouraging the practice of holistic medicine - issued a point by point rejoinder rebutting the BMA's position.[31] In terms of general criticism, the BHMA noted that the report had been compiled by hospital specialists who had no direct experience of CTs, who had a limited view of diagnostic procedure, and who seemed unaware of recent work which pointed out the limitations of the randomised clinical trial. Research, the BHMA felt, was clearly called for - but the methodology adopted had to do justice to the uniqueness of the individual patient, and the kinds of clinical settings in which complementary therapists worked.[32]

A number of points emerge from this dialogue which are worth elaborating. First, despite the fact that the BMA regarded the conventional double-blind trial as the objective arbiter of, and controlling influence on, medical judgement, it is clear that the relative <u>absence</u> of data of this kind about CTs has not prevented many practitioners from developing views about the therapeutic benefits offered by alternative practices. This in turn raises questions about why these attitudes have developed within the profession. Awareness of iatrogenic problems, and of the limitations of regular methods in coping with many contemporary ailments, is almost certainly part of the answer. But there are also suggestions that the general climate of public and patient interest in CTs, media publicity, and patient demand for these forms of treatment, have also exerted an effect.[33] Though more extensive and detailed research on this issue would be required before a more confident conclusion is possible, it is difficult not to see

a causal connection of some kind between changing therapeutic orientations among actual and potential clients, and the
new interest among general practitioners in CTs. After all, it
is doctors at the 'grass roots' level of practice, rather than
the hospital elite, who are more exposed to the views and
opinions of patients, and it is at the general practitioner level
that a revision of attitudes towards alternative methods seems
to have occurred. Given a clientele 'guaranteed' by the NHS,
there is no direct financial pressure on doctors to modify
views and practices according to the therapeutic choices made
by patients - a process clearly visible in the nineteenth
century - but there are suggestions that a measure of client
influence remains.

Secondly, it is clear that although forces promoting
changing therapeutic orientations among general practitioners
have been at work, powerful institutional and economic
factors, which help to contain their effect, remain. The
principal mechanisms adopted by the profession in the nineteenth century to limit the impact of therapeutic rivalry
within its own ranks were strategies of sectarianisation and
therapeutic reform. In the twentieth century, control of the
educational process, ensuring the production of scientifically
orientated doctors to whom the appeal of alternative therapeutic models would be limited, and the medical industries
producing the drugs and technologies of allopathic medicine,
have helped to reproduce medical consensus and uniformity of
practice among regular doctors. For much of the twentieth
century, then, the profession has been able to control therapeutic defection through the simple tactic of ensuring that it
would not occur to its members to consider it. Professional
socialisation allied with the economic power of the medical and
pharmaceutical industry have been a powerful force in the
reproduction of allopathic orthodoxy.

In the 1980s, however, many doctors are interested in
exploring and learning about CT. The forces which have
produced this change, and those that resist the expansion of
its effect, are likely to meet in a battle over the content of
medical education, and the role of lay healers in the health
services. It should not be forgotten that there are roughly as
many of these (27,800 in 1981) as there are qualified general
practitioners (29,800 in 1982).[34] Though the profession has
produced successful occupational closure as far as the
practice of medicine is concerned, no such control has been
exerted over the art of healing. Full recognition of the
existence of this duality among paid health workers, and its
possible implications as far as regular practice is concerned,
have yet to be fully incorporated into the sociology of the
medical profession.

One point which may be taken up here is that discussions of the medical profession qua profession within
sociology have often assumed that the doctor is an expert and

the patient is not.[35] What has tended to be ignored is that, although patients may not be qualified to assess the knowledge on which therapeutic decisions are based, they are expert enough in judging the results of those decisions. Patients are experts on their own bodies - at least to the extent of knowing whether they feel better for treatment or not. (There are some obvious exceptions to this - people may be 'ill', for example, and not know it, as with the diagnosis of pre-cancerous conditions.) And when patients reach conclusions about the lack of effectiveness or deleterious consequences of treatment, they are likely to seek help elsewhere. Many of the clients of alternative practitioners are indeed regular medicine's failures.

Johnson, in an influential account of the emergence of professionalism as a form of occupational control, seems to miss this issue. His basic argument is that a 'structure of uncertainty' always exists between client and practitioner, born of lay dependence on expert services.[36] For Johnson, this uncertainty needs to be managed if the relationship between producers and consumers of knowledge and services is to be stable and successful. Professionalism - which resolves the problem of uncertainty in favour of producers - is one solution. But it can only emerge where the producing group (in this context, medical practitioners) is connected with wider bases of social power and, crucially, where 'the actual consumers or clients provide a large, heterogeneous, fragmented source of demand. The polar opposite of this situation is where there is a single consumer - a patron who has the power to define his own needs and the manner in which he expects these to be catered for.'[37]

Johnson is clear that this 'large, heterogeneous, fragmented source of demand' emerged in the nineteenth century.[38] This, together with doctors' connections with the growing social importance of the middle class, created the conditions under which professionalism as a form of occupational control could emerge. In short, social and economic change had created a situation where the structure of uncertainty could be resolved in favour of practitioners rather than clients.

Unfortunately the historical record suggests that in both Britain and America the expansion and fragmentation of demand for medical services did not insulate practitioners from client influence. It is quite clear that many consumers, making judgements about the effect of regular medicine on their health, deserted regular practitioners in favour of those who offered alternative methods - such as homoeopathy - and that orthodox doctors had necessarily to change their styles of practice in order to survive.

Since it has been estimated that the number of complementary therapists is now increasing at the rate of eleven per cent a year, it is tempting to argue that history in the 1980s is repeating itself. [39] Certainly there is evidence that regular general practitioners are increasingly interested in developing expertise in one or more CTs, but how far this process will continue is partly determined by the constraints exercised by the economic interests of medical industry, elite control of medical education, and the fact that there is no direct financial incentive for doctors (in Britain) to question standard routines of practice.

Homoeopathy itself seems in a more optimistic and self-confident mood in the 1980s than for many years previously. It has certainly benefited from growing public and medical interest in CT. Nevertheless, formidable problems remain. Internal schisms persist between the lay and medically qualified, and between practitioners favouring scientific or metaphysical interpretations of homoeopathy; acceptable proof of clinical effectiveness has still to be definitively established; and a coherent theoretical explanation of potency effect to be given. The prospective legislative review of homoeopathic medicines themselves is perhaps the most immediate political threat.

But homoeopathy has a political message of its own. Philosophies usually exhibit a potential for either the consolidation or transformation of the social circumstances in which they occur. This is true for the structure of ideas and beliefs which constitute holistic medicine. While, on the one hand, its emphasis on the importance of the unique experience of sickness produces a therapeutic individualism which may inhibit the development of collective awareness of the material circumstances which determine the health of nations, on the other, the metaphors of harmony and balance, of the human organism as a delicate self-sustaining and self-correcting vitalistic system in its own right, resonate strongly with ideas informing the ecological critique of industrialism.

Holistic therapy, then, possesses a philosophical structure whose terms, while primarily representing a critique of orthodox medicine, also provide a 'green' vocabulary in which an alternative, non-aggressive, harmonious mode of economic interaction with the environment can be envisaged. In this way, the health determining material circumstances brought into focus by the development of holistic consciousness are not those of capitalism specifically, but those of the genus to which capitalism belongs - industrialism. Green medicine, then, if it breeds politics, will breed a politics that is not red: rather naturally, green medicine will cultivate a green politics. Natural-holistic therapy is thus in tune with a politics of protest that goes far beyond targets merely medical. It connects with a protest against the clinical destruction of the environment by rationalistic technology and the unsatisfiable consumption ethic of the advanced societies. The protest is worth making. But the chances of success are slim. Homoeopathy thus seems destined to be at odds with the spirit of the age for the foreseeable future.

NOTES

1. The definitive version was Ivan Illich, Limits to Medicine (Penguin Books, Harmondsworth, 1977).
2. Ibid., p. 11.
3. See Nick Black et al., (eds.). Health and Disease, A Reader (Open University Press, Milton Keynes, 1984), part 3, esp. the papers by Illich, Navarro and Oakley, and from a medical perspective, those of McKeown and Cochrane.
4. Brian Inglis, Fringe Medicine (Faber, London, 1965).
5. These survey results are reported by Ruth West, 'Alternative Medicine: Prospects and Speculations' in Nick Black et al., (eds.), op.cit., p. 343.
6. Ibid.
7. S. Fulder and R. Munro, The Status of Complementary Medicine in the United Kingdom (Threshold Foundation Bureau Ltd., London, 1982). The figures are quoted by Ruth West, op.cit., p. 343.
8. Anon., 'Magic or Medicine?', Which? (October, 1986) p. 445. Which? is published by the Consumers' Association, London.
9. Ibid., p. 443.
10. Ibid.
11. Ibid.
12. Ibid.
13. See Phillip A. Nicholls, Homoeopathy and the British Medical Profession: the Sociology of a Medical Phoenix (Unpublished Ph.D. Thesis, University of Nottingham, 1984). Table 28a, p. 364.
14. R.J. Ede, 'Chairman's Report', Homoeopathy, vol. 36 (1986), p. 143.
15. James P. Payne et al., Alternative Therapy (British Medical Association, London, 1986); Patrick C. Pietroni et al., Report on the B.M.A. Board of Science Working Party on Alternative Therapy (British Holistic Medical Association, London, 1986). See also the press reports on the latter in The Daily Telegraph, The Times, The Guardian 2 July 1986.
16. Anon., 'Editorial', The British Homoeopathic Journal, vol. LXVII (1978), p. 73.
17. See e.g., Tony Smith, 'Alternative Medicine', The British Medical Journal, vol. 287 (1983), p. 307; Richard Smith, 'Medicine and the Media', The British Medical Journal, vol. 283 (1981), p. 1460; Judith Moore et al., 'Why do People Seek Treatment by Alternative Medicine', The British Medical Journal, vol. 290 (1985), pp. 28-9.

18. These survey results are reported by Ruth West, op.cit., p. 343.
19. Sally C. Jenkins et al., 'A Survey of 500 Consecutive New Patients Attending Medical Outpatients at the Royal London Homoeopathic Hospital', The British Homoeopathic Journal, vol. 70 (1981), Table 3, p. 25.
20. Phillip A. Nicholls, op.cit., Table 26, p. 356.
21. Arabella Melville and Colin Johnson, Cured to Death (Secker and Warburg, London, 1982), p.6.
22. David Taylor Reilly, 'Young Doctors' Views on Alternative Medicine', The British Medical Journal, vol. 287 (1983), pp. 337-9.
23. Ibid., p. 337.
24. P. A. Nicholls and J. E. Luton, 'Doctors and Complementary Medicine: A Survey of General Practitioners in the Potteries', Occasional Paper, No. 2 (November 1986), Department of Sociology, North Staffordshire Polytechnic, Abstract.
25. The results of this survey are given in Anon., 'Magic or Medicine?', op.cit., p. 445.
26. David Taylor Reilly, op.cit., p. 339.
27. Ibid., p. 337.
28. James P. Payne et al., op.cit., p. 1. For the dismissive conclusions, see pp. 77-8.
29. Ibid., p. 78.
30. On this see A.L. Cochrane, 'Effectiveness and Efficiency' in Nick Black et al., (eds.), op.cit., pp. 115-121, esp. p. 117.
31. Patrick C. Pietroni et al., op.cit.
32. See the 'Press Release' of The British Holistic Medical Association, issued with the publication of its own report in July 1986, both available from the British Holistic Medical Association, 179 Gloucester Place, London NW1 6DX.
33. See Phillip A. Nicholls, Homoeopathy and the British Medical Profession, op.cit., Table 19, p. 319 and P. A. Nicholls and J. E. Luton, 'Doctors and Complementary Medicine', op.cit., p. 8.
34. S. Fulder and R. Munro, op.cit., pp. 35-7.
35. See, for example, the literature review in T. Johnson, Professions and Power (Macmillan, London, 1972).
36. Ibid., p.41.
37. Ibid., p.43.
38. Ibid., p.52.
39. S. Fulder and R. Munro, op.cit., pp. 35-7.

INDEX

decline of heroic therapy
81-2, 97-8, 103-4,
157-8, 165-9, 178-9
defences of 117-20, 127-8,
155-7
development of idea 10
difficulties of NHS practice
252-3
doctrine of signatures 261
domestic repertories 135
double-blind trials 5,
119-20, 225-6, 255
early practitioners 108-21
passim., 127-8
ecological critiques 233-4,
272-3
educational discrimination
149-51
educational struggles
219-21, 248-54
effects on regular therapy
104, 115-16, 165-79,
182, 186, 216
emanometer 223, 226-8
empiricist physicians 30
expansion of movement
103, 113-14, 122-3,
134-6
financial attractiveness to
doctors 136
first mentioned in The
Lancet 106
freemasonry 260-1
green politics 285-6
harmlessness of 152
holism 5
hostility of coroners'
courts 146-8
implications for regular
practice 120-6
improvement of
pharmacopoeia 182
internal schisms and
arguments 183-5, 221
Jungian analysis 271
Kentianism 186, 217-18,
265-6
lack of appeal to doctors
33
life assurance 179

London School of
Homoeopathy 182-3
loss of official posts 148-9
magic 5-8
Medical Act, 1858 144-5,
183, 204
medicines 4, 13n2, 81
Medicines' Act, 1968 254-5
National Insurance Bill,
1911 241-2
naturphilosophie 259-60
Nelson and Company 253
nosodes 181, 185, 228-30
obstacles to twentieth
century growth 285-6
occult 262
origin 9-10, 12-13, 14n25,
16-17, 21-7
osteopathy 246
ostracism of allopaths 149
ostracism of homoeopaths
117, 128, 133-50
passim.
Paracelsus 260-2
patient demand for 135,
254, 274, 279, 285
placebo 4-5, 119, 123,
225-6, 270
poisonings 152-3
post war WWI epidemics 245
potencies 221-28, 265, 267
evidence of action 223-8
Steiner 267
Swedenborg 265
theory of action, post
Hahnemann 221-3
practitioners as fools or
knaves 151-3
private practice 253
proposed trials 120
proving 3, 9, 31, 75-6,
179, 184-5, 224-5, 228
psoric (miasm) theory
127-8, 229, 265
public health 244-5
publicity 153
publishing discrimination
150
reasons for decline 216-18
reasons for twentieth
century popularity 280

reconciliation with allopaths
142, 178, 233-4
Reich patronage 247
rejection of fundamentalism
180-1
relations with regular
profession 40, 54,
103-5, 108-10, 114,
133-58, 165-83, 186,
219-21, 234-5
remedies used by allopaths
142, 151, 170-5
reorganisation of the NHS,
1974 253
response to developments
in allopathic science
181, 230-2
reverse dosage law 170
ridicule of 116, 121, 155
Rosicrucianism 260-2
social prejudices 243-4
masturbation 243-4
menstruation 244
feminism 244
Staines air disaster 253
Swedenborgianism 262-6
theoretical evaluations by
non-homoeopaths 106-7,
114-26 passim., 155-7
therapeutic eclecticism 119,
127-8, 152-3, 179-81,
216, 246, 253
treatment of cholera 145-6
twentieth century
iatrogenesis 232-3
veterinary failures of 153-4
World War I 242-3
World War II 247
see also BHA, BHS,
Coulter, Harris,
Forbes, Sir J.,
Hahnemann, C.F.S.,
Henderson, William,
heroic therapy,
Hippocratic medicine,
homoeopathy in
America, Royal London
Homoeopathic Hospital,
similia similibus
curentur Steiner,

Rudolf, Watson, Sir
Thomas
Homoeopathy: its Tenets and
Tendencies 155-6
Honeyman-Gillespie lectures
218
Hughes, Richard 142, 175,
180-6 passim., 220-1, 265
humour 3, 33, 179
hydrophobia (rabies) 54, 95,
229
hypertrophy 59, 95

iatrochemists 30, 33
iatromathematics 30
iatromechanism 30, 33
iliadus 261
induration 60, 96
inflammation 12, 60-2, 67-9,
71, 82-96 passim., 173
influenza 198, 245
Inquiry into the Homoeopathic
Practice of Medicine, An
118, 121, 155-6
Instructions for Surgeons
Respecting Veneral
Diseases 12
Insurance Committees 242
International Hahnemannian
Association 207, 210
International Homoeopathic
Council 242
ipecacuanha (Cephaelis
ipecacuanha) 90, 172-3,
175

jalap (Ipomoea purga) 71,
84-5, 89-94 passim.

Kent, James Tyler 186, 218,
220-1, 265-6

Lectures on Homoeopathic
Materia Medica 266
Lectures on Homoeopathic
Philosophy 266
Lectures on the Principles
and Practice of Physic 56,
63
leeches 83-96 passim.
Letter to John Forbes 127

proving 3, 9, 14n16, 31,
75-6, 104, 176, 179, 184-5,
224-5, 228
and the development of a
pharmacopoeia 31, 76
Hahnemann on 9, 31, 75-6
homoeopathic scepticism on
179, 184-5
in regular medicine 104,
176
method 3, 9, 14n16
twentieth century
developments 224-5, 228
psora 127-8, 229, 265
Public Health Service 244
purges 3, 18, 68, 71, 73,
84-96 passim.

Quin, Frederick F.H. 108-13,
116, 142, 202
quinine 10, 145, 147, 177, 204

rationalist physicians 30, 39
Reconstruction Fund 219
Regimen IV 20
Regimen for Health, A 20
Regimen in Acute Disease 25,
34
Repertory of the Homoeopathic
Materia Medica 266
rinderpest 153-4
Ringer, Sydney 169-75, 178
Royal London Homoeopathic
Hospital 110-12, 146, 182,
218, 220, 230, 242, 248-54,
280
creation of NHS 248-52
foundation 110-12
indebtedness 250
mentioned 146, 182, 218,
220, 230, 242
popular demand for
homoeopathy 280
reorganisation of NHS,
1974 253
royal patronage of 247
threat of closure 254
World War II 247

Sacred Disease, The 16, 20
scepticism 30

senna (Cassia senna) 12,
84-5, 96
serum therapy 179, 230-2
similia similibus curentur 3-27
passim., 180, 261-9
passim., 271
compared to allopathy 3-4,
16-27
curentur or curantur? 10,
190n77
development of idea 10
Hahnemann on 3, 9-10
in allopathy 3-4
in magic 5-8
Jung 271
limitations of 180
Livingston on 3
origin 9-10, 12-13, 14n25,
16-17, 21-7
Parcelsus 261
Steiner 266, 268-9
Swedenborg 263-5
theory of action 70-1
see also allopathy in
Britain (proving of
medicines), Hippocratic
medicine, proving,
serum therapy vaccine
therapy, vaccines
simillimum 5
Simpson, James Y. 133, 135,
165
smallpox 198, 228
solidism 179
Spanish fly (Cantharides
vesicatoria) 88, 94, 170,
173, 175
Steiner, Rudolf 233, 246,
261-72 passim.
sthenic 99n45
stimulants 94, 97, 145, 168,
180
strychnine (Strychnos
nuxvomica) 72, 89, 148,
170, 175, 177
Swendenborg, E. 186, 262-5,
268
syncope 82-3, 91-2
syphilis 12, 90, 114, 231, 265
System of Medicine, A 167